Societies and Political Orders in Transition

This book series presents scientific and scholarly studies focusing on societies and political orders in transition, for example in Central and Eastern Europe but also elsewhere in the world. By comparing established societies, characterized by well-established market economies and well-functioning democracies, with post-socialist societies, often characterized by emerging markets and fragile political systems, the series identifies and analyzes factors influencing change and continuity in societies and political orders. These factors include state capacity to establish formal and informal rules, democratic institutions, forms of social structuration, political regimes, levels of corruption, specificity of political cultures, as well as types and orientation of political and economic elites.

Societies and Political Orders in Transition welcomes monographs and edited volumes from a variety of disciplines and approaches, such as political and social sciences and economics, which are accessible to both academics and interested general readers.

Topics may include, but are not limited to, democratization, regime change, changing social norms, migration, etc.

All titles in this series are peer-reviewed.

This book series is indexed in Scopus.

More information about this series at http://www.springer.com/series/15626

Anna Almakaeva · Alejandro Moreno ·
Rima Wilkes
Editors

Social Capital and Subjective Well-Being

Insights from Cross-Cultural Studies

Springer

Editors
Anna Almakaeva
Higher School of Economics
National Research University
Moscow, Russia

Alejandro Moreno
Instituto Tecnológico Autónomo de México
Mexico City, Mexico

Rima Wilkes
Department of Sociology
University of British Columbia
Vancouver, BC, Canada

ISSN 2511-2201 ISSN 2511-221X (electronic)
Societies and Political Orders in Transition
ISBN 978-3-030-75812-7 ISBN 978-3-030-75813-4 (eBook)
https://doi.org/10.1007/978-3-030-75813-4

This Springer imprint is published by the registered company Springer Nature Switzerland AG
The registered company address is: Gewerbestrasse 11, 6330 Cham, Switzerland

Preface

The notion and measurement of happiness have attracted a growing attention in recent years, both from academics and policy-makers. From a policy perspective, governments and international organizations recognize that how people feel, a subjective dimension, is as important to consider for government action as their objective levels of material well-being and human development. In that sense, policy goals should aim at improving the living conditions of citizens, but take into account their sense of happiness as well. From an academic perspective, understanding and explaining the factors that foster subjective well-being may well go beyond specific governmental policies, as happiness may reflect a society's levels of economic development, its culture, its institutions, and changing conditions in each or all of them.

Ronald Inglehart, a political scientist and founding president of the World Values Survey, has proposed that happiness among the mass publics in the world is not fixed at set-points, but that it may change as a reflection of other changing circumstances and factors. "Cultural change is a process through which societies adapt their survival strategy. The process operates as if evolutionary forces were consciously seeking to maximize human happiness," he argues in *Cultural Evolution*, published in 2018. The central question is whether human happiness can be maximized, and if so, what factors contribute to it. In other words, is the pursuit of happiness possible?

This edited volume offers various analyses about how happiness may be linked to social interaction and social trust. Based on international comparative surveys, the authors look into different cultural, societal, economic, and institutional forces that may influence people's sense of well-being, but a special attention is placed on how social interconnectedness, trust in others, cooperation, and other aspects of social reciprocity, generally identified as social capital, relate to the levels of happiness. The common interest in the social components of subjective well-being that underlies these various analyses places happiness not only as an individual-level response to the environment, but as a socially shared and more collective or group-oriented phenomenon. To what extent does social capital influence the sense of well-being among the mass publics?

The book offers different ways of looking at the variation in happiness, across contexts and over time, and also as a response to shocking events like economic crises, to transforming phenomena like mass migrations, and to potentially distressing events like institutional changes, whether these be more restricting or more liberalizing in people's rights and freedoms. The central question in the book is whether social factors like interpersonal trust, social interconnectedness, and social reciprocity help individuals and societies cope differently, perhaps more adequately, to adapt to those changing circumstances, either by increasing their levels of subjective well-being, or by reducing unhappiness, if distress is a major force. The different chapters analyze the role of economic insecurities, religious beliefs, attitudes of tolerance, perceptions of freedom, recognition of individual identities, and value orientations, but most of all, the strength or weakness of social capital and social skills. The empirical bases for the analyses are a series of international comparative surveys—including the European Social Survey, the World Values Survey, regional barometers like Latinobarometer and the Americas Barometer, among others—which provide important data to the social sciences and are all available resources for public use.

One major aspect to keep in mind is the unexpected but profound impact that the COVID-19 pandemics will have—and is already having—on societies' living conditions and subjective well-being around the world. This volume began to form and was mostly written before the pandemics broke out, so the data and interpretations mark a moment of how people felt in different parts of the world before we got there. The health emergency, the high number of contagions and deaths in many countries, the deep economic and unemployment crises due partly to lockdowns, and other traumatic experiences linked to them have very likely provoked a growing sense of vulnerability, fear, discomfort, uncertainty, and pessimism. In other words, the pandemics has possibly reduced the sense of well-being globally.

One of the implications from this book is that, if the levels of happiness are linked to social capital, social interaction, social solidarity, and citizens' trust in their government institutions, it will be important to assess the impact of the pandemics on the patterns of social interconnectedness and trust in times when the central measure to face the emergency has been social distancing. We will not know for sure until the international comparative surveys offer more new data. Meanwhile, this book helps us see the extent to which our social networks, our social skills, and our trust in others influence out happiness as individuals and societies. If that is the case, building—and re-building—social capital is thus a crucial task today.

Mexico City, Mexico
February 2021

Alejandro Moreno

About This Book

This book presents a cross-cultural investigation into the interplay between social capital and subjective well-being. Based on a quantitative analysis of the latest large-N cross-cultural datasets, including the World Value Survey, European Social Survey, LAPOP, etc., and covering various countries, it offers a comparative perspective on and new insights into the determinants of social capital and well-being. By identifying both universal and culture-specific patterns, the authors shed new light on the spatial and temporal differentiation of social capital and subjective well-being.

The book is divided into two main parts, the first of which discusses mutual trust, religious and cultural tolerance, and pro-civic human values as essential dimensions of social capital. In turn, the second part studies social capital as a source of subjective well-being and life satisfaction. Given its scope, the book will appeal to scholars of sociology, social psychology, political science, and economics seeking a deeper understanding of the multifaceted nature of social capital and well-being.

Contents

Editors and Contributors

About the Editors

Anna Almakaeva (Ph.D. in Sociology) is a deputy head of the Ronald F. Inglehart Laboratory for Comparative Social Research at the Higher School of Economics (Russia). Her research interests include social capital, values, subjective well-being, and comparative studies. She is a member of the World Value Survey Russian team and the European Values Study Russian team.

Alejandro Moreno got Ph.D. from the University of Michigan in 1997. He is a professor of political science at Instituto Tecnológico Autónomo de México (ITAM) since 1996. He has served as President of the World Association for Public Opinion Research, WAPOR (2013–2014), as Vice-president for the World Values Survey Association (since 2013), and as Managing Director of the Latinobarometro surveys (2010–2017). He has also been the Director of Public Opinion Polling for newspaper Reforma (1999–2015) and currently for newspaper El Financiero (since 2016). His main research and academic interests focus on public opinion elections and voting behavior, political culture and social values, comparative politics, and survey research methodologies.

Rima Wilkes (Ph.D.) is a professor at the Department of Sociology at the University of British Columbia, Canada. In 2017–2018, she was the president of the Canadian Sociological Association. Her research interests include political sociology, race and ethnicity, trust, immigration, and social movements.

Contributors

Anna Almakaeva HSE University, Moscow, Russia

Mai Beilmann Institute of Social Studies, University of Tartu, Tartu, Estonia

Rico Bornschein HHL Leipzig Graduate School of Management, Leipzig, Germany

Kiara Castaman Department of Social Sciences, Pontificia Universidad Católica del Perú, Lima, Peru

Vladimir Gritskov St Petersburg University, St Petersburg, Russia

Muzafar Shah Habibullah Putra Business School, University Putra Malaysia, Seri Kembangan, Malaysia

Eric Holdack HHL Leipzig Graduate School of Management, Leipzig, Germany

Janine Jongbloed Institut de Recherche Sur l'Éducation: Sociologie et Économie de l'Éducation (IREDU), Université Bourgogne Franche-Comté, Dijon, France

Maricruz Lacalle-Calderon School of Economics and Business, Depament for Economic Development, Universidad Autónoma de Madrid, Madrid, Spain

Laur Lilleoja Research Centre for Survey Methodology (RECSM), Universitat Pompeu Fabra, Barcelona, Spain

Soomin Ma King's College, London, UK

Alejandro Moreno Instituto Tecnológico Autónomo de México (ITAM), Mexico City, Mexico

Isabel Neira Quantitative Economics Department, Faculty of Economics and Business Studies, Universidade de Santiago de Compostela, Santiago, Spain

Mikael Nygård Faculty of Education and Welfare Studies, Social Policy, Åbo Akademi University, Vaasa, Finland

Fredrica Nyqvist Faculty of Education and Welfare Studies, Social Policy, Åbo Akademi University, Vaasa, Finland

Jesús Peiró-Palomino Department of Applied Economics II and INTECO, University of Valencia, Valencia, Spain

Silko Pfeil HHL Leipzig Graduate School of Management, Leipzig, Germany

Marta Portela Department of Finance, Faculty of Business Administration, Universidade de Santiago de Compostela, Santiago, Spain

Ashley Pullman Education Policy Research Initiative, Graduate School of Public and International Affairs, University of Ottawa, Ottawa, Canada

Dragos Radu King's College, London, UK

Ratneswary Rasiah Taylor's University, Selangor, Malaysia

Anu Realo Department of Psychology, University of Warwick, Coventry, UK;
Institute of Psychology, University of Tartu, Tartu, Estonia

Tim Reeskens Department of Sociology, Tilburg University, Tilburg, Netherlands

Murali Sambasivan Thiagarajar School of Management, Madurai, India

Thomas Scharf Newcastle University, Population Health Sciences Institute, Newcastle upon Tyne, UK

Ekaterina Skoglund Leibniz Institute for East and Southeast European Studies, Regensburg, Germany

Sotheeswari Somasundram Taylor's University, Selangor, Malaysia

David Sulmont Department of Social Sciences, Pontificia Universidad Católica del Perú, Lima, Peru

Emili Tortosa-Ausina Departament d'Economia, Universitat Jaume I and IIDL, Castelló de la Plana, Spain

Leen Vandecasteele Institute for Social Sciences - Lifecourse and Inequality Research Centre, University of Lausanne, Lausanne, Switzerland;
LIVES Centre, Swiss Centre of Expertise in Life Course Research, Lausanne, Switzerland

Irina Vartanova Institute for Futures Studies, Stockholm, Sweden;
HSE University, Moscow, Russia

Rima Wilkes University of British Columbia, Vancouver, Canada

Abbreviations

CFI	Comparative fit index
CPI	Transparency International Perceived Corruption Index
EBRD	European Bank for Reconstruction and Development
EQI	European Quality of Government Index
ESS	European Social Survey
EVS	European Values Study
GDP	Gross domestic product
HDI	Human Development Index
LAPOP	Latin American Public Opinion Project
LFP	Labor force participation
LGBTI	Lesbian, gays, bisexual, transgender, and intersex people
LGBTQ	Lesbian, gays, bisexual, transgender, and queer people
OECD	The Organisation for Economic Co-operation and Development
OLS	Ordinary least squares
QOG	Quality of Government Institute
RMSEA	The root mean square error of approximation
SEM	Structural equation modeling
SOEP	German Socio-Economic Panel
UNDP SES	The United Nations Development Program Social Exclusion Survey
WVS	World Values Survey

Introduction: Social Capital and Subjective Well-Being: Towards a Conceptual Framework

Anna Almakaeva and Rima Wilkes

1 Introduction

Social capital and well-being have been widely recognized as important societal "common goods" that lead to social prosperity. While scholars and practitioners treat subjective well-being as the desirable outcome, they tend to treat social capital as the tool to get there or, as Portes notes, as a "cure-all for the maladies affecting society at home and abroad" (Portes, 1998, p. 2). Indeed, it is axiomatic to note the association between social capital and a set of favorable externalities which, along with economic development, health and institutional quality, also includes subjective well-being (Algan & Cahuc, 2013, 2014; Delhey & Newton, 2005; Elgar et al., 2011; Hudson, 2006; Knack & Keefer, 1997; Portela et al., 2013; Uslaner, 2013; Zak & Knack, 2001).

Earlier scholarship primarily focused on single country samples and, as a result, emphasized the role of individual-level determinants of social capital and well-being. Publicly available cross-national data launched a new era. The resulting flood of publications, on the one hand, produced mixed and inconclusive results, but, on the other hand, revealed the limited theoretical potential of single country samples. By demonstrating the spatial and temporal variability of single-country findings comparative studies raised the issue of absolute and relative individual determinants.

The scope of existing large-N comparative projects containing questions on different aspects of social capital and well-being is very broad. Scrivens and Smith (2013) counted 50 surveys that use different indicators of social capital. The largest

A. Almakaeva (✉)
HSE University, Moscow, Russia
e-mail: aalmakaeva@hse.ru

R. Wilkes
University of British Columbia, Vancouver, Canada
e-mail: wilkesr@mail.ubc.ca

A. Almakaeva et al. (eds.), *Social Capital and Subjective Well-Being*,
Societies and Political Orders in Transition,
https://doi.org/10.1007/978-3-030-75813-4_1

and the most well-known cross-national survey is the World Values Survey, established in 1981. The WVS is a global non-commercial project covering around 120 countries and 94.5% of the world population (WVS Database, n.d.). There are also a number of regional studies collecting data in Europe (European Values Study, European Social Survey, Eurobarometer, European Quality of Life Survey etc.), Latin America (Latinobarometer, LAPOP), Asia (Asian Barometer), Africa (Afrobarometer), and the Arab countries (Arab Barometer). These comparative projects, along with advanced methods of statistical data analysis, have provided a better understanding of how social capital and subjective well-being evolve, erode and interrelate under varying social, economic, institutional and cultural settings.

Figure 1 displays the growth of publications with key words "social capital" and "subjective well-being" as indexed in the Scopus database. As we see from Fig. 1 interest in these fields started around 1995 and has steadily increased. While in 1995 there were only a few papers, by 2019 there were more than 3500 manuscripts on well-being (see Fig. 1a) and more than 2000 on social capital (see Fig. 1b). The amount of papers on interconnections of social capital and well-being raised accordingly and reached around 150 publications in 2019 (see Fig. 1c). Open-access comparative projects have contributed greatly to this dramatic increase.

2 Theoretical Framework

In this section of the chapter our main aim is to provide an overview of the larger theoretical framework undergirding the chapters of the book. The construct of social capital is diverse and multidimensional. Bhandari and Yasunobu (2009, p. 486) note that social capital encompasses: "social norms, values, beliefs, trusts, obligations, relationships, networks, friends, memberships, civic engagement, information flows, and institutions that foster cooperation and collective actions". Lollo (2012) in turn, has counted 40 different definitions that have been used since Hanifan's introduction of the concept in 1916. Since social capital is an interdisciplinary and multifaceted concept, a single and universal definition is not possible. Nevertheless, the most useful approach lies somewhere between the "pragmatic" and "altruistic" extremes or, in other words, between definitions of social capital as personal and definitions of social capital as societal.

The pragmatic view interprets social capital as an individual attribute which can be converted into profitable personal outcomes and serve as important source of social support. The pragmatic tradition is grounded in the ideas of Pierre Bourdieu and James Coleman. Bourdieu differentiates between cultural, economic and social capital, defining the latter as "actual or potential resources which are linked to possession of a durable network of more or less institutionalized relationships of mutual acquaintance and recognition…or group membership" (Bourdieu, 2011, p. 21). Direct and indirect network connections constitute the volume of social capital. While direct ties refer to personal connections, indirect ties link a person to the social capital of his interconnected others. Since all forms of capital are convertible social

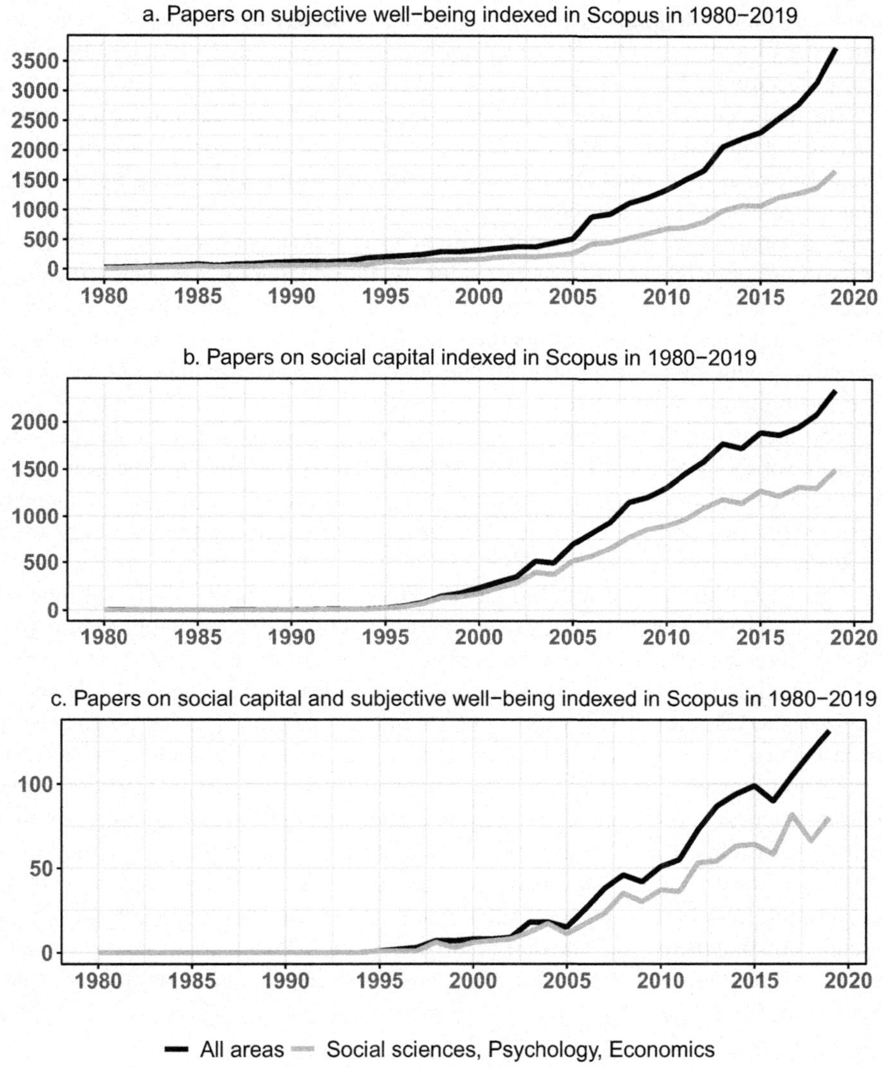

Fig. 1 Publications with key words "social capital" and "subjective well-being" indexed in Scopus in 1980–2019

capital may be transformed into cultural or economic capital. In the seminal paper "The Strength of Weak Ties" (1973) Mark Granovetter provides a brilliant example of this kind of transformation. His labor market study of blue-collar workers from Boston found out that candidates mostly used weak social ties to find potential employers.

As with Bourdieu, Coleman (1998) conceives of social capital as embedded "in the structure of relations between actors and among actors" (p. 98). It also has a productive and utilitarian nature and facilitates the achievement of specific goals and interests. Coleman sees three forms or manifestations of social capital: obligations and expectations, information channels, and social norms.

The first element refers to the mutual obligations and to a belief in a trustworthy social environment where such obligations are expected to be repaid at any time. The second element—information—is an essential but costly basis for action. Information requires attention, time and other resources which sometimes in a short supply. To gain information for personal utilitarian needs an individual can use a network of connections or, in other words, social capital. By introducing social norms as the third element Coleman goes beyond the pragmatic interpretation and links social capital to communal interests. Effective norms, in combination with external or internal sanctions, regulate behavior either by encouraging or by restricting certain actions. The most important normative manifestation is the norm that "one should forgo self-interest and act in the interests of the collectivity" (p. 104) which "leads persons to work for the public good" (p. 105). Although both Coleman and Bourdieu think of social capital as rooted in the structure of relations and obligations, Coleman emphasizes the public virtue of social capital, importance of norms and normative attitudes.

This line of theorizing was further developed by proponents of the "altruistic" paradigm. The altruistic view treats social capital as property of societies (communities) that is activated to achieve a common good. Robert Putnam, popularized the idea of social capital as a societal resource and civic virtue. Putnam and his colleagues Leonardi and Nonetti (1994) treat social capital as "features of social organization, such as trust, norms, and networks, that can improve the efficiency of society by facilitating coordinated actions" (p. 167). All elements of social capital are interconnected and interdependent. Cooperation, including cooperation in voluntary associations, breeds trust while trust "greases the wheels" of cooperation. Putnam et al. interpret trust as a prediction that another person will stick to a trustworthy behavior and abstain from opportunism. In small communities this prediction is based on an assumption that there is a context of familiarity, personal interactions and communication. More complex social environments require impersonal (social) form of trust generated through two main sources—norms of reciprocity and networks of civic engagement.

Putnam and co-authors draw a line between "balanced/specific" and "generalized/diffuse" reciprocity[1]. Specific reciprocity refers to the simultaneous equivalent exchange of values when item giving and item receiving co-occur. Generalized reciprocity is imbalanced, prolonged and requires a mutual belief that a benefit will be repaid. Effective norm of diffuse reciprocity requires dense networks of social exchange. The most important network configuration for its thriving is "horizontal" one which bridges together agents with equal status. Networks of civic engagement

[1] Putnam et al. note that this distinction was introduced in the earlier works of Marshall Sahlins (Stone Age Economics. Chicago: Aldine-Atherton, 1972), Robert O. Keohane (Reciprocity in International Organization 40 (1986)) and Robert Axelrod (An Evolutionary Approach to Norms" American Political Science Review 80 (December 1986); The Evolution of Cooperation (New York: Basic Books, 1984)) (Putnam et al. p. 243).

in the form of various formal and informal civic organizations (sport clubs, neighborhood associations, cooperatives etc.) generate such "horizontal" interactions thereby increasing the ability for cooperation in a community and stock of social capital.

Civic organizations produce this cumulative effect in several ways. First, they increase the potential costs of defection. Second, they "foster robust norms of reciprocity" (p. 173). Third, they disseminate information about trustworthiness of actors. Fourth, they store information on past success and serve as a "culturally-defined template for future collaboration" (p. 174). Conversely, "vertical" (hierarchical) networks link agents with unequal status and power resources who are unable to sustain trust due to less reliable information flows. Furthermore, sanctions against opportunism and malfeasance in "vertical" networks are less efficient since they are "likely to be imposed upwards and less likely to be acceded" (p. 174).

In *Bowling Alone* Putnam (2001) introduces the distinction between "bridging" (inclusive) and "bonding" (exclusive) social capital. "Bonding" social capital may have a "dark side" and produces negative externalities such as inequality, discrimination and intolerance. Conversely, "bridging" social capital, equality and tolerance are positive and mutually reinforcing. Szreter and Woolcock (2004) enriched this classification by adding "linking" social capital understood as relations of trust between people and power authorities. This kind of trust is most commonly measured as trust/confidence in institutions.

Debates about the diversity of social capital types, dimensions, its roots and consequences have resulted in its "wide" interpretation which encompasses tolerance, values, cooperative attitudes and other "facilitating coordinated actions" properties as its additional elements. For instance, Knack and Keefer (1997), in their seminal paper on economic payoff of social capital use several indicators. These indicators encompass trust in most people, membership in organizations and justification of immoral behavior (bribe-taking, tax-cheating, claiming illegal government benefits etc.). Nahapiet and Ghoshal (1998) distinguish between three interrelated dimensions of social capital: structural, relational and cognitive. The structural component refers to the configuration of network ties, their density, hierarchical nature etc. The relational component describes personal relations between actors in the network. Nahapiet and Ghoshal link the relational component to trust and trustworthiness, norms and sanctions, obligations and expectations, and identity. The cognitive component covers shared representations, language, system of meanings and narratives.

To keep things simple, Uphoff (2000) and later Grootaert and van Bastelaer (2001) collapse the cognitive and relational dimensions into a single element. Uphoff defines the structural component as roles (formal and informal), rules, procedures and networks which contribute to cooperation and mutually beneficial collective behavior. The cognitive/relational component refers to mental processes which result in norms, values, attitudes and beliefs that contribute to cooperative and mutually beneficial collective behavior (Uphoff, 2000). These norms, values, attitudes and beliefs as primary forms of social capital covers trust and reciprocity, solidarity, cooperation, and generosity. Table 1 provides a detailed overview of these elements.

Table 1 Structure of cognitive dimension according to Uphoff

	Norms	Values	Attitudes	Beliefs
Trust and reciprocity	Reciprocity	Being trustworthy	Trust	Others will reciprocate
Solidarity	Helping others beyond family	Maintaining solidarity within a larger group	Benevolence towards members of larger group	Others will uphold solidarity norms
Cooperation	Working together	Being cooperative	Cooperation with others	Others will cooperate
Generosity	Altruistic behavior	Acting generously	Generosity	Others will act generously Others will not take advantage of one's generosity

Adapted from Uphoff (2000), pp. 241–243

To maintain the norm of reciprocity people should value trustworthiness, be trustful and believe that others will reciprocate. Helpfulness is based on the value of solidarity with outgoups, benevolent attitudes and a belief that others will follow solidarity norms. The norm of working together requires the value of being cooperative, attitudes towards cooperation and belief that others will also cooperate. Finally, the norm of altruistic behavior has its roots in the value of acting generously, attitudes of generosity, and the belief that others will act generously and will not take advantage of that generosity.

Secondary forms of cognitive social capital such as honesty, egalitarism, fairness, participation, democratic governance, and concern for the future reinforce the primary components. Following this line, Brewer (2003) adds social altruism ("thinking and acting in helping ways"), support for equality, tolerance and humanitarism as "a sense of responsibility for other people's well-being and needs" (p. 11).

Analogously to Uphoff's interpretation of social capital, Mansbridge (1999) also acknowledge the importance of values and moral beliefs. She proposes the concept of "altruistic trust". Unlike evidence-based trust altruistic trust is not rooted in the previous experience since it is the act "for the benefit of another" (p. 292). Altruistic trust goes beyond the prediction of possible malfeasance and therefore morally praiseworthy. Mansbridge points out three possible reasons for such unwarranted but morally praiseworthy trust. First, this kind of trust can be taken as a sign of respect for other people. Second, this kind of trust demonstrates that trust can occur even at the expense of one's own interests and security. Third, this trust functions as a role model for other people.

Uslaner (2002) incorporated and further developed this approach by connecting trust to moral values. Accordingly, trust in strangers implies that one has accepted them into the "moral community" (p. 1). Strangers are trustworthy and well-intentioned because they share the same fundamental values and feeling of common fate. This default assumption reduces risk, bridges members of out-groups and make cooperation more efficient.

Modernization theory of Inglehart and Welzel (2005) continues this line of theorizing and assigns values a critical role in the formation of social capital. According to Inglehart and Welzel, the shift from survival to self-expression (postmaterialist) values catalyzed by economic growth and existential security has led to a set of transformations in many life domains. The most important consequence of such a shift is the fundamental modification of the very basis of social life. Strong in-group ties, group conformity, in-group favoritism, discrimination and authoritarianism go hand in hand with survival values as a reaction to insecurity and resource scarcity. Self-expression values liberate people from the pre-defined patriarchal ties and in-group pressure. These values lead to autonomous choice and solidarities rooted in the individual interests and preferences. In other words, a value shift results in a replacement of social capital types: "bridging ties replace bonding ties, and generalized trust replaces intimate trust" (p. 143).

This process affects not only the predominant type of trust and social ties but also another element of social capital—political and civic participation. Contra Putnam, Inglehart and Welzel do not see an erosion of voluntary membership but rather a change in its nature. While traditional membership in the "old-style hierarchical elite-directed organizations" and political participation is declining, novel forms of "elite-challenging activities" or "unconventional" participation (signing petitions, boycotts, demonstrations etc.) are increasing (Inglehart & Welzel, 2005, p. 117). Self-expression values are the key driver of such activities.

In *Freedom Rising* Welzel (2013) further develops the idea of the pro-civic character of values. He introduces a refined approach to the conceptualization and measurement of self-expression values and labels it "emancipative values". Welzel treats emancipative (self-expression) values as an individualistic orientation that is associated with unselfishness, trust and humanism but not with egoism. This interpretation of individualism sees everybody as autonomous individuals with equal rights that entail "respect and concern for others with whom there is no immediate relation" (Welzel, 2013, p. 193). To this extent such values "cut through group boundaries and make people more open to concern for remote and dissimilar others" and therefore closely related to the bridging social capital (Welzel, 2013, p. 193). This hypothesis has received strong empirical support by broad cross-cultural studies. Indeed, Welzel and his colleagues show that emancipative values have a significant and positive impact on generalized trust, benevolence and universalism. Furthermore, these links are even stronger if emancipative values prevail in a society (Welzel, 2013; Welzel & Delhey, 2015; Welzel & Deutsch, 2012).

Summarizing all existing theories, Scrivens and Smith (2013) identify four main ways of interpreting and measuring social capital: personal relationships, social network support, civic engagement, trust and cooperative norms. In the line with Uphoff, Brewer, Inglehart and Welzel they include cooperative norms as the most important values of a "good society".

The current volume also follows the broad interpretation of social capital and focuses on its three elements depicted at Fig. 2.

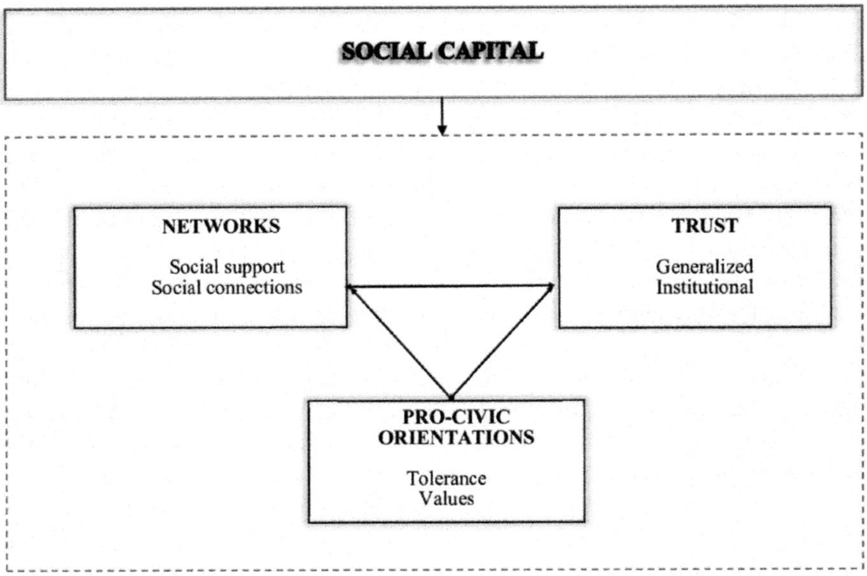

Fig. 2 The structure of social capital

Figure 2 covers: (1) networks and ties which provide social support and works as personal resource; (2) generalized and institutional trust (bridging and linking social capital); (3) human values and tolerance as pro-civic orientations which reinforce cooperative attitudes and cooperative practices. The contributors see these elements as separate but interrelated dimensions of social capital. They examine their roots in various regions of the world and their impact on subjective well-being.

3 Subjective Well-Being and Social Capital

Diener and Ryan (2009) define subjective well-being as "an umbrella term to describe the level of well-being people experience according to their subjective evaluations of their lives" (Diener & Ryan, 2009, p. 391). In other words, well-being reflects the practice of living a successful and balanced life. The history of theorizing about subjective well-being and happiness dates back to the works of ancient philosophers. Nonetheless, its active empirical exploration only began in the second half of the twentieth century by those who critiqued the idea that economy was the main indicator of human progress. Environmental problems raised the issue of more relevant and all-encompassing indicators of personal and societal development. These debates brought to the scene the concepts of "quality of life" and "subjective well-being". Today subjective well-being is a recognized and widely accepted measure of the "good life". There are several country rankings which are either completely based on subjective well-being or include its elements as a part of the overall index. Among them are the OECD's better life index (OECD Publishing, 2020), the World Happiness report (World Happiness Report, 2020), and ratings provided by the World Database of Happiness (Veenhoven, 2021a).

As with social capital, subjective well-being has a multifaceted structure. Subjective well-being is most often divided into cognitive and affective sub-dimensions. While the cognitive dimension relates to the overall life satisfaction and satisfaction with specific life domains (health, financial situation, job, social relations etc.), the affective dimension covers happiness, positive and negative affect. Veenhoven, the founder of the World Database of Happiness, counted 2839 ways of measuring subjective well-being (Veenhoven, 2021c).

The range of possible correlates of subjective well-being is also quite exhaustive (Veenhoven, 2021b). The most elaborated triggers at the individual (micro) level include genes, psychological traits, socio-demographic characteristics (age, gender, education, marriage status, children etc.), health, job characteristics, employment, income and religiosity (Clark et al., 2019; Cummins, 2000; Diener, 1999; Diener & Ryan, 2009; Diener et al., 2003; Pluess, 2015; Sonnentag, 2015; Veenhoven, 2011, 2012). The range of contextual (macro) determinants is also rather broad and encompasses climate, economic development, gender and income inequality, corruption, efficient political institutions, social policy, welfare regimes, culture and many others (Fischer & Van de Vliert, 2011; Rehdanz & Maddison, 2005; Veenhoven, 2011).

Social capital in its different interpretations and variations is considered to be one of the most important explanatory variables at the individual and country-level. A set of studies indeed demonstrate a positive association between subjective well-being, generalized trust, institutional trust, social networks, connections and social support, norms and values (Growiec & Growiec, 2014; Helliwell, 2006; Helliwell & Putnam, 2004; Hudson, 2006; Portela et al., 2013; Rodríguez-Pose & von Berlepsch, 2014; Tov & Diener, 2009). Nonetheless, these relations are relative not absolute since some scholars either fail to detect them or show that these effects are moderated by specific micro and macro-conditions and, therefore, differ in its strength, direction and significance (Burroughs & Rindfleisch, 2002; Elgar et al., 2011; Glatz & Eder, 2020; Sarracino, 2013; Schwartz & Sortheix, 2018; Sulemana, 2014; Welzel, 2013). This volume continues this line of research by investigating the limits of social capital in determining well-being across different social, economic and institutional contexts.

4 Outline of the Book

This book is organized into two sections. The first section is devoted to the trends and determinants of social capital across different regions of the world.

The first chapter is written by Mai Beilmann, Laur Lilleoja and Anu Realo. Using materials of the European Social Survey, World Values Survey and European Values

Study from 1990 to 2018 Beilmann et al. trace mutual trends of generalized, institutional trust, corruption, inequality and human development in three post-soviet Baltic countries: Estonia, Latvia and Lithuania. Their findings shed additional light on the evolution of generalized trust in the former USSR countries, its possible contextual obstacles, and triggers. The authors show that there is significant variation across three countries in terms of the shape of trust trends, speed of changes and the country-level associates.

Chapter 2 deals with emigration and trust. Although migration and its impact on receiving societies have been thoroughly explored, little is known about its influence on trust in the sending societies. Dragos Radu, Ekaterina Skoglund and Soomin Ma address this issue at the micro and macro level. Individual data obtained from six transitional countries in Eastern Europe and Central Asia (Kazakhstan, Moldova, Macedonia, Serbia, Tajikistan, Ukraine) reveals that individuals with migration experience or migration intentions have lower levels of generalized trust. At the same time, cross-sectional correlations demonstrate non-linear patterns between emigration rates and share of trusting people. Therefore, Radu et al. failed to detect a clear unidirectional impact of emigration on trust in the countries of origin.

In Chap. 3 Silko Pfeil, Rico Bornschein and Eric Holdack explore transformation of personal self-expression values in the context of migration from East to West Germany after the fall of the Berlin Wall. At the individual level values are considered to be rather stable characteristics which slowly change during the life-span. However, this stability hypothesis has insufficient empirical support since it requires a panel design with long time trends. The authors of the third chapter fill this gap incorporating longitudinal data from the German Socio-Economic Panel (SOEP) in 1996, 2006 and 2016. Their evidence favors the idea that individual values are not so stable and are likely to be adjusted to the existing social setting.

Chapter 4 continues this line of research and investigates the impact of economic hardship on values, trust, tolerance and well-being. Leen Vandecasteele and Tim Reeskens apply pseudo-panel fixed effects analysis to the data collected from 24 OECD countries participated in the European Social Survey in 2008 and 2016. They test how financial crisis of 2008 affected attitudes and values across age cohorts. Contrary to expectations, they did not find conclusive and robust evidence of the negative impact of the Great Recession on values, generalized trust and tolerance towards migrants. However, they did find a detrimental effect of economic insecurity on political trust, tolerance towards homosexuals and subjective well-being. Important to note that these effects vary across age cohorts.

Chapter 5, written by David Sulmont and Kiara Castaman, deals with tolerance to LGBTI people in Latin America. Analyzing recent changes in the legislation of the sexual and civil rights of LGBTI individuals they posit several questions. How attitudes towards LGBTI people are changing in this region? How these changes relate to the economic and cultural modernization? What are the individual drivers of the LGBTI tolerance? They show that tolerance to the LGBTI community has grown dramatically over the last 20 years. This changes co-occur with democratization and economic development but not with self-expression values. Religiosity promote intolerance to LGBTI but this effect is not universal and depend on denomination. Catholics are found to be the most tolerant religious group.

Chapter 6, authored by Sotheeswari Somasundram, Muzafar Shah Habibullah, Murali Sambasivan and Ratneswary Rasiah further investigate the impact of religiosity. They focus on religious tolerance in four countries of Southeast Asia (Malaysia, Philippines, Thailand and Singapore) and draw a line between social and individual religiosity. Their findings reveal robust positive effect of individual religiosity in Philippines, Thailand and Singapore. In Malaysia it turns to be negative. The authors assign this detrimental effect to colonial heritage and high politicization of intergroup relations.

The second section analyses the influence of social capital on different elements of subjective well-being at the individual and societal level.

Chapter 7 written by Jesús Peiró-Palomino and Emili Tortosa-Ausina examines the link between social capital as an informal institution and life satisfaction. In their study Peiró-Palomino and Tortosa-Ausina analyze the impact of social context across 166 European regions. This strategy allows them to account for within-country heterogeneity. They find evidence of a positive influence of social capital on life satisfaction but note that the strength of this effect is not universal and becomes stronger in areas where life satisfaction is lower.

Chapter 8 written by Isabel Neira, Marta Portela and Maricruz Lacalle-Calderon also considers the impact of institutions on subjective well-being. They concentrate on Latin America, which is a paradoxical region because, although there are high levels of well-being there are, at the same time, low levels of trust and satisfaction with democracy. Using multilevel regression analysis of 18 Latin America countries Neira et al. detect a positive link between subjective well-being, perceptions of democracy and institutional trust at both the individual and country-level. However, they find no impact of generalized trust on subjective well-being.

In Chap. 9 Janine Jongbloed and Ashley Pullman analyze the moderating effect of human capital on the relations between social capital and well-being. They make use of data on 27 countries from the sixth round (2012–2013) of the European Social Survey. They measure human capital as tertiary education, social capital as generalized trust and social relatedness and well-being as combination of happiness, life satisfaction and depression. Their findings show that social capital has a positive influence on subjective well-being. Education does moderate this relationship but not in all cases. The national share of people with tertiary education does not affect the link between individual social capital and well-being. Individual tertiary education reduces this positive influence and makes social capital less important in generating well-being for those who gain a university education. Therefore, Jongbloed and Pullman conclude that there is a "trade off" between human and social capital.

In Chap. 10 Irina Vartanova and Vladimir Gritskov continue investigation of human capital and its role in generating subjective well-being. They hypothesize that job-related characteristics such as salary, work-life conflict and autonomy mediate the link between knowledge work and well-being. Their study reveals significant positive impact of knowledge work on subjective well-being which is, indeed, partly explained by income. However, this positive effect is only significant in countries with less developed knowledge economy. Presumably, efficient social policy in knowledge societies mitigates the negative effect of low-skilled job on well-being.

In Chap. 11 Fredrica Nyqvist, Mikael Nygård and Thomas Scharf focus on the well-being of elderly Europeans. They examine the impact of social capital on the feeling of loneliness for people living in five welfare regions before and after Global Financial Crisis of 2008. They treat Nordic, Continental, Anglo-Saxon, Eastern-European and Southern-European welfare regimes as potential moderators affecting the link between loneliness and social capital. They confirm their hypotheses and show that the positive role of generalized trust and social contacts in overcoming alienation at an older age is not uniform across welfare regimes and time points.

The conclusion, written by Anna Almakaeva, Alejandro Moreno and Rima Wilkes, summarizes the main findings presented in all chapters of the volume. It covers several aspects which are important for better understanding of social capital and subjective well-being. First, the conclusion discusses the stability and plasticity of trust, values, tolerance and well-being. Second, it outlines the impact of cultural legacy, exogenous shocks and transition periods on social capital and well-being. Third, it analyses the roots of social capital and its influence on subjective well-being across various social, economic and institutional contexts.

Acknowledgements The work of Anna Almakaeva on this chapter and the whole volume was supported by the HSE University Basic Research Program and the Russian Academic Excellence Project '5–100'. The editors thank Francesco Sarracino for his valuable comments and suggestions.

References

Algan, Y., & Cahuc, P. (2013). Trust and growth. *Annual Review of Economics, 5*(1), 521–549. https://doi.org/10.1146/annurev-economics-081412-102108

Algan, Y., & Cahuc, P. (2014). Trust, growth, and well-being: New evidence and policy implications. In P. Aghion & S. N. Durlauf (Eds.), *Handbook of economic growth* (Vol. 2, pp. 49–120). Elsevier. https://doi.org/10.1016/B978-0-444-53538-2.00002-2

Bhandari, H., & Yasunobu, K. (2009). What is social capital? A comprehensive review of the concept. *Asian Journal of Social Science, 37*(3), 480–510. https://doi.org/10.1163/156853109X436847

Bourdieu, P. (2011). The forms of capital. *Cultural Theory: An Anthology, 1*, 81–93.

Brewer, G. A. (2003). Building social capital: Civic attitudes and behavior of public servants. *Journal of Public Administration Research and Theory: J-PART, 13*(1), 5–25.

Burroughs, J. E., & Rindfleisch, A. (2002). Materialism and well-being: A conflicting values perspective. *Journal of Consumer Research, 29*(3), 348–370. https://doi.org/10.1086/344429

Clark, A. E., Flèche, S., Layard, R., Powdthavee, N., & Ward, G. (2019). *The origins of happiness: The science of well-being over the life course*. Princeton University Press.

Coleman, J. (1998). Social capital in the creation of human capital. *American Journal of Sociology, 94*, 95–120.

Cummins, R. A. (2000). Personal income and subjective well-being: A review. *Journal of Happiness Studies, 1*(2), 133–158. https://doi.org/10.1023/A:1010079728426

Delhey, J., & Newton, K. (2005). Predicting cross-national levels of social trust: Global pattern or Nordic exceptionalism? *European Sociological Review, 21*(4), 311–327. https://doi.org/10.1093/esr/jci022

Diener, E. (1999). Subjective well-being: Three decades of progress.https://doi.org/10.1037/0033-2909.125.2.276

Diener, E., Oishi, S., & Lucas, R. E. (2003). Personality, culture, and subjective well-being: Emotional and cognitive evaluations of life. *Annual Review of Psychology, 54*(1), 403–425. https://doi.org/10.1146/annurev.psych.54.101601.145056

Diener, E., & Ryan, K. (2009). Subjective well-being: A general overview. *South African Journal of Psychology, 39*(4), 391–406. https://doi.org/10.1177/008124630903900402

Elgar, F. J., Davis, C. G., Wohl, M. J., Trites, S. J., Zelenski, J. M., & Martin, M. S. (2011). Social capital, health and life satisfaction in 50 countries. *Health & Place, 17*(5), 1044–1053. https://doi.org/10.1016/j.healthplace.2011.06.010

Fischer, R., & Van de Vliert, E. (2011). Does climate undermine subjective well-being? A 58-nation study. *Personality and Social Psychology Bulletin, 37*(8), 1031–1041. https://doi.org/10.1177/0146167211407075

Glatz, C., & Eder, A. (2020). Patterns of trust and subjective well-being across Europe: New insights from repeated cross-sectional analyses based on the European social survey 2002–2016. *Social Indicators Research, 148*(2), 417–439. https://doi.org/10.1007/s11205-019-02212-x

Granovetter, M. S. (1973). The strength of weak ties. *American Journal of Sociology, 78*(6), 1360–1380. https://doi.org/10.1086/225469

Grootaert, C., & van Bastelaer, T. (2001). *Understanding and measuring social capital: A multidisciplinary tool for practitioners*. World Bank Publications. Retrieved from http://ebookcentral.proquest.com/lib/hselibrary-ebooks/detail.action?docID=3050532

Growiec, K., & Growiec, J. (2014). Trusting only whom you know, knowing only whom you trust: The joint impact of social capital and trust on happiness in CEE countries. *Journal of Happiness Studies, 15*(5), 1015–1040. https://doi.org/10.1007/s10902-013-9461-8

Helliwell, J. F., & Putnam, R. D. (2004). The social context of well-being. *Philosophical Transactions of the Royal Society B: Biological Sciences, 359*(1449), 1435–1446. https://doi.org/10.1098/rstb.2004.1522

Helliwell, J. F. (2006). Well-being, social capital and public policy: What's new? *The Economic Journal, 116*(510), C34–C45.

Hudson, J. (2006). Institutional trust and subjective well-being across the EU. *Kyklos, 59*(1), 43–62. https://doi.org/10.1111/j.1467-6435.2006.00319.x

Inglehart, R., & Welzel, C. (2005). *Modernization, cultural change, and democracy: The human development sequence*. Cambridge University Press.

Knack, S., & Keefer, P. (1997). Does social capital have an economic payoff? A cross-country investigation. *The Quarterly Journal of Economics*, 1251–1288.

Lollo, E. (2012). *Toward a theory of social capital definition: Its dimensions and resulting social capital types*. Presented at the 14th world congress of social economics. Available at: http:/socialeconomics.orgPapersLollo1C.pdf

Mansbridge, J. (1999). Altruistic trust. In M. E. Warren (Ed.), *Democracy and trust* (pp. 290–309). Cambridge University Press. https://doi.org/10.1017/CBO9780511659959.010

Nahapiet, J., & Ghoshal, S. (1998). Social capital, intellectual capital, and the organizational advantage. *Academy of Management Review, 23*(2), 242–266. https://doi.org/10.5465/AMR.1998.533225

Pluess, M. (2015). *Genetics of psychological well-being: The role of heritability and genetics in positive psychology*. Series in Positive Psychology.

Portela, M., Neira, I., & Salinas-Jiménez, M. del M. (2013). Social capital and subjective wellbeing in Europe: A new approach on social capital. *Social Indicators Research, 114*(2), 493–511.https://doi.org/10.1007/s11205-012-0158-x

Portes, A. (1998). Social capital: Its origins and applications in modern sociology. *Annual Review of Sociology, 24*(1), 1–24. https://doi.org/10.1146/annurev.soc.24.1.1

Publishing, O. E. C. D. (2020). *How's life? 2020: Measuring well-being [Text]*. Retrieved from. https://doi.org/10.1787/9870c393-en

Putnam, R. D. (2001*). Bowling alone: The collapse and revival of American community*. Simon and Schuster.

Putnam, R. D., Leonardi, R., & Nonetti, R. Y. (1994). *Making democracy work: Civic traditions in modern Italy*. Princeton University Press.

Rehdanz, K., & Maddison, D. (2005). Climate and happiness. *Ecological Economics, 52*(1), 111–125.

Rodríguez-Pose, A., & von Berlepsch, V. (2014). Social capital and individual happiness in Europe. *Journal of Happiness Studies, 15*(2), 357–386. https://doi.org/10.1007/s10902-013-9426-y

Sarracino, F. (2013). Determinants of subjective well-being in high and low income countries: Do happiness equations differ across countries? *The Journal of Socio-Economics, 42*, 51–66. https://doi.org/10.1016/j.socec.2012.11.006

Schwartz, S. H., & Sortheix, F. (2018). Values and subjective well-being. In *Handbook of well-being. Noba Scholar*. Retrieved from https://jyx.jyu.fi/handle/123456789/56855

Scrivens, K., & Smith, C. (2013). Four interpretations of social capital: An agenda for measurement. (No. 2013/06). https://doi.org/10.1787/5jzbcx010wmt-en

Sonnentag, S. (2015). Dynamics of well-being. *Annual Review of Organizational Psychology and Organizational Behavior, 2*(1), 261–293. https://doi.org/10.1146/annurev-orgpsych-032414-111347

Sulemana, I. (2014). An empirical investigation of the relationship between social capital and subjective well-being in Ghana. *Journal of Happiness Studies*. https://doi.org/10.1007/s10902-014-9565-9

Szreter, S., & Woolcock, M. (2004). Health by association? Social capital, social theory, and the political economy of public health. *International Journal of Epidemiology, 33*(4), 650–667.

Tov, W., & Diener, E. (2009). The well-being of nations: linking together trust, cooperation, and democracy. In E. Diener (Ed.), *The science of well-being* (pp. 155–173). Springer Netherlands. Retrieved from http://dx.doi.org/https://doi.org/10.1007/978-90-481-2350-6_7

Uphoff, N. (2000). Understanding social capital: Learning from the analysis and experience of participation. *Social Capital: A Multifaceted Perspective, 6*(2), 215–249.

Uslaner, E. M. (2002). *The moral foundations of trust*. Cambridge University Press.

Uslaner, E. M. (2013). Trust and corruption revisited: How and why trust and corruption shape each other. *Quality & Quantity, 47*(6), 3603–3608. https://doi.org/10.1007/s11135-012-9742-z

Veenhoven, R. (2011). Greater happiness for a greater number: Is that possible? If so, how. In *Designing positive psychology: Taking stock and moving forward* (pp. 396–409).

Veenhoven, R. (2012). Happiness: Also known as "life satisfaction" and "subjective well-being." In *Handbook of social indicators and quality of life research* (pp. 63–77). Springer.

Veenhoven, R. (2021a). Average happiness in 162 nations 2010–2018. World database of happiness, Erasmus University Rotterdam, The Netherlands. Retrieved from worlddatabaseofhappiness-archive.eur.nl/hap_nat/findingreports/RankReport_AverageHappiness.php

Veenhoven, R. (2021b). Correlational findings on happiness. World database of happiness, Erasmus University Rotterdam, The Netherlands. Retrieved from https://worlddatabaseofhappiness.eur.nl/search-the-database/correlational-findings/

Veenhoven, R. (2021c). Happiness measures. World database of happiness, Erasmus University Rotterdam, The Netherlands. Retrieved from https://worlddatabaseofhappiness.eur.nl/search-the-database/happiness-measures/

Welzel, C. (2013). *Freedom Rising: Human empowerment and the contemporary quest for emancipation*. Cambridge University Press.

Welzel, C., & Delhey, J. (2015). Generalizing trust: The benign force of emancipation. *Journal of Cross-Cultural Psychology, 46*(7), 875–896. https://doi.org/10.1177/0022022115588366

Welzel, C., & Deutsch, F. (2012). Emancipative values and non-violent protest: The importance of 'ecological' effects. *British Journal of Political Science, 42*(2), 465–479. https://doi.org/10.1017/S0007123411000421

World Happiness Report. (2020). Retrieved from http://worldhappiness.report/
WVS Database.(n.d.). Retrieved from https://www.worldvaluessurvey.org/WVSContents.jsp.
Zak, P. J., & Knack, S. (2001). Trust and growth. *The Economic Journal, 111*(470), 295–321.

Anna Almakaeva (Ph.D. in Sociology) is a deputy head of the Ronald F. Inglehart Laboratory for Comparative Social Research at the Higher School of Economics (Russia). Her research interests include social capital, values, subjective well-being and comparative studies. She is a member of the World Value Survey Russian team and the European Values Study Russian team.

Rima Wilkes (Ph.D.) is a professor at the department of Sociology at the University of British Columbia (Canada). In 2017–2018 she was president of the Canadian Sociological Association. Her research interests include political sociology, race and ethnicity, trust, immigration and social movements.

Trust, Tolerance and Values as Dimensions of Social Capital

Learning to Trust: Trends in Generalized Social Trust in the Three Baltic Countries from 1990 to 2018

Mai Beilmann, Laur Lilleoja, and Anu Realo

1 Introduction

Generalized social trust (social trust), that is, the willingness to trust others, even total strangers, without the expectation that they will immediately reciprocate that trust or favor, is often seen as the glue that holds a society together and fosters cooperation among individuals. There is a growing amount of empirical evidence that social trust is related to many positive societal and individual outcomes, such as economic growth and good economic performance (LaPorta et al., 1997; Neira et al., 2010; Uslaner, 2002; Whiteley, 2000), reduced crime levels (Akcomak & Weel, 2011; Whiteley, 2000), higher levels of political trust (Beilmann & Lilleoja, 2017), better governance and an effective state (LaPorta et al., 1997; Uslaner, 2002; Whiteley, 2000; Zmerli & Newton, 2008), more civic participation (LaPorta et al., 1997; Putnam, 2000), better health (Knesebeck et al., 2005), and higher levels of happiness and wellbeing (Inglehart, 1999; Putnam, 2000). As a result, social trust, which is often considered one of the key elements of social capital, is extremely important for the smooth functioning of democratic societies. Even though it is still disputed whether social trust is the cause or the outcome of these desirable social

M. Beilmann (✉)
Institute of Social Studies, University of Tartu, Tartu, Estonia
e-mail: mai.beilmann@ut.ee

L. Lilleoja
Research Centre for Survey Methodology (RECSM), Universitat Pompeu Fabra, Barcelona, Spain

A. Realo
Department of Psychology, University of Warwick, Coventry, UK

Institute of Psychology, University of Tartu, Tartu, Estonia

A. Realo
e-mail: A.Realo@warwick.ac.uk

A. Almakaeva et al. (eds.), *Social Capital and Subjective Well-Being*, Societies and Political Orders in Transition,
https://doi.org/10.1007/978-3-030-75813-4_2

conditions, it appears to be an important factor for the success of a new democracy. This paper aims to analyze the trends in the levels of social trust in the three Baltic countries—Estonia, Latvia, and Lithuania—from the beginning of 1990s until the present day. The Baltic countries serve as an example of how levels of social trust can dramatically change in just a few decades alongside rapid social, economic, and political changes.

2 Sources of Social Trust

Despite extensive research, there is no consensus among scholars about the origins of social trust. Several authors have argued that prevailing values in a society are the outcome of its current political and social situation, as well as of the country's historical, cultural, and religious background (e.g., Inglehart, 1997; Schwartz, 1999). Analogously, it has been claimed that differences in social trust levels across countries may be driven by their cultural and historical differences (Bjørnskov, 2007; Halpern, 2005; Putnam, 1993; Uslaner, 2002). A nation's post-communist heritage, in particular, has been found to be a major hazard for the development and sustainability of social trust. Indeed, trust levels vary considerably between European countries (Beilmann & Lilleoja, 2015; Beilmann et al., 2018; Neller, 2008; Newton, 2004), with people in the former Eastern Bloc countries being generally less trusting than people in Western, and most notably, Northern parts of Europe (Bjørnskov, 2007).

From a theoretical perspective, there are two contrasting ways of explaining the level (and/or absence) of social trust. Social trust can be seen either as an individual trait or as an attribute of the social environment. Authors like Uslaner (2017) and Yamagishi and Yamagishi (1994) emphasize that a certain level of optimism toward the trustworthiness of others is an essential part of social trust. For them, social trust is more like an individual trait: some people just trust other people more than others because they have a trusting personality or because they were brought up that way. Another possibility is to conceptualize trust not as a characteristic of individuals, but rather as a feature of the social environment. Authors such as Putnam (2000), Whiteley (2000), Delhey and Newton (2005), Newton (2004), and Ostrom and Ahn (2009) see social trust primarily as a social norm that people can learn from their social environment over their life course. This stance is somewhat different from Uslaner's (2000, 2002) view, according to which our tendency to trust or distrust other people is learned at an early age and does not change much in our adulthood. Uslaner's view is supported by several large-scale empirical studies that have shown that social trust levels are fairly stable over time and can be thus considered as a cultural feature of a society (Bjørnskov, 2007). The latter perspective, however, does not help to explain major fluctuations in the levels of social trust in several Eastern European countries in the nearly three decades following the fall of Soviet rule. Therefore, we take a particular interest in theories which claim that social trust is primarily a norm learned from the social environment and that the surrounding social context can have a profound effect on how much people trust others around them.

A country's political and institutional setting, such as trustworthy state institutions (e.g., the police force and the legal system) and good governance, seem to be important factors in producing high levels of social trust among a country's citizens (Neller, 2008; Newton, 2004; Rothstein, 2005; Rothstein & Stolle, 2003; Stolle, 2003). Following the definition of Delhey and Newton (2005), that social trust is the belief that others will not deliberately cheat or harm us as long as they can avoid doing so, social trust can be seen as a social norm that people learn from their environment. When people see that state officials treat people equally and are not involved in corrupt activities, a highly visible example that it is reasonable to expect honesty and trustworthiness even from people whom one does not know very well is offered (Rothstein, 2005). Corrupt state institutions, on the other hand, are often considered one of the main causes of low levels of social trust, because their activities give a very strong signal that one can trust other people only very selectively (Rothstein, 2005; Uslaner, 2002). Newton (2004) even suggested that individual responses to standard trust questions are evaluations of the society in which they live, whereas Beugelsdijk (2006) argued that measures of trust are simply surrogate measures of the quality of a country's institutions, as countries with strong institutions have high levels of trust. Uslaner (2017), on the contrary, expressed very clearly that better government most definitely does not lead to greater social trust and that social trust is not based upon personal experience. According to Uslaner (2017), social trust "leads to greater institutional quality rather than stemming from structural foundations" (p. 61), and that it would be more fruitful to look at the individual characteristics of people when searching for the sources of social trust.

Indeed, there is evidence that, at the individual level, social trust is influenced by a wide range of socioeconomic and contextual factors, such as education (Hooghe et al., 2012; Neller, 2008; Putnam, 2000, 2002; Uslaner, 2017), race (Uslaner, 2017), and religion (Neller, 2008; Uslaner, 2017), among several others. However, it has been recently demonstrated that the relationship between education and social trust, for example, is in fact mediated by state efficacy. Using survey data from three continents, Güemes and Herreros, (2019) exemplified the importance of state efficacy in generating social trust by demonstrating that, in countries with high levels of state efficacy, it is the most educated (and intelligent) people who are most trusting, whereas, in countries with low state efficacy, highly educated people are the least trustful. Intuitively, this makes perfect sense, as it would be equally harmful and ignorant to place trust in others in countries with low levels of social trust (Whiteley, 2000). Therefore, it is very difficult to create social trust in places where it does not exist. These views give little hope for any rapid increase in social trust, but nevertheless suggest that there is a tiny possibility that, in societies where state institutions go through radical reforms toward more trustworthy and transparent functioning and less corruption, the citizens of these societies will eventually become more trusting towards generalized others.

Another important socioeconomic factor that has been found to affect social trust levels is social and economic (in)equality (Bjørnskov, 2007; Jordahl, 2009; Neller, 2008; Newton, 2004; Stolle, 2003; Uslaner, 2002, 2017). Uslaner (2017), for example, claims that "at the societal level, trust depends most strongly on the level of economic equality in a society. When there are high levels of inequality, the rich and the poor do not see each other as part of the same moral community" (p. 61). Yet, the mechanism of the relationship between inequality and social trust is contested and unclear, with some authors even suggesting that the relationship between inequality and social trust might only hold for countries with very high levels of income inequality (Steijn & Lancee, 2011).

3 The Aims of the Current Study

In this chapter, we will examine trends in social trust levels in the three Baltic countries—Estonia, Latvia, and Lithuania—over a period of nearly thirty years, that is, since 1991, when they regained their independence, until 2018, when the three Baltic countries celebrated the hundred year anniversary of their first declarations of independence. We will also provide some possible explanations for the changes in social trust levels in these three countries.

As the Baltic countries have gone through major social, economic, and political transitions in the last three decades, it seems plausible that explanations for changes in social trust should be primarily sought at the societal level. Therefore, our analyses will focus on examining the effects of a trustworthy state and good governance, low corruption, and social and economic equality on changes in social trust levels in the three Baltic countries. We expect to see an effect for those societal indicators on the levels of social trust. For instance, the levels of social trust and economic inequality should go hand in hand with social trust declining in the Baltic countries, as socioeconomic inequality rapidly increased after the countries regained their independence in 1991.

4 Method

4.1 Data

We were not able to find any trustworthy longitudinal studies with the *same participants being followed* continuously over a period of 30 years for all three Baltic countries. For this reason, we combined data from different cross-national and repeated cross-sectional survey programs, such as the World Values Survey (WVS), the European Values Survey (EVS), and the European Social Survey (ESS), that have measured social trust in representative samples of Estonian, Latvian, and Lithuanian inhabitants from 1990 to 2018.

More specifically, this paper draws upon six waves of WVS and EVS (1990, 1996, 1999, 2008, 2011, and 2018) and eight waves of ESS (2004, 2006, 2008, 2010, 2012, 2014, 2016, and 2018). Estonia and Lithuania have taken part in all rounds of ESS

Table 1 Overview of studies and samples used in the analyses

Study	Year	Estonia	Latvia	Lithuania
ESS	*2004*	1989	n/a	n/a
	2006	1517	1960	n/a
	2008	1661	1980	2002
	2010	1793	n/a	1677
	2012	2380	n/a	2109
	2014	2051	n/a	2250
	2016	2019	n/a	2122
	2018	1905	918	1835
WVS/EVS	*1990*	1008	903	1000
	1996	1021	1200	1009
	1999	1005	1013	1018
	2008	1518	1506	1499
	2011	1533	n/a	n/a
	2018	1308	n/a	1488

Note ESS European Social Survey, *WVS* World Values Survey, *EVS* European Values Survey

since 2004 and 2008, respectively, whereas Latvia has participated in four rounds (i.e., in 2006, 2008, 2014, and 2018) but the data for the 2014 round were never published. Therefore, for Latvia, we can only use the ESS data from 2006, 2008 to 2018. There are similar problems in WVS/EVS datasets: whereas Estonia has participated in six data collection waves since 1990, Lithuania has taken part in five and Latvia only four rounds of data collection. An overview of all studies and samples used in the analyses is shown in Table 1.

Besides social trust, which is the main interest of this study, WVS/EVS and ESS datasets also allow us to measure the levels of institutional trust across the three Baltic states from 1990 to 2018.

In order to analyze how country-level changes have affected levels of social trust, we combine individual-level survey data with several relevant country-level indexes (i.e., Transparency International Perceived Corruption Index, GINI index, and Human Development Index), as described below.

4.2 *Measures*

4.2.1 Individual-Level Indices

Social trust. Both WVS and EVS contain a dichotomous question “Generally speaking, would you say that most people can be trusted or that you need to be very careful in dealing with people?” (1 = “Most people can be trusted”, 2 = “Need to be very careful"). In ESS, social trust is measured with a similar question "Would you say that most people can be trusted, or that you can't be too careful in dealing with people?" but the answers are given on an 11-point Likert-type scale, ranging from 0 = "You can't be too careful" to 10 = "Most people can be trusted".

To make social trust variables across the different datasets comparable, the social trust variable in ESS was recoded into a binary format similar to WVS/EVS, so that 1 (values 6–10) represents respondents who would argue that "most people can be trusted" and 2 (values 0–5 and "don't knows")[1] those respondents who would rather say that one "can't be too careful" in dealing with people or who choose the answer "don't know" (Table 2). In our analyses, we use the proportion of respondents who either answered that "most people can be trusted" (as in WVS/EVS data) or who gave a score of 6–10 in ESS data.

It is clear that, due to differences in the measurement of social trust and sampling methods, social trust values across the two different datasets (i.e., WVS/EVS vs. ESS) cannot be considered 100% equivalent. However, when comparing *the trends* in social trust values in Estonia during the study period 1990–2018, we can see a very similar pattern of responses across the two surveys over time (Fig. 1). Overall, the percentage of respondents who would argue that "most people can be trusted" shows a clear increase across the study period in both surveys, yet the proportion of respondents indicating that they would trust other people seems to systematically differ between the surveys, with levels of social trust being higher in the ESS data than in the WVS/EVS data. Therefore, we acknowledge that the social trust levels in our datasets are not directly comparable, but we can assume that the relationships within each of these datasets are comparable.

Institutional trust. In WVS and EVS, the question measuring trust towards different institutions is formulated in the following way: "I am going to name a number of organizations. For each one, could you tell me how much confidence you have in them: is it a great deal of confidence, quite a lot of confidence, not very much confidence or none at all?" (1 = "A great deal", 2 = "Quite a lot", 3 = "Not very much", 4 = "None at all"). The institutions that were included in the analyses were the following: (a) the church, (b) the press, (c) the police, (d) parliament, (e) the government, f) the justice system, and g) political parties.

In ESS, the question for institutional trust is formulated in the same way as for social trust: "Using this card, please tell me on a score of 0–10 how much you personally trust each of the institutions I read out. 0 means you do not trust an institution at all, and 10 means you have complete trust." In the current study, we were interested in levels of trust in the following institutions: (a) parliament, (b) the legal system, (c) the police, (d) politicians, and (e) political parties.

A similar procedure as for social trust was applied when comparing the level of trust in different institutions across different studies (i.e., ESS and WVS/EVS). As indicated in Table 3, the variables in ESS and WVS/EVS were recoded into a binary

[1] Based on analyses for similar scales, the middle category (5) in 11-point scales tends to work also as "don't know" and, therefore, when comparing only positive responses, bias should be small (Zuell & Scholz, 2016).

Table 2 Scale transformations of social trust measures

Study	*Need to be careful or don't know* (2)							*Most people can be trusted* (1)				
ESS	DK	0 You can't be too careful	1	2	3	4	5	6	7	8	9	10 Most people can be trusted
WVS/EVS	DK	2 Need to be very careful						1 Most people can be trusted				

Note ESS European Social Survey, *WVS* World Values Survey, *EVS* European Values Survey; DK = respondents who answered "Don't know"

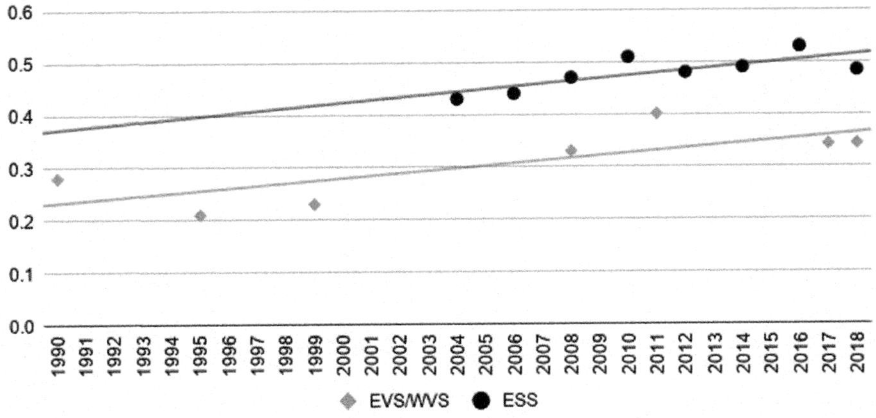

Fig. 1 The percentage of people in Estonia who would argue that most people can be trusted based on year and survey. ESS = European Social Survey; WVS = World Values Survey; EVS = European Values Survey

format similar to the social trust indicator, so that 1 (values 6–10 in ESS; values 1 and 2 in WVS/EVS) represents respondents who would argue that they trust or have confidence in different institutions and 2 (values 0 to 5 and "don't knows" in ESS; values 3, 4, and "don't knows" in WVS/EVS) those respondents who do not trust or have confidence in different institutions or "don't know."

4.3 Country-Level Indices

In our analyses, we combine individual-level survey data with several relevant country-level indices (i.e., Transparency International Perceived Corruption Index, GINI index, and Human Development Index) in order to examine how country-level changes in corruption, social inequality, and human development may have affected levels of social trust over the study period.

Transparency International Perceived Corruption Index (CPI) is an aggregate indicator that ranks countries in terms of the degree to which corruption is perceived to exist among public officials and politicians. It is a composite index drawing on corruption-related data from a variety of independent and reputable institutions that ranges from 0 ("Highly corrupt") to 1 ("Very clean"). CPI data for Estonia, Latvia, and Lithuania have been available since 1998 and are provided by Transparency International.[2]

GINI index is a measure of the income inequality or wealth inequality within a country. The index ranges from 0 to 1, with 0 representing perfect equality and 1

[2] https://www.transparency.org/research/cpi/overview.

Table 3 Scale transformations of institutional trust measures

<table>
<tr><td>Study</td><td colspan="8">Do not trust or don't know (2)</td><td colspan="5">Trust (1)</td></tr>
<tr><td>ESS</td><td>DK</td><td>0 No trust at all</td><td colspan="2">1</td><td>2</td><td>3</td><td>4</td><td>5</td><td>6</td><td>7</td><td>8</td><td>9</td><td>10 Complete trust</td></tr>
<tr><td>WVS/EVS</td><td>DK</td><td colspan="2">4 None at all</td><td colspan="5">3 Not very much</td><td colspan="4">2 Quite a lot</td><td>1 A great deal</td></tr>
</table>

Note ESS European Social Survey, *WVS* World Values Survey, *EVS* European Values Survey; DK = respondents who answered "Don't know"

representing total inequality. The GINI index values for the three countries for the study period were taken from ESS Multilevel Data.[3]

Human Development Index (HDI) is a summary measure of average achievement in key dimensions of human development: (1) a long and healthy life, (2) being knowledgeable, and (3) having a decent standard of living.[4] HDI is the geometric mean of normalized indices for each of the three dimensions, with a maximum value of 1 indicating higher human development. HDI values for the study period were taken from ESS Multilevel Data.[5]

5 Analyses

We first examine whether and how levels of social trust have changed in the three Baltic countries during the period 1990–2018. In the second part of our study, we have a closer look at trends in social trust over time, along with trends in institutional trust across the last three decades in Estonia, Latvia, and Lithuania. The third set of analyses focuses on the relationships between social trust and various indices of societal development (e.g., social inequality, human development, etc.) with particular attention on the associations between social trust and the levels of perceived corruption from 1990 to 2018.

6 Results

6.1 Changes in Social Trust Levels in the Three Baltic Countries in 1990–2018

Compared to Western democracies, levels of social trust were rather low in the Baltic countries after the collapse of the Soviet Union and during the reorganization of political and social systems in mid 1990s. However, Estonia and Lithuania were able to recover from this post-totalitarian trauma quite well, as indicated by a considerable increase in the levels of social trust from the beginning of the new millennium (Fig. 2). Nevertheless, it seems that the increase in social trust may have come to a halt in recent years, with levels of social trust dropping back to where they were around 2010. In Latvia, the levels of social trust have been historically lower than in the other two Baltic countries, and surprisingly stable since 2008.

The growth in the level of social trust has been biggest and fastest in Estonia, where, according to WVS/EVS data, the proportion of people "who trust other

[3] https://www.europeansocialsurvey.org/data/multilevel/.

[4] http://hdr.undp.org/en/content/human-development-index-hdi.

[5] https://www.europeansocialsurvey.org/data/multilevel/.

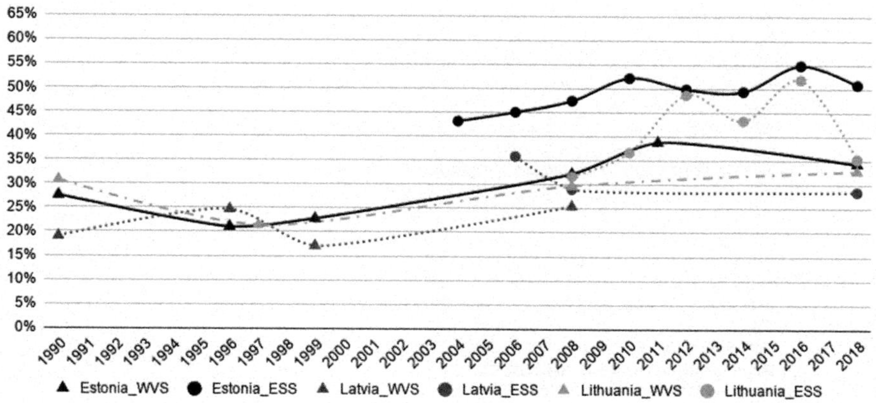

Fig. 2 The percentage of people in Estonia, Latvia, and Lithuania in 1990–2018 who would argue that most people can be trusted (*Data* ESS, WVS/EVS)

people" nearly doubled between 1996 and 2011. According to ESS data from 2018 (see Fig. 3), the proportion of Estonians (51%) who tend to trust other people is 8% higher than the European average of 43%, which ranks them 7th among 27 European countries, right after Ireland and ahead of Germany. Due to a sharp decline in their social trust levels between 2016 and 2018, Lithuanians (35.4%) have now fallen into the lower half of the European ranking, whereas levels of social trust in Latvia (28.6%), as already mentioned, were not only lower compared to its neighbor states of Estonia and Lithuania, but also well below the European average of 43% in 2018.

The growth in social trust in Estonia and Lithuania in the period 1996–2018 is rather remarkable, not only among European countries, but over the entire world. WVS/EVS data reveal that, in the period 1996–2018, the increase in social trust levels in Estonia and Lithuania was one of the greatest (13.0% and 10.4%, respectively) among the 46 countries which participated in the survey in both years (Fig. 4).

On the basis of these findings, two important conclusions can be drawn. First, the levels of social trust (especially when using ESS data) vary greatly across the three Baltic countries, with Estonia having consistently higher levels of social trust than Lithuania and, especially, Latvia. Second, while levels of social trust steadily increased in Estonia and Lithuania from 1996 to 2016, the levels of social trust in Latvia are roughly at the same level in 2018 as they were in mid-1990s.

6.2 *Social Trust and Trust in Institutions*

The different patterns and rates of change in social trust levels in the three Baltic countries raise the obvious issue of how to explain these differences. As a trustworthy state and good governance have been found to be positively associated with social

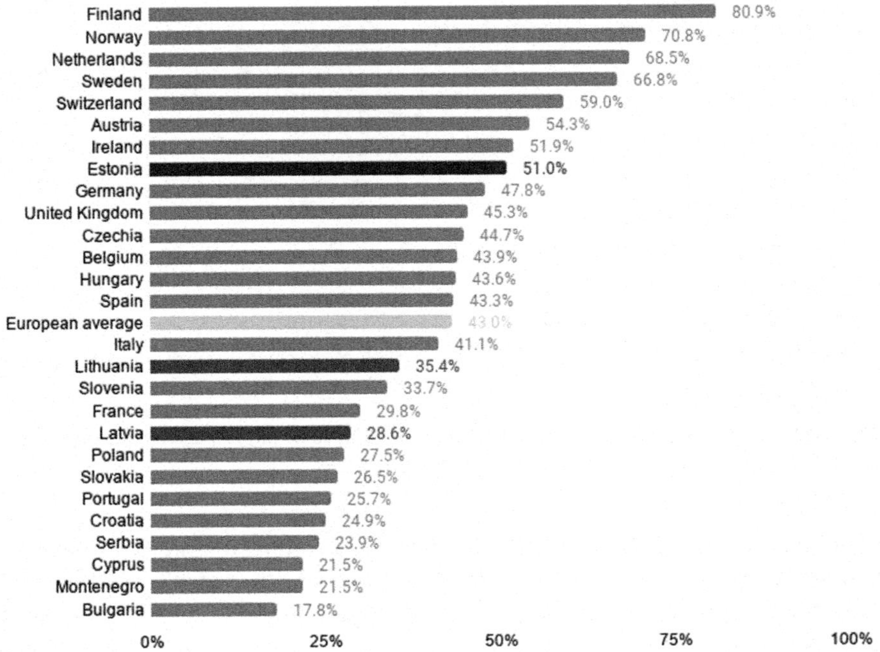

Fig. 3 Generalized social trust in European countries in 2018. The percentage of respondents who gave scores of 6 to 10 to the question "Would you say that most people can be trusted, or that you can't be too careful in dealing with people?", ranging from 0 = "You can't be too careful" to 10 = "Most people can be trusted" (*Data* ESS 2018)

trust, it is worthwhile mapping out the trends in institutional trust in the Baltic countries alongside levels of social trust from the beginning of the 1990s. Our assumption is that trustworthiness, as well as trust in state institutions, has gone through major changes since the three countries regained their independence in 1991, and these changes may contribute to changes in social trust levels, as trust and satisfaction with state institutions tend to increase levels of social trust.

Looking at the trends in social and institutional trust levels in Estonia using the WVS/EVS data, it is evident that the steady rise in social trust from 1999 is paralleled by a rapid increase in trust in non-political state institutions, such as the police and the legal system (Fig. 5). Similar growth in trust in political institutions (e.g., parliament, political parties, the government) or other major societal institutions (e.g., the press, the church) has not occurred—trust in these institutions peaked in 2011 and has steadily decreased since, reaching roughly the same level in 2018 as ten years earlier (i.e., in 2008).

In ESS data (Fig. 6), a somewhat similar pattern of rising levels of social trust and trust in non-political state institutions (e.g., police and legal system) appears. While trust in political state institutions (e.g., the government) is not as high as trust in non-political institutions, it has increased compared to the 2000s.

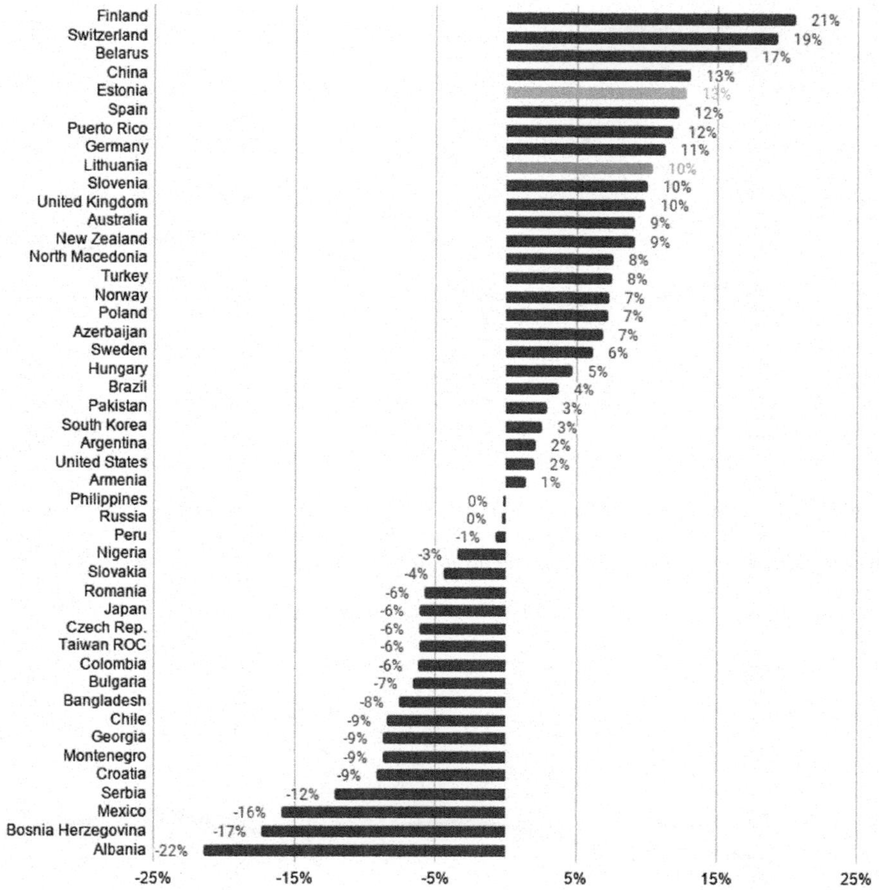

Fig. 4 Changes in the levels of generalized social trust in 46 countries in 1996–2018 (*Data* WVS/EVS). Key: scale shows how many percentage points the levels of generalized social trust have increased (the positive side of the scale) or decreased (the negative side of the scale) over the study period. Only the countries that participated in WVS/EVS survey rounds both in 1996 and 2018 are included in the analysis

In order to further analyze the relationships between the levels of social trust and trust in different institutions across time, we examined the profile correlations of trust levels in the Estonian and Lithuanian data. Table 4 describes the intraclass correlations between the levels of social trust and institutional trust across time, calculated as a Spearman correlation. As can be seen in Table 4, in Estonia, social trust was positively and significantly correlated with trust in the police in WVS/EVS data, and with confidence in the police, the justice system, the parliament, politicians, and political parties in ESS data. In Lithuania, social trust was positively and significantly correlated only with confidence in the justice system in WVS/EVS data. Latvia was excluded from this analysis due to the small number of data points.

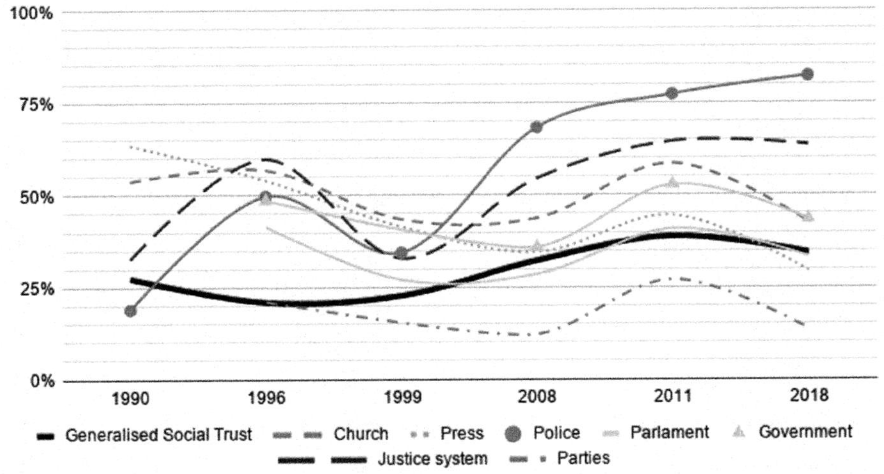

Fig. 5 Percentage of people in Estonia in 1990–2018 who believe that other people can be trusted (social trust) and who trust the following institutions: the church, the press, the police, parliament, the government, the justice system, and political parties (*Data* WVS/EVS)

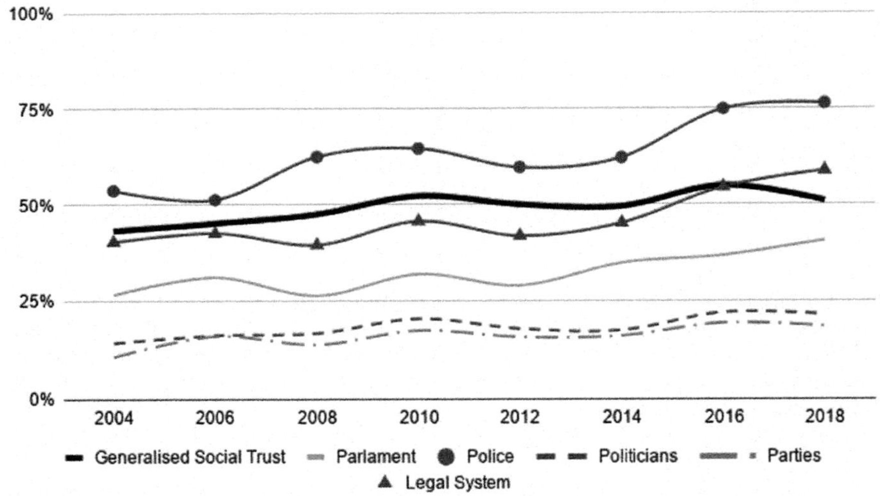

Fig. 6 Percentage of people in Estonia in 2004–2018 who believe that other people can be trusted (social trust) or who trust the following institutions: parliament, the police, politicians, and political parties (*Data* ESS)

Therefore, the Estonian data seem to provide some support for the claim that social trust goes hand in hand with trust in non-political state institutions. As the legal system and the police force have gone through major changes and reforms since the turbid nineties, the systems have become more trustworthy in the eyes of citizens. At the same time, we can see a steady rise in social trust, although it is not

Table 4 Intraclass correlations (Spearman's Rho) between the levels of social trust and institutional trust across the period of study

Study		The church	The press	The police	Parliament	The government	The justice system	Politicians	Parties
Estonia	WVS 1990–2018 (n = 6)	0.03	−0.43	*0.71**	0	0.40	0.60		0.40
	ESS 2004–2018 (n = 8)			*0.83***	*0.69**		*0.76**	*0.95***	*0.76**
Lithuania	WVS 1990–2018 (n = 4)	0.40	−0.40	0.80			1**		
	ESS 2008–2018 (n = 5)			0.60	0.71		0.48	0.71	0.71

Note *WVS/EVS* World Values Survey and European Values Survey, *ESS* European Social Survey
$^{*}p < 0.05$, $^{**}p < 0.01$

as fast as the increase in trust in the police and the legal system. The trend lines of social trust and non-political state institutions diverge from 2016, when trust in the police and legal system stay steady, while social trust is in decline along with trust in some political state institutions, the press, and the church. If the growth in trust in non-political state institutions and the decline in social trust continue in the coming years, this trend would contradict our assumption about the relationship between social trust and trust in non-political state institutions. However, it should be made quite clear that we cannot claim any causality based on those trends.

Even though the increase in social trust since 1990s has been more modest in Lithuania, there are similar trends of increasing trust in the police and the legal system (Fig. 7). In the case of Lithuania, trust in the police started to increase rapidly from 1996, while trust in the legal system started to increase in the second half of the 2000s. Compared to Estonians, Lithuanians put much more trust in the church and press: until 2010, the press was considered more trustworthy than the police in Lithuania, and the church remained the most trusted institution at the end of study period. As social trust was positively and significantly correlated with trust in the justice system in Lithuania (Table 4), this lends some support to our earlier conclusion that trust in non-political state institutions (at least partly) contributes to growth in social trust.

The ESS data provide some further insight into the trends in social and institutional trust in Lithuania from 2008 to 2018 (Fig. 8). Broadly speaking, the profiles of social trust as well as of institutional trust in the parliament, politicians, and political parties follow very similar trends across the study period. First, there is a steady increase in the levels of social and institutional trust in the parliament, politicians, and political parties from 2008 to 2016, followed by a decline between 2016 and 2018. Only

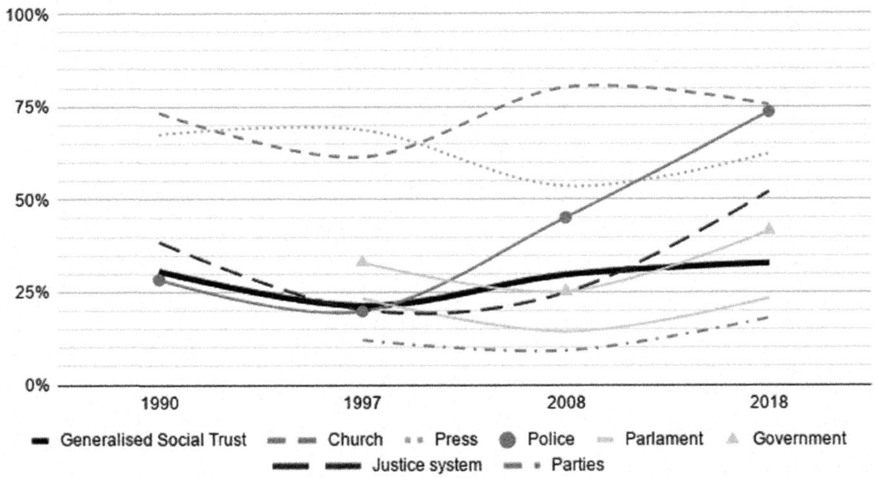

Fig. 7 Percentage of people in Lithuania in 1990–2018 who believe that other people can be trusted (social trust) or who trust the following institutions: the church, the press, the police, parliament, the government, the justice system, and political parties (*Data* WVS/EVS)

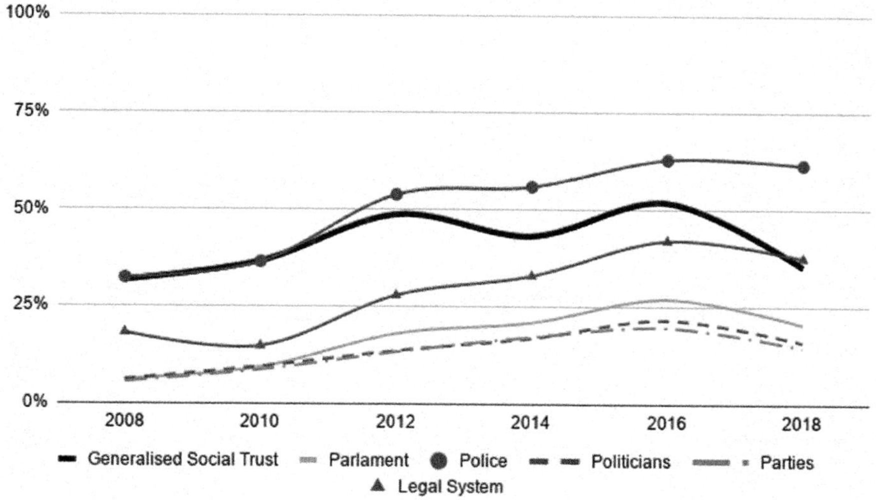

Fig. 8 Percentage of people in Lithuania in 2008–2018 who believe that other people can be trusted (social trust) or who trust the following institutions: parliament, the police, the legal system, politicians, and political parties (*Data* ESS)

trust in the police has consistently increased throughout the whole observed period. However, these trends do not offer much evidence to support our assumption of a link between social trust and trust in institutions, as the levels of social trust and trust in different institutions across time are not significantly correlated in the Lithuanian ESS data (Table 4).

In Latvia, social trust, as well as trust in different political and non-political institutions, tends to be lower than in their northern and southern neighbor countries (Fig. 9). However, there are some similarities with Lithuania in the general trust trend lines. In both countries, the church is the institution with the highest trust scores throughout the study period, followed by trust in the press throughout the nineties and first half of 2000s. From the middle of 2000s, trust in the police became higher than trust in the press. At the same time, the percentage of people who believe that other people can be trusted has stayed at around 20–25% throughout the study period. Therefore, Latvian trends in social and institutional trust do not lend any support to our assumption that trust in non-political state institutions leads (at least partly) to growth in social trust.

6.3 *Social Trust and Societal Development*

Our final analyses focus on examining changes in the level of social trust in the context of wider societal indicators, such as levels of corruption, human development, and social inequality across the study period.

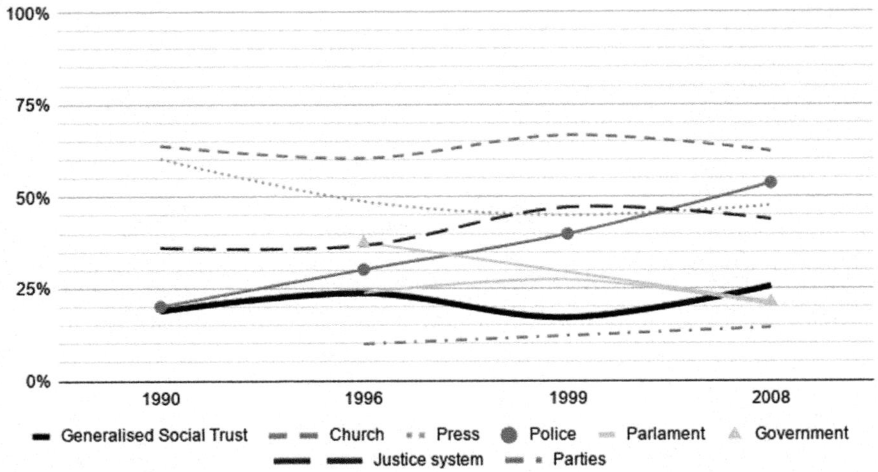

Fig. 9 Percentage of people in Latvia in 1990–2008 who believe that other people can be trusted (social trust) or who trust the following institutions: the church, the press, police, parliament, the government, the justice system, and political parties (*Data* WVS/EVS)

As it has been suggested that corruption has a negative effect on social trust levels, we also looked at the trends in perceived corruption in Estonia, Latvia, and Lithuania in the period 1998–2018. Indeed, in Estonia and Lithuania, CPI scores followed very similar general trends as social trust levels during the period under consideration, with the decrease in perceived corruption being accompanied by an increase in social trust (Figs. 10 and 12). In Latvia, on the other hand, decreasing levels of corruption do not seem to lead to higher levels of social trust, as social trust levels remain surprisingly stable over the ten years from 2008 to 2018 (Fig. 11). A possible explanation for this unexpected finding may be that, even though the levels of political corruption in Latvia, as measured by CPI, have dramatically decreased since 2011, there are other studies that indicate that the average Latvian still believes that Latvia is one of the most corrupt countries in Europe (European Commission, 2017). Thus, if people in Latvia still feel that way, then Latvian social trust patterns fit our theoretical assumption that social trust levels are affected by perceived corruption rather well—it is not wise to become more trusting towards other people if you believe that you live in a highly corrupt country. However, there are no grounds for drawing any far-reaching conclusions from these results, as the levels of social trust and CPI across time are not significantly correlated in any of the three countries (Table 5).

Human Development Index may be a rather poor proxy for welfare state development, but it nevertheless provides at least some insight into the improving living standards in the Baltic countries since the early nineties. Figures 10, 11, and 12 demonstrate that the levels of HDI have been rising steadily in the Baltic countries from the mid-nineties. In Estonia and Lithuania, it has been followed by an increase in social trust (with the exception of a couple of recent years, which witness some decline in social trust levels), but, in Latvia, we cannot see any positive effect for

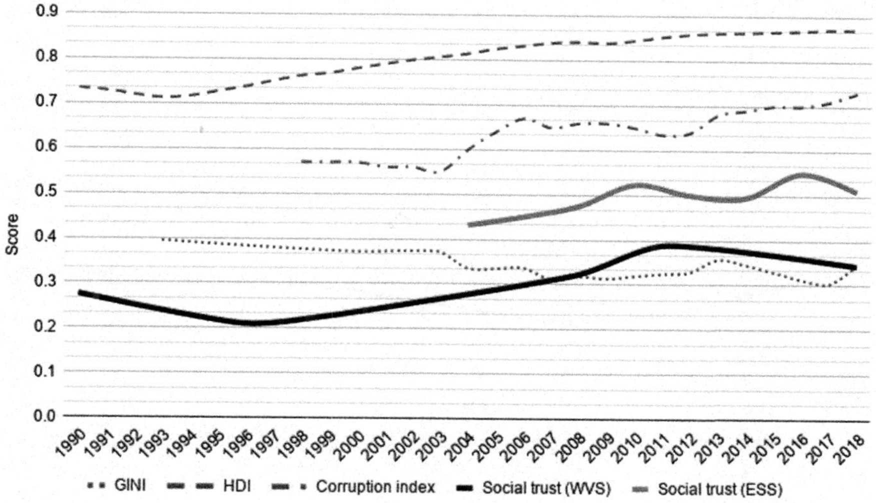

Fig. 10 Changes in levels of social trust and the three indicators of societal development in Estonia in 1990–2018. GINI = GINI index on a scale from 0 (total inequality) to 1 (total inequality); HDI = Human development index on a scale from 0 (least developed) to 1 (most highly developed); corruption index = transparency international perceived corruption index score on a scale from 0 (highly corrupt) to 1 (very clean); social trust: percentage of people who believe that most people can be trusted (WVS/ESS)

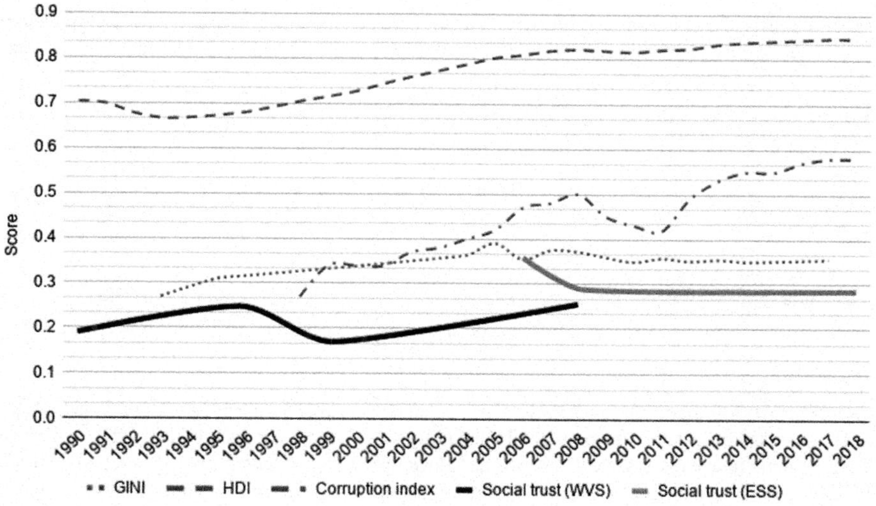

Fig. 11 Changes in levels of social trust and the three indicators of societal development in Latvia in 1990–2018. GINI = GINI index on a scale from 0 (total inequality) to 1 (maximal inequality); HDI = Human development index on a scale from 0 (least developed) to 1 (most highly developed); Corruption index = transparency international perceived corruption index score on a scale from 0 (highly corrupt) to 1 (very clean); trust: percentage of people who believe that most people can be trusted (WVS/ESS)

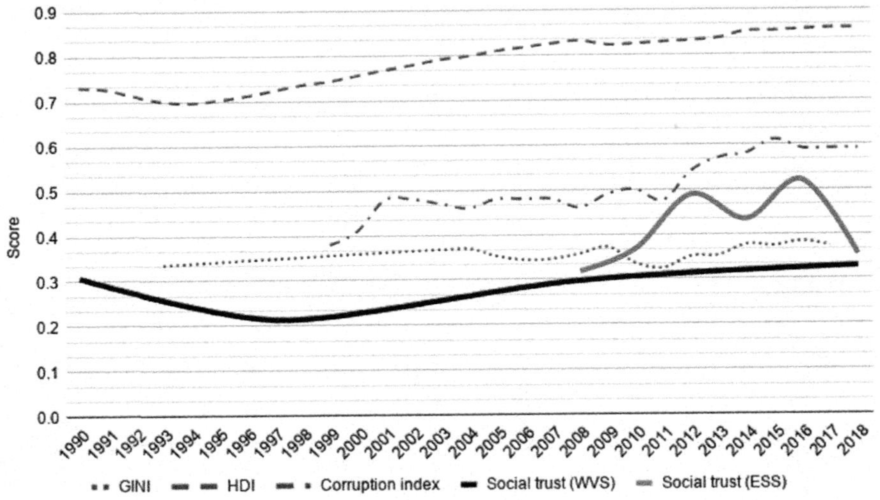

Fig. 12 Changes in levels of social trust and the three indicators of societal development in Lithuania in 1990–2018. GINI = GINI index on a scale from 0 (total inequality) to 1 (maximal inequality); HDI = Human development index on a scale from 0 (least developed) to 1 (most highly developed); corruption index = transparency international perceived corruption index score on a scale from 0 (highly corrupt) to 1 (very clean); trust: percentage of people who believe that most people can be trusted (WVS/ESS)

Table 5 Intraclass correlations (Spearman's Rho) between the levels of social trust and indicators of societal development across WVS/EVS (1990–2018) and ESS (2004–2018) data sets. Number of cases added in brackets

Country	Study	GINI	HDI	CPI
Estonia	ESS	0.17(8)	0.78^{*}(8)	0.48(8)
	WVS	0.8(4)	0.77^{*}(6)	0.4(4)
Latvia	ESS	–	–	–
	WVS	0.22(4)	0.43(4)	–
Lithuania	ESS	0.43(6)	0.29(6)	0.59(6)
	WVS	−0.05(4)	0.71(4)	0.8(4)
Average		*0.32*	*0.59*	*0.57*

Note WVS World Values Survey, *EVS* European Values Survey, *ESS* European Social Survey. GINI = GINI index on a scale from 0 (total inequality) to 1 (maximal inequality); HDI = Human Development Index on a scale from 0 (least developed) to 1 (most highly developed); CPI = Transparency International Perceived Corruption Index score on a scale from 0 (highly corrupt) to 1 (very clean); Trust: percentage of people who believe that most people can be trusted
$^{*}p < 0.05$, $^{**}p < 0.01$

increasing HDI on social trust. As can be seen in Table 5, levels of social trust are significantly correlated with HDI over time only in Estonia.

However, considering the potential link between social and economic inequality and social trust, it is probably more important to look at the trends in social trust together with the GINI index (Figs. 10, 11, and 12). In Estonia, the increase in inequality (operationalized via the GINI index) was accompanied by falling levels of social trust in the early nineties (Fig. 10). Since then, economic inequality in Estonia has remained rather stable. However, since the new millennium, the general trend is toward a modest decline in inequality. At the same time, social trust levels have increased since the late nineties. The increase in economic inequality was less sharp in Latvia after regaining independence (Fig. 11). Levels of social trust, too, did not drop very rapidly. However, increasing economic inequality was accompanied by rising levels of social trust from 1999 to 2004. Since then, levels of both economic inequality and social trust have been rather stable. In Lithuania, the increase in inequality was not as rapid as in Estonia, but sharper than in Latvia (Fig. 12). Increasing inequality was followed by decreasing levels of social trust. Since the early nineties, economic inequality has remained fairly stable in Lithuania, with minor ups and downs in the GINI index. However, social trust levels have been less stable, demonstrating a rather fluctuating trend line. Furthermore, intraclass correlations between the levels of social trust and GINI index across time do not allow us to attribute any changes in social trust to the changes in economic inequality (Table 5).

In sum, our analyses did not provide support for the theoretical assumption that changes in levels of social trust may be triggered by changes in levels of corruption, human development, or social inequality. While HDI was positively correlated with levels of social trust in Estonia, correlations were non-significant in Latvia and Lithuania (Table 5). Furthermore, social trust levels seemed to have nothing to do with the levels of economic inequality and perceived corruption in the Baltic countries (Table 5).

7 Conclusion

Several large-scale studies have shown that generalized trust does not change much over time (Bjørnskov, 2007; Uslaner, 2017; Volken, 2002). However, this may only hold true for stable democracies and not for societies that have gone through major political, economic, or social transitions. The fast change in social trust levels in two of the Baltic countries—Estonia and Lithuania—during the last decades is rather unprecedented in international comparison, especially when considering that countries from the former Eastern bloc are generally believed to have less social trust than stable Western democracies (e.g., Bjørnskov, 2007; Neller, 2008; Newton, 2004). Even if the low levels of social trust in the Baltic countries in the early 1990s can be easily explained by the countries' Soviet past, it is a more difficult task to explain the fast growth of social trust in Estonia and Lithuania, but not in Latvia, from the end of 1990s until the middle of the last decade. Unlike its southern and northern neighbors, Latvia meets the general expectation for the former Eastern bloc country, with rather low social trust levels. Therefore, Latvia seems to fit the presumptions shared by several authors (e.g., Uslaner, 2000, 2002; Whiteley, 2000), that social trust is rather stable over time and extremely difficult to create in places where it does not exist. Rather rapid changes in social trust in the other two Baltic countries are much more difficult to explain and are at odds with the theoretical claims of relative stability in social trust levels over time. In this chapter, we tried to shed some light on the possible factors that may have helped Estonia and Lithuania recover from their post-totalitarian trauma and demonstrate levels of social trust comparable with established democracies.

Looking for possible explanations, we relied on theories that conceptualize trust as a feature of the social environment, suggesting that individuals become more trusting by experiencing trustworthy behavior in their daily life (Delhey & Newton, 2005; Newton, 2004; Ostrom & Ahn, 2009; Putnam, 2000; Rothstein, 2005; Whiteley, 2000). According to these theories, social trust can be seen as a social norm that individuals learn from their social environment. Trustworthy state institutions (such as the police force and the legal system, in particular) and good governance, seem to be especially important factors for producing high levels of social trust among a country's citizens. When people see that state officials treat people equally and are not involved in corrupt activities, a highly visible example that it is reasonable to expect honesty and trustworthiness even from people whom one does not know very well is offered. Corrupt state institutions, on the other hand, are often considered one of the main causes for low levels of social trust, because people learn from these that they can trust people only very selectively. The results presented in this chapter partially support the hypothesis that a trustworthy state and good governance (as suggested by Newton, 2004; Rothstein, 2005; Rothstein & Stolle, 2003; Stolle, 2003) play some role in generating social trust. However, this only applies to Estonia and, to a considerably lesser extent, Lithuania. Furthermore, EVS/WVS and ESS data from the Baltic countries do not demonstrate any link between social trust and low corruption in state institutions (as suggested by Rothstein, 2005; Uslaner, 2002).

We are, of course, fully aware that our analyses hardly let us make any claims about the direction of the causality between the changes in social trust and perception of state institutions. Nevertheless, our results do not offer support to Uslaner's (2017) claim that there is hardly any evidence that democratization after the fall of Communism has been followed by increasing levels of social trust and "where trust is low, institutional change does not seem to be the route to increase it" (p. 73). Estonia and Lithuania present a case where, despite increased socioeconomic inequalities, the process of democratization has been accompanied by a significant increase in social trust, and it seems plausible that, in this case, the increasing levels of social trust followed the institutional changes, rather than other way around. However, it may be too early to celebrate high social trust levels in Estonia and Lithuania given that the last couple of years have seen some decrease in those levels.

In sum, our analysis demonstrates that social trust levels have not followed identical patterns in the three Baltic countries, indicating that both their starting point after the collapse of Soviet Union as well as the social and political choices in the subsequent decades have been different and yielded different levels of social trust. The high levels of social trust in Estonia and (to a somewhat lesser extent in) Lithuania indicate that people living in those two Baltic countries have indeed learned that, in general, most people can be trusted. However, it seems that the experiences of Latvians have been remarkably different, as social trust levels have remained low throughout the three decades since regaining independence. Furthermore, it is yet to be seen whether the other two Baltic countries—Estonia and Lithuania—can maintain their high levels of social trust despite any economic and political changes, or if the slight decrease in social trust levels in recent years is the beginning of a downward trend.

References

Akcomak, S., & ter Weel, B. (2011). The impact of social capital on crime: Evidence from the Netherlands. *Regional Science and Urban Economics, 42*, 323–340.

Beilmann, M., & Lilleoja, L. (2015). Social trust and value similarity: The relationship between social trust and human values in Europe. *Studies of Transition States and Societies, 7*, 19–30.

Beilmann, M., & Lilleoja, L. (2017). Explaining the relationship between social trust and value similarity: The case of Estonia. *Juridica International, 25*, 14–21.

Beilmann, M., Kööts-Ausmees, L., & Realo, A. (2018). The relationship between social capital and individualism-collectivism in Europe. *Social Indicators Research, 137*(2), 641–664.

Beugelsdijk, S. (2006). A note on the theory and measurement of trust in explaining differences in economic growth. *Cambridge Journal of Economics, 30*, 371–387.

Bjørnskov, C. (2007). Determinants of generalized trust: A cross-country comparison. *Public Choice, 130*, 1–21.

Delhey, J., & Newton, K. (2005). Predicting cross-national levels of social trust: Global patterns or Nordic exceptionalism. *European Sociological Review, 21*, 311–327.

European Commission (2017). Special Eurobarometer 470. Corruption. http://ec.europa.eu/commfrontoffice/publicopinion/index.cfm/ResultDoc/download/DocumentKy/81007

ESS round 2: European social survey round 2 data (2004). Data file edition 3.5. NSD—Norwegian Centre for Research Data, Norway—Data Archive and distributor of ESS data for ESS ERIC. https://doi.org/10.21338/NSD-ESS2-2004

ESS round 3: European social survey round 3 data (2006). Data file edition 3.6. NSD—Norwegian Centre for Research Data, Norway—Data Archive and distributor of ESS data for ESS ERIC. https://doi.org/10.21338/NSD-ESS3-2006

ESS round 4: European social survey round 4 data (2008). Data file edition 4.4. NSD—Norwegian Centre for Research Data, Norway—Data Archive and distributor of ESS data for ESS ERIC. https://doi.org/10.21338/NSD-ESS4-2008

ESS round 5: European social survey round 5 data (2010). Data file edition 3.3. NSD—Norwegian Centre for Research Data, Norway—Data Archive and distributor of ESS data for ESS ERIC. https://doi.org/10.21338/NSD-ESS5-2010

ESS round 6: European social survey round 6 data (2012). Data file edition 2.3. NSD—Norwegian Centre for Research Data, Norway—Data Archive and distributor of ESS data for ESS ERIC. https://doi.org/10.21338/NSD-ESS6-2012

ESS round 7: European social survey round 7 data (2014). Data file edition 2.1. NSD—Norwegian Centre for Research Data, Norway—Data Archive and distributor of ESS data for ESS ERIC. https://doi.org/10.21338/NSD-ESS7-2014

ESS round 8: European social survey round 8 data (2016). Data file edition 1.0. NSD—Norwegian Centre for Research Data, Norway—Data Archive and distributor of ESS data for ESS ERIC. https://doi.org/10.21338/NSD-ESS8-2016
ESS round 9: European social survey round 9 data (2018). Data file edition 2.0. NSD—Norwegian Centre for Research Data, Norway—Data Archive and distributor of ESS data for ESS ERIC. https://doi.org/10.21338/NSD-ESS9-2018
EVS: European Values Study Longitudinal Data File 1981–2008 (EVS 1981–2008) (2020a). GESIS Data Archive, Cologne. ZA4804 Data file Version 3.1.0. https://doi.org/10.4232/1.13486
EVS: European Values Study 2017: Integrated Dataset (EVS 2017) (2020b). GESIS Data Archive, Cologne. ZA7500 Data file Version 3.0.0. https://doi.org/10.4232/1.13511
Güemes, C., & Herreros, F. (2019). Education and trust: A tale of three continents. *International Political Science Review, 40*(5), 676–693.
Halpern, D. (2005). *Social capital*. Polity Press.
Hooghe, M., Marien, S., & de Vroome, T. (2012). The cognitive basis of trust. The relationship between education, cognitive ability, and generalized and political trust. *Intelligence, 40*, 604–613.
Inglehart, R., Haerpfer, C., Moreno, A., Welzel, C., Kizilova, K., Diez-Medrano J., Lagos, M., Norris, P., Ponarin, E., & Puranen, B., et al. (Eds.). (2020). World Values Survey: All Rounds—Country-Pooled Datafile. Madrid, Spain & Vienna, Austria: JD Systems Institute & WVSA Secretariat. http://www.worldvaluessurvey.org/WVSDocumentationWVL.jsp
Inglehart, R. (1997). Modernization and postmodernization: Cultural, economic and political change in 43 societies. Princeton University Press.
Inglehart, R. (1999). Trust, well-being and democracy. In M. E. Warren (Ed.), *Democracy and trust* (pp. 88–120). Cambridge University Press.
Jordahl, H. (2009). Economic inequality. In G. T. Svendsen & G. L. H. Svendsen (Eds.), *Handbook of social capital: The Troika of sociology, political science and economics* (pp. 323–336). Edward Elgar.
LaPorta, R., Lopez-Silanes, F., Schleifer, A., & Vishney, R. W. (1997). Trust in large organizations. *American Economic Review Papers and Proceedings, 87*, 333–338.
Neira, I., Portela, M., & Vieira, E. (2010). Social capital and growth in European regions. *Regional and Sectoral Economic Studies, 10*, 19–28.
Neller, K. (2008). Explaining social trust: What makes people trust their fellow citizens. In H. Meulemann (Ed.),*Social Capital in Europe: Similarity of Countries and Diversity of People? Multi-Level Analysis of the European Social Survey 2002* (pp. 103–133). Leiden & Boston: Brill.
Newton, K. (2004). Social trust: Individual and cross-national approaches. *Portuguese Journal of Social Science, 3*, 15–35.
Ostrom, E., & Ahn, T. K. (2009). The meaning of social capital and its link to collective action. In G. T. Svendsen & G. L. H. Svendsen (Eds.), *Handbook of social capital: The Troika of sociology, political science and economics* (pp. 17–35). Edward Elgar Publishing.
Putnam, R. D. (1993). *Making democracy work. Civic traditions in modern Italy*. Princeton University Press.
Putnam, R. D. (2000). *Bowling alone: The collapse and revival of american community*. Simon and Schuster.
Putnam, R. D. (2002). *Democracies in flux: The evolution of social capital in contemporary society*. Oxford University Press.
Rothstein, B. (2005). *Social traps and the problem of trust*. Cambridge University Press.
Rothstein, B., & Stolle, D. (2003). Social capital, impartiality, and the welfare state: An institutional approach. In M. Hooghe & D. Stolle (Eds.), *Generating social capital: civil society and institutions in comparative perspective* (pp. 191–209). Basingstoke: Palgrave.
Schwartz, S. H. (1999). A theory of cultural values and some implications for work. *Applied Psychology: An International Review, 48*, 23–47.

Steijn, S., & Lancee, B. (2011). Does income inequality negatively affect general trust?*Examining three potential problems with the inequality-trust hypothesis*. Amsterdam, AIAS, GINI Discussion Paper 20. http://www.gini-research.org/system/uploads/274/original/DP_20_-_Steijn_Lancee.pdf

Stolle, D. (2003). The sources of social capital. In M. Hooghe & D. Stolle (Eds.), *Generating social capital. Civil society and institutions in comparative perspective* (pp. 19–42). Palgrave Macmillan.

Uslaner, E. M. (2000). Producing and consuming trust. *Political Science Quarterly, 115*, 569–590.

Uslaner, E. M. (2002). *The moral foundations of trust*. Cambridge University Press.

Uslaner, E. M. (2017). The roots of trust. In Y. Li (Ed.), *Handbook of research methods and applications in social capital* (pp. 60–75). Edward Elgar Publishing.

von dem Knesebeck, O., Dragano, N., Siegrist, J. (2005). Social capital and self-rated health in 21 European countries. *GMS Psycho-Social-Medicine, 2*, 1–9.

Whiteley, P. F. (2000). Economic growth and social capital. *Political Studies, 48*, 443–466.

Yamagishi, T., & Yamagishi, M. (1994). Trust and commitment in the United States and Japan. *Motivation and Emotion, 18*, 129–165.

Zmerli, S., & Newton, K. (2008). Social trust and attitudes toward democracy. *Public Opinion Quarterly, 72*, 706–724.

Zuell, C., & Scholz, E. (2016). 10 points versus 11 points? Effects of left-right scale design in a cross-national perspective. *ASK: Research and Methods, 25*, 3–16.

Mai Beilmann (Ph.D. in Sociology) is a Research Fellow in Sociology at the Institute of Social Studies, University of Tartu, Estonia. Her research interests include social capital, (social) trust, cultural values, social and political participation, with a special focus on youth and childhood studies. She is a member of The European Network for Social Policy Analysis Baltics Network and the President of the Estonian Association of Sociologists (2018–2022).

Laur Lilleoja (Ph.D. in Sociology) is an independent consultant for survey methodology. He has developed himself at Tallinn University, Pompeu Fabra University and the Autonomous University of Barcelona. He is a member of the European Survey Research Association (ESRA) and author of more than 20 articles and book chapters on social psychology and survey methodology. His primary research interests are basic human values and, more broadly, the development of methodology for studying values.

Anu Realo is Professor of Psychology at the University of Warwick, United Kingdom. Her background is in personality and cross-cultural psychology and she has conducted considerable research on the fundamental nature of personality traits, the definition and conceptualisation of subjective wellbeing, and on the nature of cultural characteristics, such as individualism-collectivism, social capital, and tightness-looseness. She is the principal investigator for the World Values Survey in Estonia, the President of the European Association for Personality Psychology (2020–2022), and a member of the Estonian Academy of Sciences.

Emigration and Trust: Evidence from Eastern Europe and Central Asia

Dragos Radu, Ekaterina Skoglund, and Soomin Ma

1 Introduction

There is surprisingly little evidence on whether and in which way large-scale emigration feeds back on the formation of attitudes and social capital (generalised trust) in countries of origin. Do large emigration flows have a detrimental effect on levels of institutional and generalised trust "back home"? What are the main social mechanisms through which emigration impacts upon levels of trust among those who remain in sending areas? Answering such questions is crucial for understanding the long-term effects of emigration upon living conditions in transition and developing countries.

This chapter addresses these questions for a set of representative transition countries in Eastern Europe and Central Asia. Previous literature documented the two great divides between major sending and receiving countries of intensifying migration flows in Europe: the income differential and the divide in levels of trust and social capital due to the communist legacy (e.g., Bartolini et al., 2015; Fidrmuc & Gërxhani, 2008; Kornai et al., 2004).

Compared to previous studies, the original contribution of our analysis is to provide a descriptive perspective and to propose explanatory mechanisms linking emigration to levels of generalised and institutional trust in the sending countries. By focusing on the effects of emigration on trust, we believe our chapter adds a novel perspective to the literature on emigration and modernization (e.g., De Haas, 2010; Faist et al., 2011; Okólski, 2012; Skeldon, 2014; Zelinsky, 1971).

D. Radu (✉) · S. Ma
King's College, 30 Aldwych, WC2B 4BG London, UK
e-mail: dragos.radu@kcl.ac.uk

S. Ma
e-mail: soomin.ma@kcl.ac.uk

E. Skoglund
Leibniz Institute for East and Southeast European Studies, Landshuter Str. 4, 93047 Regensburg, Germany
e-mail: skoglund@ios-regensburg.de

A. Almakaeva et al. (eds.), *Social Capital and Subjective Well-Being*, Societies and Political Orders in Transition,
https://doi.org/10.1007/978-3-030-75813-4_3

In the next section we motivate our research question and discuss the role trust plays in processes of development and modernization in general and of post-communist transition in particular. We also briefly describe some main features of migration flows from our countries of interest which are relevant to our question. Section 3 sketches a conceptual framework we propose to look at the mechanisms/channels through which large scale emigration can affect institutional and generalised trust in the sending countries. These help us to formulate some testable hypotheses about the impacts of emigration on trust among non-migrants in the communities of origin. Section 4 presents the sources of data and describes the variables used in our empirical analysis. We discuss our results at the micro/individual level in Sect. 5.

The main challenge for our empirical analysis is to identify which mechanisms/channels or combination thereof is the most likely suspect to explain the effect of emigration on social attitudes and trust. This is a difficult task given that most of the available variables are endogenous in explaining trust, or as Putnam (2001, p. 145) puts it: "The causal arrows among civic involvement, reciprocity, honesty, and trust are as tangled as well-tossed spaghetti". We discuss the shortcomings of our proposed explanations and the limitations of our data in the concluding section of the chapter.

2 Previous Research and the Relevance of Trust

The conceptualization of trust and the empirical investigations of the role of trust in development have led to a very fruitful agenda in current social science research. The initial focus of this research was on the powerful and popular metaphor of social capital. Ever since it was introduced in the literature by Loury (1977) and Coleman (1988), social capital became an important input in explaining processes of economic growth, development and state-building (see e.g., Durlauf & Fafchamps, 2005; Portes, 1998, for comprehensive surveys). For the purpose of our chapter, we refer mainly to this literature which identifies the lack of social capital as a major impediment for economic development and democratization. Studies belonging to this tradition (e.g., Putnam et al., 1994; Woolcock, 1998) define social capital as a type of (positive) group externality and highlight its impact on social aggregates. Social capital can therefore be validly construed as "resources embedded in social networks and accessed and used by actors for action" (Lin, 2001, p. 25).

Despite its shortcomings, such a definition helps to illustrate how geographic mobility and migration can hamper social capital, since networks depend on the (future) presence of their members (see e.g., Glaeser et al., 2002). Fafchamps and Minten (2002) coined the term "social network capital" in this context and various studies used this "social networks" lens when analyzing international migrants (e.g., Banerjee, 1983; Gallego & Mendola, 2013; Munshi, 2003).

2.1 Why (Generalized) Trust?

From the perspective of empirical work, several studies confirmed that one "essential component of social capital" (Putnam et al., 1994, p. 170)—social trust—is a fundamental cultural value that could explain economic development (Algan & Cahuc, 2014) and an important determinant of a number of economic and political outcomes, including governance and life satisfaction (see e.g., Bjørnskov, 2006; Selezneva, 2015). Trust has been broadly defined as a cooperative attitude outside the family circle which "facilitates coordinated actions" (Putnam et al., 1994, p. 167) or more succinctly by Fafchamps (2002) as an optimistic expectation regarding the behavior of others. Social trust entered the mainstream economic literature as one of the key measures of the quality of 'the social fabric' (Helliwell et al. 2014) and the 'lubricant' of social interactions (Arrow, 1974; Dasgupta, 2000; Putnam, 2001).

While quantifying trust is a problematic endeavour, the measure that has been typically implemented in quantitative research is the fraction of people that think most people can be trusted. Using this measure, a growing number of studies shows that trust is a significant causal component of growth (starting with the seminal paper by Knack and Keefer (1997). Recent studies suggest that it is the level of trust, rather than other elements of social capital, are robust determinants of economic growth (Bartolini et al., 2015; Beugelsdijk et al., 2004; Bjørnskov, 2012; Whiteley, 2000; Zak & Knack, 2001).

Several of the available studies on trust addressed also the potential mechanisms linking trust to economic growth and some tried to deal with the inherent causality problems. However, most of these studies did so only implicitly (Beugelsdijk et al., 2004; Whiteley, 2000; Zak & Knack, 2001) and only few tried to make the transmission mechanism of the trust-growth relation explicit (e.g. Bjørnskov, 2012). Algan and Cahuc (2010) found a sizeable causal impact, isolated from the insittutional and geographical factors, of (inherited) trust on economic development.

Three types of transmission mechanisms from social trust to economic growth have been outlined in the literature. The first one can be traced back to Coleman (1988) seminal paper where he argued that trust (social capital) is a factor in the creation of human capital. The argument is that higher levels of trust imply more certainty about a fair return on investments into education, and will thus result in higher levels of schooling (Papagapitos & Riley, 2009). This is why trust can be conducive to human capital accumulation (Dearmon & Grier, 2011) and has a positive impact on human development (Özcan & Bjørnskov, 2011).

The second mechanism discussed in the literature is the positive relation between trust and investment (Bjørnskov, 2012; Carlin et al., 2009; Zak & Knack, 2001). In his classic sociological analysis of trust, Luhman (1979) defines trust as a complexity reducing device. Zak and Knack 2001 use this argument to model an economic choice between productive activities and activities related the verification of others' behavior. In such a setting, high levels of trust lower transaction cost and stimulate economic exchange and investment.

The third mechanism links trust to economic development via its impact of governance. This trust-governance link was documented e.g. by Helliwell and Putnam (1995) who showed that different levels of social capital led to differences in the quality of governance across regions in Italy and by Knack (2002) who shows that higher levels of generalized trust lead to more reform prone policies across US regions.

2.2 *Trust in Post-socialist Countries*

Given the extensive literature on the relationship between trust and economic development[1] discussed above, it is important to understand what factors determine the level of trust in the first place. This seems even more urgent for countries undergoing periods of crisis and social and economic transformation, where trust appears to be a powerful resource (Helliwell et al., 2014). Understanding what factors contribute to the creation of trust in post-socialist countries (see also Kornai et al., 2004) is particularly relevant in this context because trust "touches on issues central to the transition process and its eventual outcome" (Rose-Ackerman, 2001, p. 415), and can be "seen as an essential component of a successful market economy" (Rebmann, 2015, p. 523).

Trust is a necessary condition for both functioning democracy and civil society (Rose, 1994) as well as a succesful transition to a market economy (Raiser, 2003). However, the communist system left a pervasive legacy of distrust (Rebmann, 2015). The collapse of the communist system revealed very low levels of trust across transitional countries. The East-West trust divide in Europe is argued to persist even nowadays (Bartolini & Sarracino, 2014; Fidrmuc & Gërxhani, 2008). The EBRD report, based on the 2016 wave of the Life in transition survey,[2] highlights that only 31 per cent of respondents from transitional countries—which is 3% points lower than in 2010—had at least "some trust" in other people. Among the transition countries, the highest trust levels are in Estonia, Poland and Tajikistan, while figures for Kazakhstan, Kosovo and Russia demonstrated a pronounced decline.

While the persisting differences in the level of trust between the "East" and the "West" constitute a well-established evidence, we know relatively little about the prospects for bridging this gap. Is a legacy of distrust amenable to reversals in socio-economic conditions, does trust respond to policy changes or economic shocks? Most of the existing studies would suggest a rather pessimistic answer. Following Putnam et al. (1994), empirical research accumulates which shows that social attitudes are persistent over time and determined by the past—the communist past (Alesina & Fuchs-Schündeln, 2007; Pop-Eleches & Tucker, 2011) or even earlier legacies of empires (Becker et al., 2016) or pre-modern political institutions. Algan and Cahuc

---

[1] However, the relationship between trust and economic growth is rarely studied for the subset of transition countries, despite the extensive literature on social and institutional trust in Eastern Europe (see also Bartolini et al., 2015).

[2] European Bank for Reconstruction and Development (EBRD) (2016).

(2014) make a distinction between the implications of Putnam et al. (1994), i.e. that trust is determined by history and remains stable over time, for which they coined the label 'Putnam I' and those of Putnam (2001), i.e. that trust can in fact change over relatively short periods of time, for which they use the label 'Putnam II'. Recent research by Ananyev and Guriev (2019) is the first credible attempt to quantify the magnitude of 'Putnam II'. Using data on the 2009 economic crisis in Russia and a very careful empirical strategy, they are able to identify a substantial change in social trust over a very short period of time in response to an income shock. This result lends support also to the relevance of our research question since it proves there are legitimate reasons to analyze factors that impact on trust in the short run. Our contribution is in the tradition of 'Putnam II': we attempt to uncover the potential for emigration shocks to influence the levels of trust in the sending communities.

2.3 *Relevant Migration Patterns for Selected Countries*

We discuss here briefly some of the main features of recent migration flows from the six East European and Central Asian countries on which we focus in this chapter: Kazakhstan, Moldova, Macedonia, Serbia, Tajikistan and Ukraine. Recent migration flows from these countries encompass the representative patterns of migration from transition and developing countries and more specifically of East-West migration in Europe after the demise of the communist regimes, several waves of EU enlargements and the 2008 financial crisis (see e.g. Kaczmarczyk & Okólski, 2008; O'Reilly et al., 2015, for overviews).

These six countries vary greatly both in term of the level of trust and in the composition and volume of out-migration flows they experienced in recent decades. Moldova, Macedonia and Serbia are the least trusting while Ukraine and Kazakhstan are the most trusting countries (we discuss in details the data for this in Sect. 5.1, see also Fig. 2). The countries also differ significantly in terms of population,[3] the average levels of schooling, prevalence of remittances and migration. Table 1 provides an overview of these main country characteristics. The variety of exposure to emigration is also reflected in the three measures we discuss in detail in Sect. 5.2 and report in Table 4.

Macedonia, the smallest country in our sample, experienced big population outflows at the beginning of the 1990s during a harsh economic and political crisis that hit the countries of the former Yugoslavia (Dietz, 2010). The emigration flow, first of unskilled and then of skilled workers, resulted in a stock of more than half-a-million Macedonians residing abroad at the beginning of the 2000s (Nikolovska, 2004). The emigration rate remains roughly at 12% since the 1990s, the female emigration rate

[3] According to the World Bank, at the level of 2019 the population figures are: 2.08 million in Macedonia, 2.66 million in Moldova, 6.94 million in Serbia, 9.32 million in Tajikistan, 18.51 million in Kazakhstan, and 44.39 million in Ukraine. World Bank, Total population, available at https://data.worldbank.org/indicator/SP.POP.TOTL.

Table 1 Selected characteristics of countries included in the UNPD SES survey

	Kazakhstan	Macedonia	Moldova	Tajikistan	Serbia	Ukraine
Population in thousands[a]	16,321.87	2070.74	2861.49	7527.39	7291.44	45,870.74
Human capital average years of schooling[b]	11.4	9.1	11.1	10.9	10.4	11.3
Emigration rate (stock)[c]	23.6	21.90	21.50	11.2	18.00	14.40
GDP PPP per capita[d]	15,112.25	10,827.92	3326.73	2018.79	12,108.22	8298.32
Remittances as a percentage of GDP[e]	0.2	4.1	25.1	35.8	9.8	4.8
Gini coefficient[f]	28.0	40.2	32.1	30.8	39.5	24.8
Ethnic fractionalisation index[g]	0.565	0.556	0.448	0.392	0.404	0.379

Sources

[a]Data for 2010 from the United Nations Population Division, World Population Prospects

[b]Average number of years of total schooling across all education levels, for the population aged 25 and above, taken from the UNDP, HDR

[c]Stock of emigrants as percentage of the total population at the level of 2010 from the World Bank Migration and remittances factbook 2011

[d]Calculated from Penn World Table (PWT9.1) using Real GDP expenditure-based PPP (in 2011 $) and population size

[e]2010 data from the World Bank

[f]Inequality measure, from World Development Indicator (2010 data for all, but 2013 for Serbia)

[g]Presents the probability of two randomly drawn individuals within a country are from different ethnic groups, 2010 data from the HIEF dataset

lagging only one p.p. behind that of males (e.g., 11.5% and 12.5%, respectively, in 2010). The biggest loss of the labour market potential is among those with low (29.8%) and high (32.0%) education (Brücker et al., 2013). The increasing outflow of highly educated youth is also growing, though low educated might be on average even more prone to emigrate (Petreski & Petreski, 2015). Officially recorded remittances account for 2.5% of GDP,[4] while the total amount of private transfers oscillates in the range from 13 to 21% of GDP. This is comparable to the country's trade deficit (Former Yugoslav Republic of Macedonia, 2014; Nikolovska, 2004). Previous studies found a positive correlation between receiving remittances and emigration intentions Petreski and Petreski (2015).

Another former Yugoslavian country that experienced significant emigration flows is Serbia: it lost about 18% of its population in the mid-1990s. 2010, the emigration rate is estimated at 10.2% (Brücker et al., 2013), with 14.0 and 14.8% emigration rate among those with low and high education in 2010, respectively. Emigration

[4] World Bank estimate.

intentions are remain high among the younger population and in particular among those with IT and medical training (Bobić & Anđelković, 2019). More than 80% of medical undergraduates consider emigration as an option (Santric-Milicevic et al., 2014) and emigration is predicted to accelerate in the coming years (Petreski et al., 2018).

The four remaining countries are the former Soviet Union Republics. Kazakhstan is the only country in our sample that can be classified as a receiving country of labor migrants (Ryazantsev & Korneev, 2013). It experienced a significant outflow during the 1990s, loosing 1.4 of the 16.4 million people in 1992 alone,[5] while over the last 15 years the migration balance remained predominantly positive. By 2010, the total emigration rate only slightly exceeded 1.1% (Brücker et al., 2013). The country has an intensive bilateral migration flows with the Russian Federation. Russia, Uzbekistan, and Ukraine are among the top-5 areas of origin of migrants (stock) in Kazakhstan and at the same time among the top-5 countries of destination in 2013. According to the UN Migration Report (2017), 2.4 million migrants from Kazakhstan reside in Russia: the seventh largest stock of international migrants from a single country or area of origin living in a single destination.

The other countries in our sample, Ukraine, Moldova and Tajikistan are countries of emigration but Moldova and Ukraine experience large transit migration flows towards the European Union (Ryazantsev & Korneev, 2013).

About a fifth of the working age population of Ukraine lives abroad, which makes it one of the top-10 sending countries in the world. Ukrainian migrants are usually working on a temporary basis either in countries of the former Soviet Union or in the European Union, in particular in Italy and Germany (VanMol et al., 2018). Migrants with higher levels of education move to Russia, while those with lower education migrate to the EU (Danzer & Dietz, 2014). The EUMAGINE survey in 2010, found a high share of the youth—up to 40–54% among those aged 18–39, and up to 41–61 among those aged 18–24—planning to move abroad to live or for work (Carling & Schewel, 2018).

Moldova and Tajikistan, the countries with the lowest well-being index included in our sample (Richardson et al., 2008), display also the highest emigration intentions. From 1995 to 2010, emigration rates quadrupled in Moldova up to about 3.5%, and the country experience between the two last censuses—2004 and 2014—a population decline from 3.3 to 2.8 million.[6] Top destination countries are Russia, Ukraine, Kazakhstan, but also EU countries (Romania, Italy, Germany).[7] The remittances flow, in 2009, accounted for 1,211 million US dollars (GNI of 5.8 billion US$s), or nearly 25% of the GDP. In Moldova, receiving remittances was found to be associated with a 7.0% points increase in the probability of not working and with a 7.4% points decrease in probability of a formal employment (Ivlevs, 2016).

---

[5] UNDP, World Population Prospects, Revision 2019.

[6] https://www.statistica.md/category.php?l=en&idc=103, https://esa.un.org/miggmgprofiles/indicators/files/Moldova.pdf.

[7] http://siteresources.worldbank.org/INTPROSPECTS/Resources/334934-1199807908806/Moldova.pdf.

The poorest of the former Soviet republics, Tajikistan, is also one of the most remittance-dependent economies in the world.[8] Estimates of the migration stock abroad differ from 26.4 to 43.9% of working population—with Russia, Kazakhstan, Uzbekistan, and Ukraine as main destinations ((Ryazantsev & Korneev, 2013). The majority of migrants are men of working age (Kumo, 2012) driven abroad by socio-economic insecurity and low wages (Dietz et al., 2015). This induced a "missing men" phenomenon and major gender imbalances in the country (Malyuchenko, 2015). In their destination countries, migrants from Tajikistan are often linked to poor working conditions, marginalization and negative public opinion—due their grey economy employment, especially in Russia (Zotova & Cohen, 2016). Migrant networks play a major role for Tajik migration (Kumo, 2012) while migration to Russia is facilitated by a dual citizenship agreement.[9] Unlike the case of Moldova, remittances to Tajikistan appear to stimulate households to invest in the education of their children rather than to fuel consumption (Yamada, 2016).

These are some of the main features of migration from our sampled countries which we believe are relevant to understand the links between emigration and trust. We fist discus the ways in which we can conceptualise this link and return to the evidence we collated for this chapter in Sect. 5.

3 Emigration and Trust

Our argument in this chapter is that large emigration flows, like those experienced by post-socialist countries after 1990, signal uncertainty and negative assessments of the trustworthiness of individuals and institutions. We hypothesize therefore that the out-migration of fellow citizens lowers a person's generalized trust and can lead to a decline in the overall level of trust in the communities of origin. Using a simple conceptual framework we try to uncover the potential mechanisms via which emigration is conducive to such negative externalities. We start by distinguishing between direct and indirect mechanisms linking emigration to generalized trust. The direct linkages are due to the scale and composition of emigration flows: who's leaving will change the balance between those trusting and not-trusting among stayers, while how many move will influence trust via signalling and transmission effects. The indirect linkages are due first to emigration affecting (i) economic development in the sending area and (ii) inequality among non-migrants in the sending community and second, because both (i) and (ii) will in turn impact on levels of generalized trust.

---

[8] According to the World Bank database, the received personal remittances to the GDP hit the massive share of 49.29% in 2008, and has never gone under 26% ever since. For more details, see http://data.worldbank.org/indicator. Official statistics account only for the formal channels of money transfer and underestimate actual remittances (Malyuchenko, 2015).

[9] "Treaty on the settlement of issues of dual citizenship between the Republic of Tajikistan and the Russian Federation" September 7, 1995, Bulletin of international agreements of the Russian Federation 2, 1997.

For our purposes, the direct mechanisms derive directly from two main characteristics of international migration which are salient in the recent migration flows from post-communist countries in Eastern Europe and Central Asia. These are: the (self)selective nature of migration and the salience of social networks and herd effects in migration decisions. We claim that both of these features of migration directly affect the evolution of generalized trust among stayers in sending communities. The first one works via the self-selection of migrants, the second via the transmission of norms and attitudes.

The new economics of migration predicts that a desire to improve the (relative) social and economic status (in comparison to a reference group) is one of the most important drivers of migration (Stark & Taylor, 1991). Recent research has documented the self-selection of migrants from Eastern Europe and the former Soviet Union not only on economic variables but also on values, beliefs and attitudes. Berlinschi and Harutyunyan (2019) find that persons with high levels of generalized trust and low levels of risk aversion have higher propensities to emigrate, while Dustmann and Okatenko (2014) and Lam (2002) identify political and institutional trust, i.e. confidence in the home country's government and judicial system as a major determinant of migration decisions. Since migration intentions are strong predictors of actual migration choices, the positive selection of emigrants in terms of their levels of generalized trust can represent a source of "trust drain": the higher the emigration rates, the lower the levels of trust among non-migrants who remain in the sending communities. We can test the validity of this hypothesis by determining if prospective migrants display levels of trust that are significantly different than those of non-migrants (prospective channel).

The second direct effect, the transmission channel, can be best construed in reference to the role of migrant social networks—which are both a conduit of information about migration opportunities abroad and provide a safety net of social trust and support. According to Tilly (2007), migrant trust network play an important part in the solidarity between people at origin and destination. Migrant trust networks bind members over the long term and operate simultaneously as social insurance and as social control. These networks create and depend "on boundaries that separate members from outsiders" (Tilly, 2007, p. 6). Apart from Tilly's "trust network", migration scholars developed and employed various other concepts to capture similar facts and arguments, like Alejandro Portes' "social capital", Douglas Massey's "culture of migration" or Robert Sampson "collective efficacy" (see also Lamela, 2014, for anoverview). For our research question, the 'stake of migration-trust networks' is twofold. First, migration-trust networks create boundaries which separate their members from outsiders, mainly at destination but also at origin. As social ties in the sending communities are broken, one can expect the level of generalize trust to be hit by a negative shock after episodes of large emigration, especially if these were initiated and perpetuated by trust networks. Second, migrant-trust networks help to transmit not only remittances but also norms, attitudes and political information. This last aspect is particularly relevant for our quest for the direct linkages between emigration and trust. It implies that emigration can have two types of impacts on trust, defined either as attitude or as relationship with practices attached

(Tilly, 2007). On the one hand, in the presence of migrant networks, emigrants and in particular returning migrants, can serve as a transmission channel for civic values from a host to the sending country (Chauvet & Mercier, 2014; Nikolova et al., 2017; Spilimbergo, 2009). In this case, we would expect an improvement of levels of trust in sending society. On the other hand and in a complementary way, migrant networks also contribute to the diffusion of civic attitudes and political information about the functioning of institutions, political parties and the trustworthiness of the government of the origin country (e.g., Barsbai et al., 2017). Since emigrants tend to be by definition dissatisfied with the performance of existing institutions at origin (see Moses, 2017, for a recent overview) the two effects might in fact reinforce each other resulting in a compounded negative effect of emigration on trust: migrant networks help the transmission of civic values from more advanced democratic systems at destination and at the same time signal political dysfunction in the countries of origin (Moses, 2017). This means that due to emigration communities at origin become more active (e.g. Gallego & Mendola, 2013) and vigilant and a more sophisticated citizenry might emerge with lower levels of political trust (Catterberg & Moreno, 2006). The lower level of political trust leads in turn to lower levels of generalized trust (Rothstein & Eek, 2009).

While not easy to operationalise in our analysis, we summarize the two linkages discussed above using a simple diagram as in Fig. 1. Based on an exit-voice framework as proposed by Hirschman (1970), dissatisfaction with the functioning of home institutions can lead to either exit or voice. Expressing voice can in turn lead to more active political participation and control over government thus improving institutional quality and increasing political trust. Emigration (exit) on the other side first impacts social trust via the selection effect and second via its effect on institutional trust via the signalling effect in the presence of migrant-trust networks.

We discuss briefly also the two indirect linkages between emigration and trust. The first one can be best understood using the 'modernization hypothesis': due emigration (brain gain) and the effects of remittances and return migration, economic conditions in the sending countries can improve. This economic development can lay the preconditions for political development (Lipset, 1959) and improvement in

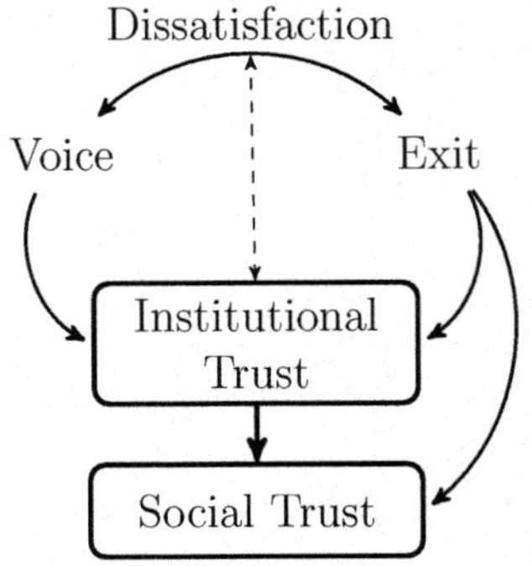

Fig. 1 The interplay between exit, voice and forms of trust

the quality of government and the performance of home country institutions. Once these improvements materialize, the levels of both institutional and social trust will rise.

The second indirect effect is the compositional effect due to the selection of migrants. Since migrants are not a random group in the population of the country of origin with respect to their individual characteristics like: education, earning abilities, wealth, norms, political attitudes and electoral preferences, large emigration flows with always lead to changes in the distribution of these characteristics and therefore to changes in inequality and potentially to distributional conflicts. A similar argument to that put forward by Rodrik (1997) in relation to international trade can be formulated with regard to the impacts of emigration: "Nations do have legitimate reasons for worrying about what globalization does to their norms and social arrangement" (Rodrik, 1997, p. 733). In the same vein, we argue that large and highly selective emigration flows can affect inequality in the home country creating the conditions for uprooting social values and for what Rodrik (1997) calls "social disintegration". Emigration rates above a certain threshold would in that case lead to a negative emigration- social trust relationship similar to the one identified by Chan (2007) between trade and generalized trust.

Due to the limitations of available data, we cannot account for these two indirect effects of emigration on trust in our empirical analysis. However, given the large heterogeneity among the countries included in our sample, we will used them when discussing the cross-country differences in our results.

4 Estimation Strategy and Data Sources

Based on the potential relations between emigration and trust discussed above, our empirical analysis will test the presence of three types of effects. More specifically, we look at social trust as well as at trust in selected institutions and use a definition of migration that includes persons who migrate (and return) but also persons who intend to migrate and those who have migrants in their households and receive remittances from abroad. This broader definition of migration (see e.g. Weiß, 2017, for a similar perspective) allows us to analyse three channels via which migration impact on trust. First, for what we call the prospective channel, we estimate the individual level effect of emigration plans on interpersonal trust. This will shed some light on the potential role played by selection into migration levels of generalized trust. Second, we test whether return migrants display different levels of generalized trust compared to non-migrants (returnee channel). Third, we will test if remittances received from households members residing abroad impact on the interpersonal trust of those receiving them. The first step of our empirical analysis is to characterise the relationship between emigration and trust at aggregate level. We then look in more detail at the potential effects of emigration on trust using individual level data from selected countries of origin.

4.1 Macro-Level Data

The first descriptive evidence we provide about the relationship between trust and emigration is at aggregate country-level. We extract a measure of generalised trust from six waves of the World Values Survey and the European Values Study for the period 1981 to 2014.[10]

Generalised trust is the proportion in the population who consider that "Most people can be trusted" when answering the question: "Generally speaking, would you say that most people can be trusted or that you need to be very careful in dealing with people?". We include only those aged 21–54 from the merged WVS/EVS data.

To these data we match emigration rates by country from the IAB Brain Drain Database.[11] In each source country, the emigration rates are defined as the proportion of migrants—to OECD countries—over the pre-migration population (Brücker et al., 2013). We merge the emigration rates to the corresponding years available is the WVS-EVS waves.[12]

We also use a set of covariates extracted from the World Development Indicators database.[13] In line with previous studies on the determinant of trust, we include the Gini coefficient, the real GDP per capita (in constant 2010 US$ prices), expenditure on education as % of total government expenditure, internet users (per 100 people), rural population (% of total population), smoking prevalence, males (% of adults), labor force participation rate for ages 15–24.

4.2 Micro-Level Data

As discussed above, we use micro-level data to analyze how three measures of migration are related to interpersonal and institutional trust: (i) emigration intentions, (ii) return migration, i.e. having work experience abroad followed by return migration, and (iii) receiving remittances from households members abroad.

Our data are from the United Nations Development Program Social Exclusion Survey (UNDP SES) for 2009–2010. These data offer at least two advantages for our research question. First, the country samples of about 2700 observations are large

---

[10] Inglehart, R., C. Haerpfer, A. Moreno, C. Welzel, K. Kizilova, J. Diez-Medrano, M. Lagos, P. Norris, E. Ponarin and B. Puranen et al. (eds.). 2014. World Values Survey: All Rounds—Country-Pooled Datafile 1981–2014. http://www.worldvaluessurvey.org/WVSDocumentationWVL.jsp.
EVS (2011): European Values Study 2008: Integrated Dataset (EVS 2008). GESIS Data Archive, Cologne. ZA4800 Data file version 3.0.0, doi:10.4232/1.11004.

[11] Brücker H., Capuano, S. and Marfouk, A. (2013). Education, gender and international migration: insights from a panel-dataset 1980–2010, mimeo. Available at: http://www.iab.de/en/daten/iab-brain-drain-data.aspx.

[12] The emigration rates from 1980 are matched with the Wave 1 (1981–1984), those from 1990 to Wave 2 (1989–1993), from 1995 to Wave 3 (1994–1998), from 2000 to Wave 4 (1999–2004), from 2005 to Wave 5 (2005–2009), and from 2010 to Wave 6 (2010–2014).

[13] Available at: http://data.worldbank.org/data-catalog/world-development-indicators.

enough to cover a sufficient number of potential emigrants and of returnees (both groups usually difficult to sample) residing in Kazakhstan, Moldova, Macedonia, Serbia, Tajikistan, and Ukraine. Second, the survey collected information on migration (including migration intentions, reasons for migration, migration experience, remittances received from abroad) as well as on trust and social inclusion. These variables allow us to control for usual socio-demographics as well as for attitudes towards institutions, social norms, civic engagement and perceptions of democratic processes in these six former communist countries. We base our measure of general trust on the binary answer to the question "Generally speaking, do you think most people can be trusted?". We include also indicators of institutional trust such as trust in judiciary, health, pension, and social security systems.

The survey also includes rich information on migration choices, our variable of interest. It covers migration intentions, reasons for migrating abroad, and a subjective evaluation of the likelihood of migration ("What is the probability for you to move abroad?"). We can identify the groups that are potentially planning to migrate either for education, or for work, or to emigrate to live abroad.Return migrants are defined as those who report at least one episode of working abroad for more than three months. We consider a household exposed to emigration if it receives remittances from abroad.

The list of control variables includes gender, age, belonging to country majority group with regard to ethnicity, language or religion, marital status, having children, health status (1 = "poor", 5 = "excellent"), education (0 = "no education", 9 = "Ph.D."), income quantile, labour market status (private employee, state employee, self-employed, unemployed), internet access, land ownership, used subsistence farming 25 years ago to provide food to the household, neighbourhood type (1 = "slam", 5 = "elite"), conditions of the property, size of municipality, size of the ethnic group, rural area, as well as county and regional dummies.

For both the macro- and the micro-level, we estimate models of the following type:

$$\text{Generalized Trust}_i = \beta_0 + \beta_1 \cdot \text{emigration}_i + \mathbf{X}_i' \cdot \gamma + \phi_c + \varepsilon_i \tag{1}$$

where the level of observation (**i**) corresponds to an individual respondent at micro-level, and to a country at macro-level. The outcome variable is the individual response of person **i** to the question if most people an be trusted—or the measure of institutional trust—in our individual survey data. As explained above, we use three measures of exposure to migration at individual level: migration plans, work experience abroad (returnee) and remittances. $\mathbf{X}_i$ is a vector of personal characteristics predicting migration in the individual level analysis. $\phi_\mathbf{c}$ captures country random effects in macro-level models.

5 Discussion of Results

5.1 Macro-Level Evidence

We start with a visual investigation of the relationship between emigration rates and the (weighted) means of generalized trust. For the counties covered by the World Value and European Value Survey over the period 1981–2014 this is depicted in (Fig. 2). The mean trust—as the original variable is binary—can be interpreted as a share of population that is prone to trust other people in a society. Figure 2 suggests a possible negative—and non-linear—relation between trust and emigration rate. However, the result might be driven by outliers with the very high emigration rates. As the sample in the consideration includes a very heterogeneous set of countries, the drivers of emigration and the channels through which emigration affects trust might vary significantly.

To better link the figure to the micro-level analysis, we highlight in Fig. 2 the six relevant countries. These also differ significantly, with Kazakhstan being the country with the highest mean levels of generalized trust and low emigration rates, and Macedonia at the opposite end.

Because education correlates with trust, a brain drain is potentially leading to a trust drain. We therefore plot the means of generalized trust against the emigration

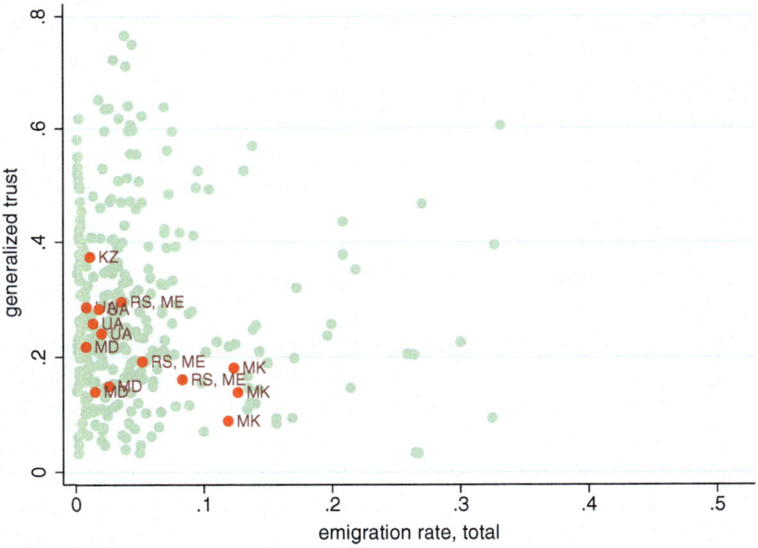

Fig. 2 Emigration and trust: evidence at macro-level. *Source* Own calculation using WVS-EVS (1989–2014) and IAB Brain Drain database. *Note* MD—Moldova, KZ—Kazakhstan, RS, ME—Serbia and Montenegro, UA—Ukraine

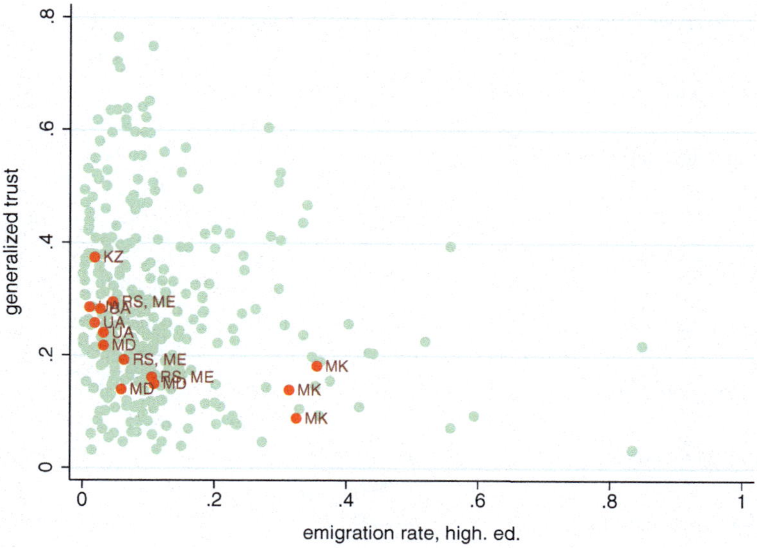

Fig. 3 Emigration of highly-educated and trust: evidence at macro-level. *Source* Own calculation using WVS-EVS (1989–2014) and IAB Brain Drain database. *Note* MD—Moldova, KZ—Kazakhstan, RS, ME—Serbia and Montenegro, UA—Ukraine

rates of those with higher education only (Fig. 3). The negative relation between the two variables appears visually stronger, though still potentially driven by the outliers.

We estimate simple random effects[14] models with the total emigration rate and the set of emigration rates by levels of education, in both absolute value and as logs. The results are consistent with those from the visual representation: they support a non-linear negative relationship between the two variables of interest (see Table 9, Model 4). We do not claim any causality between emigration and trust, but interpret our findings in terms of the partial correlations.

In order to control for the country heterogeneity, we further include some of the characteristics that can impact the trust levels at the macro-levels. To reduce possible multicollinearity issues, the pairs of variable with very high correlation should be excluded (see Table 9 in the Appendix). We can see that the GDP per capita indicator is significantly and positively correlated to the share of internet users (correlation coefficient of 0.601), and negatively to the share of rural population (correlation coefficient of −0.608). We refrain from the inclusion of the respective variables in our model simultaneously.[15]

[14] As it follows from the results of the Hausman test, the H0 cannot be rejected and thus the random effects model is more efficient. Similarly, a higher 'between' variation in comparison to the 'within' variation, also suggests we use the random effects specification. The Breusch and Pagan Lagrangian multiplier test for random effects rejects the H0, thus making a simple OLS regression inappropriate.

[15] Models 5 and 6 in Table 10 and 6 in Table 11 in Appendix, demonstrate only a change in the magnitude of the coefficients of interest but not of their significance in case when the controls

Table 2 Overview of country level evidence: emigration and trust

	Model 1	Model 2	Model 3	Model 4	Model 5
Emig. rate, total	−0.194 (0.150)		−0.454 (0.281)		−0.464 (0.303)
Ln(Emig. rate, total) logtot		−0.011 (0.008)		−0.024* (0.012)	
	Model 6	Model 7	Model 8	Model 9	Model 10
Emig. rate, low. educ.	0.075 (0.075)		0.148 (0.122)	0.029 (0.126)	
Emig. rate, med. educ.	0.085 (0.232)		0.081 (0.414)	0.170 (0.612)	
Emig. rate, high. educ.	−0.255** (0.104)		−0.363* (0.209)	−0.322 (0.271)	
ln(Emig. rate, low. edu.)		0.014 (0.008)			−0.020 (0.016)
ln(Emig. rate, med. edu.)		−0.003 (0.013)			0.002 (0.029)
ln(Emig. rate, high. edu.)		−0.031** (0.014)			−0.003 (0.028)
Additional controls[1]	No	No	Yes	Yes	Yes
Additional controls[2]	No	No	No	Yes	Yes

Standard errors in parentheses.
Models in the same column have the same controls
$***p < 0.01$, $**p < 0.05$, $*p < 0.1$
Additional controls[1]: GDP, Gini coefficient, LFP
Additional controls[2]: Expenditure on education

The signs of the control variables align with findings from the previous literature, namely a negative significant coefficients for Gini coefficient, share of rural population, and positive significant for real GDP per capita (in constant 2010 US$ prices), share of expenditure on education in total government expenditure, share of internet users in the population, labor force participation rate for ages 15–24; the coefficient for smoking prevalence among men is insignificant, so we exclude this variable from the analysis.

The various specifications of the model (see Tables 2, 10 and 11 in Appendix) suggest that only the coefficient for emigration rate of highly educated migrants in the log-form becomes significantly negative when the country-specific controls are introduced (Models 6–8). The other coefficients for emigration rate of those with low and medium, as well as total emigration rate remain insignificant in both absolute and log-form regardless the presence of absence of the country-level controls. The negative effect of (logarithm of) emigration in case of highly educated migrants

are present in the specifications. Nevertheless, we refrain from interpreting the above-mentioned models.

outflow, however, becomes insignificant when we control for the share of education expenditures in total government spending.

We derive two main findings from the cross-country analysis: (i) the negative relationship between (log) mean emigration rates and the levels of generalised trust, and (ii) this negative relationship is likely driven by the highly educated group of emigrants, so that the selection of migrants likely plays an important role for our question.

5.2 *Individual Level Evidence*

We we complement the findings discussed in the previous section with more detailed evidence by using micro data from the six Eastern-European countries included in our sample. Table 3 presents some descriptive statistics for the variables we use in the analysis and Table 4 the means of our variables of interest: migration plans, return migration and remittances, by country. We also summarise the mean levels of trust by migration status and country in Table 5.

We start the discussion of the results with the two former Yugoslav countries included in our sample: Macedonia and Sebia. The UNDP SES data suggest that only 8% of respondents in Macedonia report to receive remittances, while emigration intentions are expressed by 29% of those included in the sample (Table 4). Returnees who also receive remittances are the least trusting, in particular when they do not have further emigration plans: only 23.1% of the latter report trusting others compared to 47.8% among those with no migration experience, intentions or remittances received (Table 5). The lower generalized trust among the prospective emigrants appears along distrust in institutions such as the judiciary and social assistance systems but no relative distrust in the health system (Tables 6 and 12). This might suggest that trust (in its various forms) belongs to traits on which emigrants self-select in Macedonia. This is consistent with the findings of Dustman and Okatenko Dustmann & Okatenko (2014), who underline the importance of satisfaction with local amenities and institutions to prevent population from emigration. The lower levels of trust in the group with migration intentions, however, would not lead to the "trust drain" if the intentions are realized.

In Serbia 18.5% of respondents declare plans to migrate for work, study, or long term emigration, while 7.5% report to already have work experience abroad, i.e. are return migrants (Table 4). Migration status is not systematically related to social trust and trust in the judiciary. However, compared to non-migrants (no intentions and no work experience abroad), potential migrants have significantly higher levels of trust in the Serbian welfare state (pensions and social assistance systems) (Tables 6 and 12). Individuals who receive remittances and also plan to emigrate for the first time are the most trusting (29.0%) group while returnees who receive no remittances and have no further intention to emigrate, are the least trusting group of the population (15.2%; see Table 5).

Table 3 Individual level analysis: summary statistics for all countries

Variable	Obs	Mean	Std. Dev.	Min	Max
Social trust	14,748	0.408	0.492	0	1
Migration plans	14,865	0.22	0.414	0	1
Returnee	15,334	0.087	0.282	0	1
Remittances	15,901	0.125	0.33	0	1
Plan_migrate	15,121	0.246	0.431	0	1
Male	15,901	0.46	0.498	0	1
Age	15,901	42.238	17.379	15	105
Secondary ed.	15,901	0.577	0.494	0	1
Tertiary ed.	15,901	0.186	0.389	0	1
Income	14,900	1.654	1.429	0	5
Married	15,148	0.678	0.467	0	1
Small town	15,901	0.191	0.393	0	1
Big town	15,901	0.198	0 0.398	0	1
Capital	15,901	0.127	0.332	0	1
Ethnic majority	15,901	0.742	0.437	0	1
Religious majority	15,901	0.794	0.405	0	1
Corruption score	12,892	1.423	2.632	0	9
Trust judiciary	14,434	1.294	0.921	0	3
Trust health system	15,356	1.617	0.885	0	3
Trust pension system	14,472	1.39	0.956	0	3
Trust social assistance system	14,365	1.264	0.935	0	3

Source Own calculation, UNDP-SES data

Among the four former Soviet Republics included in our sample, Kazakhstan stand out as the one country in which both migration intentions and work experience abroad (return migration) seems associated with lower levels of all forms of trust we consider (Table 4). After controlling for covariates, the negative signs remain but the coefficients are not statistically significant (Table 6). Nevertheless, even the migration intentions do not prevent those with no emigration experience but receiving remittances from being the most trusting—towards the others—group (60.0%; Table 5). We observe also lower levels of trust among returnees who plan to emigrate again (only 50.0% in this group declare trusting others).

Table 4 Migration intentions, returnees and remittances, shares by country

Country	Migration plans[a]	Returnees[a]	Remittances[b]
Kazakhstan	0.121	0.015	0.023
	2571	2682	2700
Macedonia	0.290	0.0759	0.081
	2386	2463	2700
Moldova	0.337	0.185	0.258
	2640	2684	2700
Serbia	0.185	0.075	0.053
	2271	2159	2401
Tajikistan	0.265	0.134	0.299
	2454	2665	2700
Ukraine	0.120	0.036	0.025
	2543	2681	2700
Total	0.220	0.087	0.125
	14,865	15,334	15,901

Source Own calculation, UNDP-SES data
[a]shares in the total population
[b]share of households receiving remittances

In Ukraine, where only 12% elicit migration intentions, the shares of returnees and those receiving remittances are under 4% (Table 4). Like in Kazakhstan, migration intentions are systematically associated with lower levels of social trust and trust in the pension system (Table 6). The lowest levels of trust can be observed among those who receives remittances, have no previous migration experience but make plans to emigrate (33.0%; Table 5).

In our data, Moldova and Tajikistan display not only contain the highest share of returnees (18.5 and 13.4% accordingly), but also the highest exposure to emigration through ratio of households receiving remittances from abroad (25.8 and 29.9%) (Table 4). They are also the only two countries in our sample in which emigration plans are associated with significantly lower social trust in both the overall population and among younger respondents (Table 6). In both countries, the least trusting groups are returnees with further emigration plans, receiving remittances (21.0% trusting others in Moldova) and not receiving remittances (31.9% in Tajikistan, Table 5).

Like in the case of our tentative macro-level analysis, the results at individual level should be treated as descriptive rather than causal. Both migration and trust are notoriously difficult to define and instrument in quantitative analyses. However, we find a systematic pattern which suggest that the negative association between migration and social trust implied by our macro results is mirrored at individual level: most of the coefficients reported in our overview table (Tabe 6) are negative and some of them robust to the introduction of a large set of control variables. The differences

Table 5 Mean levels of trust (proportions) by migration status and country

Country	Kazakhstan	Macedonia	Moldova	Serbia	Tajikistan	Ukraine	Total
No migration plans, non-returnee without remittances	0.579	0.478	0.288	0.215	0.431	0.551	0.446
No migration plans, non-returnee with remittances	0.571	0.404	0.275	0.177	0.385	0.641	0.358
No migration plans, returnee without remittances	0.545	0.433	0.264	0.152	0.524	0.412	0.339
No migration plans, returnee with remittances		0.231	0.152	0.231	0.516	n.a.	0.288
Migration plans, non-returnee without remittances	0.552	0.424	0.239	0.202	0.392	0.461	0.371
Migration plans, non-returnee with remittances	0.600	0.421	0.223	0.290	0.427	0.333	0.323
Migration plans, returnee without remittances	0.500	0.379	0.233	0.200	0.319	0.583	0.306
Migration plans, returnee with remittances	0.500	0.357	0.210	0.200	0.451	0.500	0.333
Total	0.575	0.454	0.264	0.210	0.413	0.541	0.414

Source Own calculation, UNDP-SES data

we observe across countries can be traced back to differences in institutional settings and to a different evolution of migration patterns after the demise of the communist regime.

6 Conclusions

This chapter is a first attempt to analyze and quantify the effects of international migration on social trust in sending countries. Research related to ecological factors that shape the evolution of trust in the short rather than the long run, i.e. social or economic shocks, institutions or public policies, is still very limited. A consensus is emerging that both of the two conflicting views illustrated by the 'Putnam I' versus 'Putnam II' hypotheses have an element of truth (Algan & Cahuc, 2014). One part of trust is determined by history and hardly malleable, which leaves little room for action ('Putnam I'). But another part of trust does change quickly in response to changes in the current environment. Our chapter contributes to this second stream

Table 6 Overview of regressions coefficients: forms of trust on migration plans

	Predicted sign	Kazakhstan	Macedonia	Moldova	Serbia	Tadjikistan	Ukraine
Social trust (all age groups)[a]	–	−0.026 (0.038)	−0.033 (0.035)	−0.055** (0.025)	0.003 (0.030)	−0.076** (0.034)	−0.095** (0.044)
Social trust (age below 35)[b]	–	−0.068 (0.052)	−0.104* (0.062)	−0.091** (0.037)	0.040 (0.043)	−0.090* (0.048)	−0.067 (0.060)
Trust in the judiciary	–	−0.059 (0.069)	−0.225*** (0.066)	−0.072 (0.048)	0.094 (0.062)	−0.225*** (0.061)	0.009 (0.069)
Trust in the health system	–	−0.093 (0.065)	−0.110* (0.058)	0.122 (0.047)	0.047 (0.063)	−0.157*** (0.054)	0.050 (0.076)
Trust in the pension system	–	−0.118 (0.072)	−0.157*** (0.066)	−0.133*** (0.048)	0.217*** (0.070)	−0.078 (0.055)	−0.149*** (0.072)
Trust in social assistance system	–	−0.099 (0.072)	−0.143** (0.068)	−0.084* (0.048)	0.129* (0.069)	−0.112* (0.059)	−0.106 (0.070)

All regressions use the full specification (the covariates are listed in Table 8)
[a]model 4, [b]model 5 in the country regressions reported in the online appendix
Standard errors in parentheses
Robust standard errors across clusters (counties)
Based on the full sample of the UNDP Social Exclusion Survey
$^{*}p < 0.10$, $^{**}p < 0.05$, $^{***}p < 0.01$

of the literature (‘Putnam II’) by showing that trust does adjust to changes in the environment, namely to large emigration shocks.

The evidence we present at both macro and micro level is in line with the argument that horizontal transmission channels (Bisin & Verdier, 2001) from contemporaneous changes in society are at work in formation of trust. Although our results are only descriptive, they are in line with the findings of e.g. Nikolova et al. (2019) and Ananyev and Guriev (2019) who find causal impacts on trust from two different episodes in Russia’s recent history and of Bai and Wu (2020) who identify significant effects of political movement on trust formation in the context of China’s Cultural Revolution. This stream of emerging literature in economics supports the view that levels of trust can change even over short periods of time in response to shock and that these changes can persist in the long run.

The common thread of the different parts of our empirical analysis is the uncovered negative relationship between emigration and the levels of trust in the sending community. We find negative signs in both macro and micro models estimated using various measures of migration: emigration rates (aggregate and by skill level), migration intentions, migration experience (return migration) and remittances from household members abroad.

Because of inherent limitations in the data and due to the complex relationship between emigration and trust, our analysis is of descriptive nature and we cannot uncover the actual channels though which emigration affects trust among non-migrants who stay in the sending countries. The heterogenity of the countries included in our sample and the different measures of migration we use allow us however to formulate some tentative conclusions about the potential ways in which emigration affects trust.

First, our results suggest that while migrants are highly selected in terms of trusting others, selection is not the mechanism driving the negative relationship between emigration and levels of trust. Large emigration outflows do not imply a direct 'trust drain', rather the opposite. Which also means that not being able to account for selection leads to underestimation of the other channels via which emigration impacts on trust. Future research will need to reconcile this finding with our result at aggregate level that even after controlling for country fixed effects, the rate of high skilled emigration (ration of highly educated among emigrants) has the strongest negative effect on trust.

Second, the effects of emigration on trust among stayers seems to kick in after a certain threshold (as the "social disintegration" hypothesis also predicts). In countries with lower levels of emigration we find weaker effects in the individual level models. This applies to both migration intentions and migration experience (return migration) and has implication for the way in which large emigration flows contribute to social traps—setting in which due to the lack of coordination individuals act independently and are unable to cooperate to achieve joint benefits (Rothstein, 2005).

Third, the type of migration (temporary versus permanent), the motives for migrating (work versus study) and the selection on age (under versus over 35) do play a role in mediating the impact of emigration on trust. All results should be interpreted as correlations and not the causation. Further research, that explores some other measures of emigration (bilateral stocks and flows) and application of gravity-type models of migration could shed more light on the structure and causal direction of these relationships. Similarly, at least some of the characteristics of destination countries could arguably be exogenous for interpersonal trust among those who remain in countries of origin and could be used to instrument of emigration in models estimating levels of trust at individual or aggregate level.

Appendix

See Tables 7 and 8.

List of countries included in the IAB-Data:

Albania, Algeria, Andorra, Azerbaijan, Argentina, Australia, Austria, Bangladesh, Armenia, Belgium, Bosnia Herzegovina, Brazil, Bulgaria, Belarus, Canada, Chile, China, Taiwan, Colombia, Croatia, Cyprus, Czech Rep., Denmark, Dominican Rep., Ecuador, El Salvador, Ethiopia, Estonia, Finland, France, Georgia, Palestine, Germany, Ghana, Greece, Guatemala, Hong Kong, Hungary, Iceland, India, Indonesia,

Table 7 Macro-level variables

Variable	Description
Emigration rate[a]	Ratio of migrants over the pre-migration population by skill level
Control variables[b]	
GDP	Real GDP per capita in 2010 USD
Gini coefficient	
Expend. on education	As percentage of government spending
LFP	Labour force participation, age 15–24
Rural population	Percentage of total population

[a]from the IAB brain-drain data
[b]from the World Development Idicators database

Table 8 Variables from the UNDP social exclusion survey

Variable	Description
Migration plans	= 1 if respondent plans to move abroad for work, study or permanently
Return migrant	= 1 if respondent has spells of work abroad and returned
Remittances	= 1 if respondent's household receives remittances from abroad
Age	Constructed using the self-reported year of birth
Woman	Dummy based on self reported gender
Education	Self-reported level of education
Income	Self-reported level of income
State employee	Employed in state/municipal firm or organisation
Private employee	Employed in private firms
Self-employed	Self-employed/business owner/member of production cooperative
Unemployed	Unemployed based on self-reported activity status
Ethnicity	Dummy based on self-reported ethnicity
Religion	Dummy based on self-reported affiliation to religious group
Language	Dummy based on self-reported language that is spoken in the household

Iran, Iraq, Ireland, Israel, Italy, Japan, Kazakhstan, Jordan, South Korea, Kuwait, Kyrgyzstan, Lebanon, Latvia, Libya, Lithuania,Luxembourg, Malaysia, Mali, Malta, Mexico, Moldova, Morocco, Netherlands, New Zealand, Nigeria, Norway, Pakistan, Peru, Philippines, Poland, Portugal, Qatar, Romania, Russia, Rwanda, Saudi Arabia, Serbia and Montenegro, Singapore, Slovakia, Viet Nam, Slovenia, South Africa, Zimbabwe, Spain, Sweden, Switzerland, Thailand, Trinidad and Tobago, Tunisia, Turkey, Uganda, Ukraine, Macedonia, Egypt, United Kingdom, Tanzania, United States, Burkina Faso, Uruguay, Uzbekistan, Venezuela, Yemen, Serbia and Montenegro, Zambia, North Ireland (Tables 9, 10 and 11).

Table 9 Correlation matrix, macro variables

		(1)	(2)	(3)	(4)	(5)	(6)	(7)
(1)	Gini coefficient	1						
(2)	GDP p.c. (in 2010 USD)	−0.369***	1					
(3)	Expend. on education (% of gov. spending)	0.230**	−0.259***	1				
(4)	Internet users (per 100 people)	−0.478***	0.601***	−0.235***	1			
(5)	Rural population (% of total)	0.0847	−0.608***	0.233***	−0.417***	1		
(6)	Smoking prevalence (males, %)	−0.243**	−0.155***	−0.204***	−0.109*	−0.0176	1	
(7)	Labour force participation, age 15–24	0.228***	−0.00941	0.120*	−0.140***	0.307***	−0.176***	1

$^{*}p < 0.05$, $^{**}p < 0.01$, $^{***}p < 0.001$

Table 10 Cross-country results: generalized trust, total emigration rate

	Model 1	Model 2	Model 3	Model 4	Model 5	Model 6
Emig. rate, total	−0.194 (0.150)		−0.454 (0.281)		−0.464 (0.303)	
Ln(Emig. rate, total) logtot		−0.0114 (0.00855)		−0.0243* (0.0129)		−0.0274* (0.0141)
Gini coefficient			−0.00608*** (0.00184)	−0.00599*** (0.00181)	−0.00860*** (0.00197)	−0.00888*** (0.00194)
GDP p.c. (in 2010 USD)			5.29e−06*** (8.27e−07)	5.60e−06*** (8.60e−07)		
Labour force participation, age 15–24			0.00277** (0.00120)	0.00235* (0.00123)	0.00487*** (0.00115)	0.00449*** (0.00117)
Expend. on education (% of gov. spending)			0.00598* (0.00360)	0.00592* (0.00357)	0.00655* (0.00385)	0.00671* (0.00380)
Internet users (per 100 people)					0.00187*** (0.000533)	0.00194*** (0.000534)
Rural population (% of total)					−0.00226** (0.000993)	−0.00270*** (0.000993)
Constant	0.269*** (0.0158)	0.217*** (0.0343)	0.192** (0.0862)	0.0958 (0.0904)	0.292*** (0.108)	0.211* (0.110)
Observations	315	315	77	77	76	76
Number of s003	105	105	52	52	52	52
Wald test Chi2(3)	1.683	1.767	113.1	116.9	95.16	100.4
R-sq. between	0.00617	0.00258	0.715	0.715	0.678	0.687
R-sq. within	0.00519	0.0114	0.0827	0.110	0.132	0.132
R-sq. overall	0.00268	0.00285	0.664	0.671	0.656	0.672

Standard errors in parentheses
$^{***}p < 0.01$, $^{**}p < 0.05$, $^{*}p < 0.1$

Table 11 Cross-country results: generalized trust, emigration rates by educational levels

	Model 1	Model 2	Model 3	Model 4	Model 5	Model 6
Emig. rate, low. educ.	0.075 (0.075)		0.148 (0.122)	0.029 (0.126)		
Emig rate, med. educ.	0.085 (0.232)		0.081 (0.414)	0.170 (0.612)		
Emig. rate, high. educ.	−0.255** (0.104)		−0.363* (0.209)	−0.322 (0.271)		
Ln(Emig. rate, low. edu.)		0.014 (0.008)			−0.021 (0.016)	−0.015 (0.017)
Ln(Emig. rate, med. edu.)		−0.003 (0.013)			0.002 (0.029)	0.011 (0.031)
Ln(Emig. rate, high. edu.)		−0.031** (0.014)			−0.003 (0.028)	−0.024 (0.030)
Constant	0.285*** (0.0170)	0.223*** (0.034)	0.228*** (0.082)	0.194** (0.098)	0.164 (0.128)	0.258* (0.148)
Observations	315	315	116	77	77	76
Number of s003	105	105	68	52	52	52
Wald test Chi2(3)	8.359	8.663	82.70	106.1	110.8	96.48
R-sq. between	0.057	0.080	0.587	0.716	0.717	0.692
R-sq. within	0.0106	0.005	0.008	0.070	0.093	0.112
R-sq. overall	0.046	0.053	0.493	0.663	0.671	0.670

Standard errors in parentheses
Additional controls: Gini coefficient (models: 3–6), GDP (models: 3–5)
labour force participation (models: 3–6), expenditure on education (models: 4–6)
internet users (per 100, model 6), rural population (%, model 6)
$^{***}p < 0.01$, $^{**}p < 0.05$, $^{*}p < 0.1$

Table 12 Social and other forms of trust by migration plans and country

	Migration plans	Non migrants	Difference	t-value
Social trust				
Kazakhstan	0.520	0.575	−0.055	−1.548
Macedonia	0.404	0.479	−0.075	−2.815
Moldova	0.221	0.268	−0.047	−2.107
Serbia	0.205	0.208	−0.003	−0.128
Tadjikistan	0.373	0.415	−0.042	−1.527
Ukraine	0.450	0.539	−0.088	−2.301
Trust judiciary				
Kazakhstan	1.246	1.413	−0.167	−2.576
Macedonia	1.011	1.239	−0.228	−4.387
Moldova	1.267	1.352	−0.085	−2.018
Serbia	1.485	1.430	0.054	1.004
Tadjikistan	1.499	1.695	−0.196	−3.880
Ukraine	0.820	0.797	0.023	0.367
Trust health system				
Kazakhstan	1.518	1.630	−0.112	−1.841
Macedonia	1.800	1.937	−0.136	−3.028
Moldova	1.420	1.491	−0.071	−1.742
Serbia	1.894	1.865	0.028	0.518
Tadjikistan	1.509	1.622	−0.113	−2.574
Ukraine	1.308	1.245	0.063	0.928
Trust pension system				
Kazakhstan	1.293	1.500	−0.206	−3.077
Macedonia	1.580	1.738	−0.158	−3.061
Moldova	1.168	1.347	−0.179	−4.240
Serbia	1.384	1.234	0.150	2.445
Tadjikistan	1.411	1.496	−0.085	−1.898
Ukraine	0.662	0.825	−0.163	−2.543
Trust social assistance				
Kazakhstan	1.250	1.362	−0.112	−1.660
Macedonia	1.331	1.512	−0.180	−3.369
Moldova	1.240	1.373	−0.133	−3.155
Serbia	1.292	1.182	0.109	1.823
Tadjikistan	1.286	1.373	−0.087	−1.822
Ukraine	0.657	0.768	−0.111	−1.782

Source Own calculation, UNDP-SES data

Table 13 Social and other forms of trust by return migration and country, UNPD SES data

	Returnee	Non-returnee	Difference	t-value
Social trust				
Kazakhstan	0.455	0.568	−0.113	−1.299
Macedonia	0.405	0.458	−0.053	−1.116
Moldova	0.230	0.255	−0.025	−0.981
Serbia	0.161	0.212	−0.051	−1.132
Tadjikistan	0.405	0.397	0.008	0.265
Ukraine	0.459	0.528	−0.069	−1.046
Trust judiciary				
Kazakhstan	1.281	1.389	−0.108	−0.673
Macedonia	0.984	1.161	−0.178	−1.956
Moldova	1.256	1.336	−0.080	−1.700
Serbia	1.381	1.452	−0.070	−0.769
Tadjikistan	1.618	1.652	−0.034	−0.579
Ukraine	0.588	0.808	−0.220	−2.158
Trust health system				
Kazakhstan	1.457	1.615	−0.158	−1.091
Macedonia	1.784	1.889	−0.105	−1.329
Moldova	1.362	1.492	−0.130	−2.868
Serbia	1.705	1.861	−0.156	−1.687
Tadjikistan	1.594	1.599	−0.005	−0.102
Ukraine	1.361	1.255	0.106	0.982
Trust pension system				
Kazakhstan	1.400	1.463	−0.063	−0.396
Macedonia	1.521	1.694	−0.173	−1.937
Moldova	1.179	1.305	−0.126	−2.669
Serbia	1.043	1.301	−0.258	−2.433
Tadjikistan	1.402	1.494	−0.092	−1.793
Ukraine	0.507	0.819	−0.311	−2.996
Trust social assistance				
Kazakhstan	1.200	1.339	−0.139	−0.874
Macedonia	1.295	1.467	−0.172	−1.870
Moldova	1.173	1.370	−0.197	−4.234
Serbia	0.933	1.251	−0.319	−3.037
Tadjikistan	1.290	1.361	−0.071	−1.283
Ukraine	0.486	0.770	−0.285	−2.798

Source Own calculation, UNDP-SES data

Table 14 Social and other forms of trust by remittances and country, UNPD SES data

	Remittances	No remittances	Difference	t-value
Social trust				
Kazakhstan	0.500	0.566	−0.066	−0.857
Macedonia	0.400	0.448	−0.048	−1.118
Moldova	0.231	0.254	−0.023	−0.906
Serbia	0.214	0.204	0.010	0.231
Tadjikistan	0.390	0.400	−0.009	−0.357
Ukraine	0.581	0.524	0.057	0.628
Trust judiciary				
Kazakhstan	1.122	1.393	−0.271	−1.903
Macedonia	0.971	1.149	−0.177	−2.073
Moldova	1.351	1.304	0.047	0.998
Serbia	1.506	1.434	0.072	0.738
Tadjikistan	1.508	1.705	−0.197	−4.080
Ukraine	0.821	0.799	0.022	0.163
Trust health system				
Kazakhstan	1.171	1.622	−0.452	−3.376
Macedonia	1.827	1.870	−0.043	−0.590
Moldova	1.486	1.448	0.039	0.846
Serbia	1.953	1.855	0.098	1.004
Tadjikistan	1.573	1.606	−0.033	−0.791
Ukraine	1.421	1.255	0.166	1.125
Trust pension system				
Kazakhstan	1.415	1.460	−0.045	−0.307
Macedonia	1.556	1.674	−0.119	−1.400
Moldova	1.294	1.266	0.028	0.596
Serbia	1.381	1.248	0.133	1.201
Tadjikistan	1.464	1.486	−0.022	−0.509
Ukraine	1.079	0.795	0.284	2.048
Trust social assistance				
Kazakhstan	1.268	1.335	−0.066	−0.451
Macedonia	1.357	1.446	−0.089	−1.046
Moldova	1.315	1.322	−0.007	−0.155
Serbia	1.247	1.198	0.050	0.462
Tadjikistan	1.373	1.339	0.035	0.760
Ukraine	0.821	0.751	0.070	0.516

Source Own calculation, UNDP-SES data

References

Alesina, A., & Fuchs-Schündeln, N. (2007). Goodbye lenin (or not?): The effect of communism on people's preferences. *American Economic Review, 97*(4), 1507–1528.

Algan, Y., & Cahuc, P. (2010). Inherited trust and growth. *American Economic Review, 100*(5), 2060–2092.

Algan, Y., & Cahuc, P. (2014). Trust, growth, and well-being: New evidence and policy implications. In *Handbook of economic growth* (Vol. 2, pp. 49–120). Elsevier.

Ananyev, M., & Guriev, S. (2019). Effect of income on trust: Evidence from the 2009 economic crisis in russia. *The Economic Journal, 129*(619), 1082–1118.

Arrow, K. J. (1974). *The limits of organization.* WW Norton & Company.

Bai, L., & Wu, L. (2020). Political movement and trust formation: Evidence from the cultural revolution (1966–76). *European Economic Review, 122.*

Banerjee, B. (1983). Social networks in the migration process: Empirical evidence on chain migration in India. *The Journal of Developing Areas, 17*(2), 185–196.

Barsbai, T., Rapoport, H., Steinmayr, A., & Trebesch, C. (2017). The effect of labor migration on the diffusion of democracy: evidence from a former Soviet Republic. *American Economic Journal: Applied Economics, 9*(3), 36–69.

Bartolini, S., & Sarracino, F. (2014). Happy for how long? how social capital and economic growth relate to happiness over time. *Ecological Economics, 108*, 242–256.

Bartolini, S., Mikucka, M. & Sarracino, F. (2015). Money, trust and happiness in transition countries: evidence from time series. In *Social indicators research* (pp. 1–20).

Becker, S. O., Boeckh, K., Hainz, C., & Woessmann, L. (2016). The empire is dead, long live the empire! long-run persistence of trust and corruption in the bureaucracy. *The Economic Journal, 126*(590), 40–74.

Berlinschi, R., & Harutyunyan, A. (2019). Do migrants think differently? evidence from Eastern European and post-Soviet states. *International Migration Review, 50*(3), 831–868.

Beugelsdijk, S., De Groot, H. L., & Van Schaik, A. B. (2004). Trust and economic growth: A robustness analysis. *Oxford Economic Papers, 56*(1), 118–134.

Bisin, A., & Verdier, T. (2001). The economics of cultural transmission and the dynamics of preferences. *Journal of Economic Theory, 97*(2), 298–319.

Bjørnskov, C. (2006). The multiple facets of social capital. *European Journal of Political Economy, 22*(1), 22–40.

Bjørnskov, C. (2012). How does social trust affect economic growth? *Southern Economic Journal, 78*(4), 1346–1368.

Bobić, M., & Anđelković, M. V. (2019). Skilled youth outmigration from Serbia in a developmental perspective. *Southeastern Europe, 43*(3), 255–276.

Brücker, H., Capuano, S., & Marfouk, A. (2013). *Education, gender and international migration: Insights from a panel-dataset 1980–2010.* The research institute of the federal employment agency, IAB Nuremberg. Technical report.

Carlin, B. I., Dorobantu, F., & Viswanathan, S. (2009). Public trust, the law, and financial investment. *Journal of Financial Economics, 92*(3), 321–341.

Carling, J., & Schewel, K. (2018). Revisiting aspiration and ability in international migration. *Journal of Ethnic and Migration Studies, 44*(6), 945–963.

Catterberg, G., & Moreno, A. (2006). The individual bases of political trust: Trends in new and established democracies. *International Journal of Public Opinion Research, 18*(1), 31–48.

Chan, K. S. (2007). Trade, social values, and the generalized trust. *Southern Economic Journal,* 733–753.

Chauvet, L., & Mercier, M. (2014). Do return migrants transfer political norms to their origin country? evidence from mali. *Journal of Comparative Economics, 42*(3), 630–651.

Coleman, J. S. (1988). Social capital in the creation of human capital. *American Journal of Sociology, 94*, S95–S120.

Danzer, A. M., & Dietz, B. (2014). Labour migration from Eastern Europe and the EU's quest for talents. *JCMS: Journal of Common Market Studies, 52*(2), 183–199.

Dasgupta, P. (2000). Trust as a commodity. *Trust: Making and breaking cooperative relations* (Vol. 4, pp. 49–72).

De Haas, H. (2010). Migration and development: A theoretical perspective 1. *International Migration Review, 44*(1), 227–264.

Dearmon, J., & Grier, R. (2011). Trust and the accumulation of physical and human capital. *European Journal of Political Economy*, *27*(3), 507–519.
Dietz, B. (2010). *Migration and remittances in macedonia: A review*. Available at SSRN 1713747.
Dietz, B., Gatskova, K. & Ivlevs, A. (2015). *Emigration, remittances and the education of children staying behind: Evidence from Tajikistan*.
Durlauf, S., & Fafchamps, M. (2005). Social capital. In P. Aghion & S. Durlauf (Eds.), *Handbook of Economic Growth* (Vol. 1, part B, pp. 1639–1699). Elsevier.
Dustmann, C., & Okatenko, A. (2014). Out-migration, wealth constraints, and the quality of local amenities. *Journal of Development Economics*, *110*(C), 52–63.
Fafchamps, M. (2002). Spontaneous market emergence. In *Topics in Theoretical Economics*.
Fafchamps, M., & Minten, B. (2002). Returns to social network capital among traders. *Oxford Economic Papers*, *54*(2), 173–206.
Faist, T., Fauser, M., & Kivisto, P. (2011). *The migration-development nexus: A transnational perspective*. Springer.
Fidrmuc, J., & Gërxhani, K. (2008). Mind the gap! Social capital, East and West. *Journal of Comparative Economics*, *36*(2), 264–286.
Former Yugoslav Republic of Macedonia. (2014). Technical report, International Monetary Fund.
Gallego, J. M., & Mendola, M. (2013). Labour migration and social networks participation in southern mozambique. *Economica*, *80*(320), 721–759.
Glaeser, E. L., Laibson, D., & Sacerdote, B. (2002). An economic approach to social capital. *The Economic Journal*, *112*(483), F437–F458.
Helliwell, J. F., & Putnam, R. D. (1995). Economic growth and social capital in Italy. *Eastern Economic Journal*, *21*(3), 295–307.
Helliwell, J. F., Huang, H., & Wang, S. (2014). Social capital and well-being in times of crisis. *Journal of Happiness Studies*, *15*(1), 145–162.
Hirschman, A. O. (1970). *Exit, voice, and loyalty: Responses to decline in firms, organizations, and states* (Vol. 25). Harvard university press.
Ivlevs, A. (2016). Remittances and informal work. *International Journal of Manpower*, *37*(7), 1172–1190.
Kaczmarczyk, P., & Okólski, M. (2008). Demographic and labour-market impacts of migration on Poland. *Oxford Review of Economic Policy*, *24*(3), 599–624.
Knack, S. (2002). Social capital and the quality of government: Evidence from the States. *American Journal of Political Science*, *46*(4), 772–785.
Knack, S., & Keefer, P. (1997). Does social capital have an economic payoff? A cross-country investigation. *The Quarterly Journal of Economics*, *112*(4), 1251–1288.
Kornai, J., Rothstein, B., & Rose-Ackerman, S. (2004). *Creating social trust in post-socialist transition*. Springer.
Kumo, K. (2012). Tajik labour migrants and their remittances: is Tajik migration pro-poor? *Post-Communist Economies*, *24*(1), 87–109.
Lam, K.-C. (2002). Interaction between economic and political factors in the migration decision. *Journal of Comparative Economics*, *30*(3), 488–504.
Lamela, C. (2014). *Migration-trust networks: Social cohesion in Mexican US-bound emigration*.
Lin, N. (2001). *Social capital: A theory of social structure and action* (Vol. 19). Cambridge university press.
Lipset, S. M. (1959). Some social requisites of democracy: Economic development and political legitimacy. *American Political Science Review*, *53*(1), 69–105.
Loury, G. C. (1977). A dynamic theory of racial income differences. *Women, Minorities, and Employment Discrimination*, *153*, 86–153.
Luhman, N. (1979). *Trust and power: Two works*.
Malyuchenko, I. (2015). *Labour migration from Central Asia to Russia: Economic and social impact on the societies of Kyrgyzstan, Tajikistan, and Uzbekistan*. Central Asia Security Policy Briefs.
Moses, J. W. (2017). Sparrows of despair: Migration as a signalling device for dysfunctional states in Europe. *Government and Opposition*, *52*(2), 295–328.

Munshi, K. (2003). Networks in the modern economy: Mexican migrants in the US labor market. *The Quarterly Journal of Economics*, *118*(2), 549–599.

Nikolova, M., Popova, O. & Otrachshenko, V. (2019). *Stalin and the origins of mistrust*.

Nikolova, M., Roman, M., & Zimmermann, K. F. (2017). Left behind but doing good? Civic engagement in two post-socialist countries. *Journal of Comparative Economics*, *45*(3), 658–684.

Nikolovska, M. (2004). Employment, education, and emigration: The FYR of Macedonia. *Higher Education in Europe*, *29*(3), 319–328.

Okólski, M. (2012). Modernising impacts of emigration. *Studia Socjologiczne*.

Özcan, B., & Bjørnskov, C. (2011). Social trust and human development. *The Journal of Socio-Economics*, *40*(6), 753–762.

O'Reilly, J., Eichhorst, W., Gábos, A., Hadjivassiliou, K., Lain, D., Leschke, J., et al. (2015). Five characteristics of youth unemployment in Europe: Flexibility, education, migration, family legacies, and EU policy. *SAGE Open*, *5*(1), 2158244015574962.

Papagapitos, A., & Riley, R. (2009). Social trust and human capital formation. *Economics Letters*, *102*(3), 158–160.

Petreski, M., & Petreski, B. (2015). Dissatisfied, feeling unequal and inclined to emigrate: Perceptions from Macedonia in a MIMIC model. *Migration Letters*, *12*(3), 300.

Petreski, M., Petreski, B., Tumanoska, D., Narazani, E., Kazazi, F., Ognjanov, G., et al. (2018). The size and effects of emigration and remittances in the Western Balkans:A forecasting based on a Delphi Process. *Südosteuropa*, *65*(4), 679–695.

Pop-Eleches, G., & Tucker, J. A. (2011). Communism's shadow: Postcommunist legacies, values, and behavior. *Comparative Politics*, *43*(4), 379–408.

Portes, A. (1998). Social capital: Its origins and applications in modern sociology. *Annual Review of Sociology*, *24*(1), 1–24.

Putnam, R. D. (2001). *Bowling alone: The collapse and revival of American community*. Simon and Schuster.

Putnam, R. D., Leonardi, R., & Nanetti, R. Y. (1994). *Making democracy work: Civic traditions in modern Italy*. Princeton University Press.

Raiser, M. (2003). Trust in transition. In F. Bonker, K. Muller & A. Pickel, (Eds.), Postcommunist transformation and the social sciences: Cross-disciplinary approaches(pp. 77–96). Rowman & Littlefield.

Rebmann, A. (2015). Trust. In *Palgrave dictionary on Emerging markets and transition economics* (pp. 522–544).

Richardson, D., Hoelscher, P., & Bradshaw, J. (2008). Child well-being in Central and Eastern European countries (CEE) and the Commonwealth of Independent States (CIS). *Child Indicators Research*, *1*(3), 211–250.

Rodrik, D. (1997). *Has globalization gone too far?* Institute for International Economics.

Rose-Ackerman, S. (2001). Trust and honesty in post-socialist societies. *Kyklos*, *54*(2–3), 415–443.

Rose, R. (1994). Postcommunism and the problem of trust. *Journal of Democracy*, *5*(3), 18–30.

Rothstein, B. (2005). *Social traps and the problem of trust*. Cambridge University Press.

Rothstein, B., & Eek, D. (2009). Political corruption and social trust: An experimental approach. *Rationality and Society*, *21*(1), 81–112.

Ryazantsev, S. & Korneev, O. (2013). *Russia and Kazakhstan in Eurasian migration system: Development trends, socio-economic consequences of migration and approaches to regulation*. Technical report.

Santric-Milicevic, M. M., Terzic-Supic, Z. J., Matejic, B. R., Vasic, V., & Ricketts, T. C, I. I. I. (2014). First-and fifth-year medical students' intention for emigration and practice abroad: A case study of Serbia. *Health Policy*, *118*(2), 173–183.

Selezneva, E. (2015). Happiness in transition. In *Palgrave dictionary on Emerging markets and transition economics* (pp. 545–564).

Skeldon, R. (2014). *Migration and development: A global perspective*. Routledge.

Spilimbergo, A. (2009). Democracy and foreign education. *American Economic Review*, *99*(1), 528–43.

Stark, O. & Taylor, J. E. (1991). *Relative deprivation and migration: Theory, evidence, and policy implications* (Vol. 656). World Bank Publications.
Tilly, C. (2007). Trust networks in transnational migration. In *Sociological forum* (Vol. 22, pp. 3–24). Wiley Online Library.
Van Mol, C., Snel, E., Hemmerechts, K., & Timmerman, C. (2018). Migration aspirations and migration cultures: A case study of Ukrainian migration towards the European Union. *Population, Space and Place, 24*(5).
Weiß, A. (2017). Inequality and migration. In *Inequality in economics and sociology: New perspectives* (p. 122).
Whiteley, P. F. (2000). Economic growth and social capital. *Political Studies, 48*(3), 443–466.
Woolcock, M. (1998). Social capital and economic development: Toward a theoretical synthesis and policy framework. *Theory and society, 27*(2), 151–208.
Yamada, D. (2016). *Negative effect of past migration experience on education investment: Evidence from Tajikistan.* Available at SSRN 2568964.
Zak, P. J., & Knack, S. (2001). Trust and growth. *The Economic Journal, 111*(470), 295–321.
Zelinsky, W. (1971). The hypothesis of the mobility transition. *Geographical Review,* 219–249.
Zotova, N., & Cohen, J. H. (2016). Remittances and their social meaning in Tajikistan. *Remittances Review, 1*(1), 5–16.

Dragos Radu is Assistant Professor in Economics at King's College London. He is a research fellow of the Leibniz Institute of East and Southeast European Studies (Regensburg). His research interests are in labour and international economics. He works on the economic and political impacts of international migration and participated in policy evaluation studies.

Ekaterina Skoglund holds a Ph.D. from the University of Turin (Italy) (2009) on the topic of "Subjective well-being in Russia". She is Management Research and dissertation coordinator at the EU Business School in Munich. She is associated researcher at the Leibniz Institute for East and Southeast European Studies and at the international Research Network of the Ronald F. Inglehart Laboratory for Comparative Social Research at the Higher School of Economics (Russia). Her scientific and professional interests include applied research related to labour market and gender economics topics, and in particular, those which involve the usage of subjective measures.

Soomin Ma is a research assistant in the Economics Department, King's College London.

Cultural Transition of Human Values—A Longitudinal Study on East–West Migration in Germany

Eric Holdack, Rico Bornschein, and Silko Pfeil

1 Introduction

From an economic, political, and business perspective, change in personal values is a promising area of research because it represents both the conditions for and consequences of economic development and thus, of modernization and social capital (Dalton & Welzel, 2014; Inglehart & Welzel, 2005). Post-industrial modernization and the associated value change towards post-materialism came with mass demands for democracy and changes in political, religious, social, and sexual norms (Inglehart & Welzel, 2005). The impact of value change is found to be prevalent in all areas of life, ranging from mental health (Maercker et al., 2015), subjective well-being (Delhey, 2010), public opinion (Kilburn, 2009), to vocational preferences (Sagiv, 2002) and consumer choice (Pepper et al., 2009).

Peoples' values determine the level of collaboration in society and thus, ultimately, social capital. In particular, it explains why individuals in a society cooperate without knowing each other in the first place. Post-materialistic values are found to be associated with higher levels of trust (Uslaner, 2001a, b, 2002), which in turn, fosters collaboration and accumulates social capital (Putnam, 1993).

Conversely, post-materialism is dependent on the provision of certain collective goods (i.e., social networks). A society's capability to provide those goods comes with its ability to overcome barriers to collective action, that is, its available social capital. In the words of Maslow (1987), "higher needs require better outside conditions [and

E. Holdack (✉) · R. Bornschein · S. Pfeil
HHL Leipzig Graduate School of Management, Leipzig, Germany
e-mail: Eric.Holdack@hhl.de

R. Bornschein
e-mail: Rico.Bornschein@hhl.de

A. Almakaeva et al. (eds.), *Social Capital and Subjective Well-Being*, Societies and Political Orders in Transition,
https://doi.org/10.1007/978-3-030-75813-4_4

at the same time] have desirable civic and social consequences" (p. 58). Therefore, the present study understands social capital and post-materialism as mutually reinforcing.

On a personal level, values are assumed to be relatively stable over time (Welzel & Inglehart, 2010). They instead evolve on a societal level (Inglehart, 1977). Considering that formative conditions change only gradually, the level of post-materialism is said to change slowly over time from generation to generation. However, one could argue that drastic changes to a person's economic, political, and cultural environment provoke alternative logics of value change (Mishler & Rose, 2007; Sapiro, 2004; Tormos, 2012). In other words, sudden and dramatic institutional changes, affecting a person's everyday life, might thwart the stable nature of individual values and lead to accelerated value change.

In this context, the existence of two diametrically opposed political and economic systems in Germany after World War II with different levels of social capital and the dramatic turnaround in East Germany after the fall of the Berlin Wall can be considered as a unique quasi-experimental setting for value research (Frijters et al., 2004; Lenhart, 2018; Vogel et al., 2017). The German reunification has not only dramatically changed the social and political institutions, but also the living conditions of citizens residing in East Germany (Lenhart, 2018). Beyond that, one can argue that moving from East to West Germany has led to an even more drastic change in living conditions and thus in the circumstances for value transition.

Over the last decades, several empirical studies have contrasted the paths of value change in East and West Germany (e.g., Schnabel et al., 1994; Strohschneider, 1996; Trommsdorff, 1999). Extant research, however, has neglected the idea of value change on a personal level because of inward migration from East to West Germany. To the best of our knowledge, no longitudinal or repeated cross-sectional study has ever examined the value change of East–West movers compared to those who chose to stay.

Besides, existing studies examining value change in East and West Germany do not allow an interpretation of value transition related to the fall of the Berlin Wall. As personal values gradually change over time, they have a cumulative character (Inglehart & Welzel, 2005). By contrast, so-called break variables like a regime change and migration become manifest only at a certain point in time. Apart from these manifestations, there are no changes in a break variable. Hence, the relationship between a cumulative and a break variable cannot be continuous. Standard time-series techniques, which researchers often use to analyze value transition, treat each time interval equally. They mix blips of the break variable with prolonged periods of staying completely unchanged. As a result, they are not adequate to analyze individual value change related to the fall of the Berlin Wall (Inglehart & Welzel, 2005).

The current study addresses the outlined research gap by conducting a discrete-time survival analysis with a unique longitudinal dataset. It compares the change in post-materialist values of East–West-migrants with people who continuously stayed in East or West Germany. It does so to sharpen the understanding of how different environments drive modernization in post-Soviet times. At the same time, it contributes to the discussion about the extent to which critical life events can alter an individual's value orientation even at later stages in life. To this end, we investigate the following research question: How does migration from East to West Germany after the fall of the Berlin Wall impact the adoption of post-materialist values on an individual level?

2 Theoretical Background

2.1 Post-Materialism and the Persistence of Traditional Values

Classical theories of modernization build on the idea that socio-economic developments come with significant social changes. Specifically, they are said to come with rising rates of elite-challenging mass activities in Western countries (Inglehart, 1977, 1990, 1997). One reason for this argumentation is the intergenerational shift from materialist to post-materialist values. While materialists focus more on the satisfying survival needs, post-materialists feel relatively secure about the latter.

Younger generations tend to have higher levels of political skills and access to informational resources, leading to a process of cognitive mobilization (Dalton, 2006; Inglehart, 1977, 1990). In addition to being socialized with less material scarcity and a sense of security, this leads to capacity for non-material matters (Dalton & Welzel, 2014; Inglehart, 2008; Inglehart & Welzel, 2005). Hence, with technological progress, rising levels of education, and increased labor productivity comes a reliably predictable cultural change towards values of self-expression, and with it comes post-materialism (Inglehart, 2008; Inglehart & Baker, 2000; Inglehart & Welzel, 2005).

Some researchers, in the tradition of classical modernization theorists, argue that globally rising socio-economic standards, therefore, will lead to a cross-national convergence of values (Meyer et al., 1997; Stevenson, 1997). However, researchers have not observed such a convergence yet. Cross-national differences in post-materialism seem to be robust and enduring. Cultural peculiarities and, associated with that, different baselines of post-materialism persist. Even when exposed to the same forces of socio-economic development, societies will follow different paths of value change.

Moreover, the progress towards post-materialism is neither linear nor inevitable. When it comes to economic downturns, cultural changes tend to develop in the opposite direction. A society's culture is shaped by its entire historical heritage, thus forming a unique path towards post-materialism (Inglehart & Welzel, 2005).

One of the most profound historical changes in the twentieth century was the rise and fall of the Soviet Union (Inglehart & Baker, 2000; Inglehart & Welzel, 2005). Its fall caused a period of rapid political, economic, and social upheavals. Post-Soviet countries suffered considerable economic hardships, a collapse of the known order, and a loss of security, as there was no experience in transforming a planned economy into a market economy (Haerpfer & Kizilova, 2014; Mishler & Rose, 2007). This heritage left a clear imprint on people's value orientation (Haerpfer & Kizilova, 2014; Inglehart & Baker, 2000; Pacheco & Owen, 2015).

2.2 *Personal Value Change in East and West Germany*

Concerning value differences between post-Soviet and Western countries, the German separation can be considered an exceptional case (Frijters et al., 2004; Lenhart, 2018; Vogel et al., 2017). After the collapse of the Soviet Union and the abolition of the one-party rule in East Germany, both the German states signed a Unification Treaty in 1990 (Lenhart, 2018). Until then, the government banned freedom of movement and settlement between East and West Germany and citizens in comparable geographic and historical contexts were exposed to vastly diverging living conditions (Frijters et al., 2004; Vogel et al., 2017). As a result, both regions differ in the diffusion of post-materialism.

West Germany, concerning post-materialism, was characterized by its National Socialist past up into the 1950s (Kielmansegg, 2000; van Deth, 2001). Less than two decades later in the 1970s, it reached post-materialism levels of other Western countries, but only within younger birth cohorts, while older generations still showed disproportionately high levels of materialism. This situation can be considered a specific West German value fracture between generations (Kielmansegg, 2000; van Deth, 2001). Following a period of relative stability, the proportion of post-materialists made another leap in the mid-1980s. Between 1987 and 1988, West Germany even showed the highest levels of post-materialism among Western industrialized countries (van Deth, 2001).

There exist no reliable data for the value structure in East Germany until 1990. During this time, the productivity level in East Germany equaled one-third of the level of West Germany. Socio-economic inequalities had accumulated over time and resonated throughout history (Diener, 2000; Ferraro & Shippee, 2009; Vogel et al., 2017). Still today, the average income in West Germany is about 20 percent higher than in East Germany. East German citizens face a higher risk of suffering from old-age poverty and needing care (Frommert & Himmelreicher, 2010; Kumpmann et al., 2012). Correspondingly, they report more social losses, more worries about their economic situation, and worse perceived health (Motel-Klingebiel et al., 2010).

At the same time, there has been evidence suggesting that the national funds invested in East Germany steadily lead to a harmonization of the living conditions in East and West Germany (Vogel et al., 2017). Investments were made to upgrade the healthcare services to state-of-the-art levels, and East German pensions have been up-valued by law (Frommert & Himmelreicher, 2010). The German well-developed welfare system provides financial security to East German citizens experiencing difficulties with integrating into the market economy (Hall & Ludwig, 1994; Lenhart,

2018). However, the share of post-materialists in East Germany—despite the alignment process in living conditions—has been inferior at all times (Kielmansegg, 2000; Sortheix & Lönnqvist, 2014; van Deth, 2001).

2.3 *Agency and Individual Value Transition*

Within the specific paths of value development at the societal level, individuals are supposed to internalize a big part of their respective value structures in an unconscious and unquestioned manner (Kluckhohn, 1951; Rokeach, 1968; Schwartz, 2007). The resulting personal values that evolve throughout the impressionable pre-adult years are perceived to remain relatively stable throughout one's life (Inglehart, 1997). However, several studies have shown that the current environment of an individual—rather than his/her formative conditions—shape the degree to which post-materialist values are adopted (Clarke & Dutt, 1991; Clarke et al., 1997; Duch & Taylor, 1993, 1994; Trommsdorff, 1999). For example, adults in the post-Soviet period in Russia are observed to acquire values coherent with democracy (Mishler & Rose, 2007). Contrary to that, evidence suggests that significant cultural changes toward post-materialism among Western industrialized countries reflect a process of intergenerational change, with rather stable values on a personal level (Abramson & Inglehart, 1995; Inglehart, 2008; Inglehart & Welzel, 2005).

In an attempt to reconcile these divergent views, one could argue that personal value change is indeed possible, but it depends on 'agency' (Welzel & Inglehart, 2010). Agency refers to the capability of an individual to act expediently to his/her advantage (Guisinger & Blatt, 1994; McAdamy, 1997).

The process of socialization gives individuals an understanding of socially accepted behavior in their social stratum. In this context, refusing to act by certain norms is socially sanctioned (Tooby & Cosmides, 2005; Welzel & Inglehart, 2010). Through socialization, societies reproduce ideologies for specifying and legitimizing the places and expected life strategies of each in a stratified society. Moreover, stratification limits the horizon within which humans search for role models. Stricter social norms and stratification increasingly limit individuals in terms of social learning, role model diffusion, and positive selection, impeding the alternation of personal values (Welzel & Inglehart, 2010).

However, social environments may drastically change, diminishing the usefulness of old strategies and related value orientations to the extent that they are no longer beneficial (Welzel & Inglehart, 2010). Thus, the experience of rapid upheavals, like the collapse of the Soviet Union, may lead to people experimenting with new lifestyles and related values (Flanagan & Lee, 2000; Inglehart & Welzel, 2005; Sapiro, 2004; Tormos, 2012; Welzel & Inglehart, 2010).

More specifically, migrating to West Germany is such a rapid upheaval or critical life event. Compared to staying in an East German community, migration leads to an accelerated alternation of living conditions. We assume the confrontation with unknown socio-economic conditions and norms of reciprocity for migrants to be less gradual and more drastic. Moreover, such a move can be associated with an abrupt loss of social approval, social control, and attachment in informal systems related to GDR-specific stratification. We presume this disentanglement to result in a higher level of individual adaptability. This adaptability, in turn, may result in a fundamental alteration of an individual's life model and personal value orientation. Experiencing potentially less scarcity and a higher sense of security may expand the focus from satisfying survival needs to other non-material matters.

Based on these reflections, we frame the following hypothesis: *Migrating from East to West Germany after the fall of the Berlin Wall compared to staying in East Germany is associated with an accelerated shift toward post-materialist values on an individual level.*

3 Method

3.1 Study Design and Sample

Accounting for the assumable stable nature of post-materialist values, one needs longtime observational data on an individual level to address the outlined hypothesis. The German Socio-Economic Panel (SOEP) constitutes a unique dataset that satisfies this condition by surveying more than 25,000 individuals yearly. It continuously tracked approximately 3000 panelists in West Germany from 1984 to 2016. Individuals from East Germany, the former German Democratic Republic (GDR), joined the SOEP after the German reunification in 1990. Data about people's post-materialist value orientations, measured with Inglehart's (1977) four-item ranking scale, are available at three points in time after the fall of the Berlin Wall: 1996, 2006, and 2016. All analyses were limited to those 3413 panel members that continuously took part in these three SOEP waves. Furthermore, individuals with missing or inconsistent data for the measure of post-materialistic values were excluded ($n = 989$). The vast majority of inconsistent answers were equally ranked items. Additionally, information on respondents' place of residence in 1989 was utilized to drop remaining SOEP participants who lived outside Germany in 1989 ($n = 45$).

Among the remaining participants ($n = 2379$), 52% were female and 48% male, aged between 37 and 96 in 2016 (average age of 59.5). 59% of the respondents were married, and 41% were in work (full-time or part-time) in 2016. In 1989, 65% of the respondents in our final sample lived in West Germany and 35% in East Germany. In 2016, these values changed to 68% and 32% respectively, with 175 respondents (7%) moving at least once between East and West Germany. The group of people moving from West to East Germany was extremely small ($n = 39$). Therefore, the authors excluded it from for further analysis. Instead, the focus was on the comparison of people moving from East to West Germany with those who lived continuously in East or West Germany.

With three observation points (1996, 2006, and 2016), the years between 1989 and 2016 can be divided into three distinct time intervals (1989–1996, 1996–2006, 2006–2016).[1] Although a transition to post-materialism may occur in continuous time, we only know the time interval within which a potential transition occurred. Later, we use both time-constant and time-varying person-specific independent variables to model a person's propensity of transitioning to post-materialism.

3.2 *Measures*

3.2.1 Dependent Variable

In terms of post-materialist value orientations, Inglehart's (1977) four-item ranking scale constitutes the only measure that has been collected for a sufficiently long period to address our hypothesis. Several international surveys, including the SOEP, have implemented this ranking scale. The latter presents the scale as follows:

> You can't have everything at once – and that applies to politics, too. In the following, we will state four possible goals that politicians might pursue. If you had to choose, which of these goals would be most important? Please rank them in order of importance, starting with the first.
>
> Maintaining peace and order in this country
>
> Increasing citizen influence on government decisions
>
> Fighting inflation
>
> Protecting the right to free speech

Based on their stated priorities, respondents are commonly classified as 'post-materialists', 'materialists', or 'mixed types'. In an attempt to reduce model complexity at a later stage, these categories were collapsed into 'post-materialists' (1) and 'non-post-materialists' (0).

3.2.2 Independent Variables

To model a person's propensity of transitioning to post-materialistic values throughout each time interval, we use both time-constant and time-varying person-specific independent variables.

The focal independent variable of this study is the migration status of a respondent, which the authors computed as a conjunction of past and current place of residence (East vs. West Germany). That is, both a respondent's current place of residence,

[1] The dates of each respondent's interviews—that took place at some point in time in 1996, 2006, and 2016—serve to map time into disjoint intervals (1989–1996, 1996–2006, 2006–2016). Interval 1989–1996 spanned from the fall of the Berlin Wall to the date of a respondent's interview in 1996. Interval 1996–2006 comprises the time after the interview date in 1996 until and including the interview date in 2006. Interval 2006–2016 is defined accordingly.

which the SOEP collected on a yearly basis, and a respondent's place of residence in 1989, before the fall of the Berlin Wall, served as input to classify respondents into

(a) people residing continuously in West Germany (West Stayers),
(b) people residing continuously in East Germany (East Stayers),
(c) people that moved from East to West Germany (East–West Movers).

In particular, the authors coded respondents as (a) or (b) for the respective time interval, only if their place of residence in 1989 was identical with every yearly-observed place of residence within the corresponding time interval. Once respondents classified as East–West Movers, they retained this migration status for later time intervals, because the experience they made during their sojourn in West Germany may resonate and affect their post-materialistic value orientation even after a potential return.

In addition to the respondents' migration status, we considered variables that were both available in the SOEP and known to affect a respondent's post-materialistic value orientation. First, a person's value priorities are assumed to shift through psychosocial or biological maturation and the associated gain in experience (Johnson, 2001; Prince-Gibson & Schwartz, 1998). Commonly, aging is viewed to be negatively associated with a post-materialistic value orientation because younger people are more likely to possess an attitude which the literature often refers to as 'youthful idealism' and they have fewer social obligations (Pavlović, 2009).

Second, education fosters cognitive capabilities, knowledge, and skills, and thereby shapes the standards by which people evaluate themselves as well as the world around them (Pallas, 2000). An increase in education is thought to be associated with an increase in post-materialistic values (Inglehart, 1997; Nový et al., 2017). Consequently, a person's education, measured as cumulative years of education, was included as a control variable.

Third, the adoption of specific family roles, including marriage, is assumed to be negatively associated with post-materialism, as they are institutions based on sexual and familial norms (Inglehart, 2008). For each time interval, respondents were classified into people who were married and those who were not. The former were coded as 1, the latter as 0. Fourth, in line with the notion that a perceived satisfaction of essential material and security needs should translate into an increasing emphasis on post-materialistic values (Inglehart, 1997, 2008), respondents' satisfaction with their household income was utilized as another control variable. Persons' satisfaction with their household income was collected yearly and recoded as an average satisfaction score for each of the time intervals. Fifth, religion teaches believers a unique system of moral values, which may also interfere with the post-materialistic value dimension (Rokeach, 1968). In principle, many religions imply restraining from the earthy pleasure and depreciate the idea of pursuing personal (materialistic) wealth. As a result, religion should be positively associated with a post-materialistic value orientation (Masoom & Sarker, 2018). Participants' self-reported religious confession is utilized to classify them as theists, coded as 1, and atheists, coded as 0, for each of the time intervals. Finally, early gender-specific socialization is known to lead to differences in personal values (Gouveia et al., 2015; Schwartz & Rubel, 2005). Commonly, women exhibit a greater emphasis on materialistic values than men because their socialization into economic prosperity occurred later. Even today, it is more difficult for women to develop their proficiency in careers outside the household (Inglehart, 1977, 2008). Gender constituted a time-constant independent variable and was coded as 1 (female) or 0 (male).

In this study, the fall of the Berlin Wall, which abruptly enabled free personal and cultural exchange between East and West Germany, is viewed as the start of a quasi-natural experiment. Borrowing from experimental language, leaving East Germany to live in West Germany (East–West Movers) can be understood as receiving a 'migration' treatment, while their counterparts who stayed in East Germany (East Stayers) represent the control group. We are particularly interested in the post-Berlin-Wall treatment effect of migration on the pace of embracing post-materialistic values. In other words, this study is concerned with the question of whether East–West Movers passed through an accelerated shift to post-materialist values after the fall of the Berlin Wall, that is, they were prone to manifest post-materialist values at a faster rate than East Stayers. From this perspective, the hypothesis suggests that the duration spent in an origin state, here non-post-materialism, until a transition to a destination state, here post-materialism, is shortened for East–West Movers compared to East Stayers.

In order to address this hypothesis, this study draws on event-history analysis, also referred to as failure-time, duration data, or survival data analysis. The event-history analysis is a class of established statistical methods that are commonly applied in a variety of disciplines to model transition data, which describe the length of time from an original state to an endpoint or destination state (McCullagh & Nelder, 1999). Aside from its natural fit with the outlined research question, event-history analysis is capable of dealing with a property of the data at hand, that is, right censoring. Right censoring occurs, if throughout the time of observation the relevant event (transition to post-materialism) had not yet occurred, therefore the spell end date is unknown, and so the total length of time spent in the origin state (non-post-materialism) is unknown. It represents a considerable problem to other commonly used methods, such as Ordinary Least Squares regression (Allison, 1982; Jenkins, 2005).

4 Results

4.1 Descriptive Indications

When exploring a plot of the time-varying proportions of respondents holding post-materialist values across the groups of East Stayers, West Stayers, and East–West Movers (Fig. 1), two observations are salient. First, there exists an absolute difference in the proportions of post-materialists across East–West Movers and East Stayers, with the latter showing lower proportions throughout all observation points. Second, the absolute difference follows a reversed U-shape over time; that is, it increases

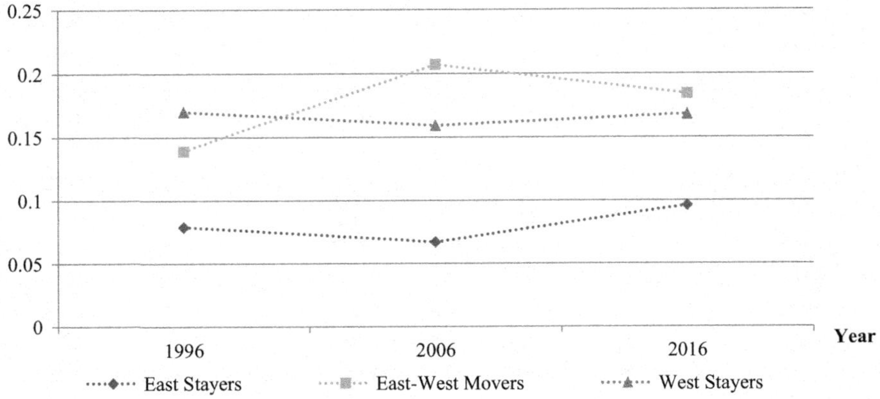

Fig. 1 Time-varying proportions of post-materialists across migration status

from 1996 to 2006 and decreases from 2006 to 2016. The difference increase from 1996 to 2006 is equivalent to varying average gradients for both groups, represented by the dotted lines. The difference in average gradients serves as a first indication that transition to post-materialism, also on a micro-level, takes place at a faster rate within the group of East–West Movers compared to East Stayers, at least for the interval 1996–2006. To examine this point, we now turn to a discrete-time event-history analysis. For reasons of simplicity, in the following, we will refer to the time interval between 1996–2006 as period 1 and to the time interval 2006–2016 as period 2.

4.2 *Discrete-Time Event-History Analysis*

Because we only know the time interval within which a potential transition to post-materialism occurred, we conduct a discrete-time event-history analysis (Cleves et al., 2016). To considerably reduce model complexity, Inglehart's (2008) macro-perspective notion of the unidirectionality of the post-materialistic value development, given a favorable socio-economic development, is transferred to a micro perspective. That is, we assume that once respondents reached post-materialism (destination state), they will not fall back into non-post-materialism (origin state). The data from 1996 only served to conduct left truncation, meaning to exclude respondents ($n = 329$) who had already experienced the event, meaning a transition to post-materialism, at the beginning of the observational study (Rabe-Hesketh & Skrondal, 2012). Discrete-time logit models were then specified to obtained estimates of the discrete-time hazards (period 1 and period 2) and the effects of the covariates on these hazards. Also, cloglog-based discrete-time models were specified but led to similar results, so only results of the logit models are reported (Table 1). All final

Table 1 Maximum likelihood estimates for logistic discrete-time hazards model for post-materialism

	Model 1			Model 2			Model 3		
	Logit coefficient	P > |z|	Odds ratio	Logit coefficient	P > |z|	Odds ratio	Logit coefficient	P > |z|	Odds ratio
Period 2	0.217 (0.124)*	0.081	1.242	0.192 (0.125)	0.124	1.212	0.594 (0.251)**	0.018	1.811
Migration status (reference: east stayers)									
East–West movers	–	–	–	0.654 (0.252)***	0.009	1.924	1.144 (0.336)***	0.001	3.139
West stayers	–	–	–	0.985 (0.167)***	<0.001	2.677	1.228 (0.228)***	<0.001	3.413
Control variables									
Age	−0.017 (0.005)***	<0.001	0.983	−0.015 (0.005)***	0.002	0.985	−0.015 (0.005)***	0.002	0.985
Education	0.087 (0.022)***	<0.001	1.091	0.111 (0.022)***	<0.001	1.117	0.112 (0.022)***	<0.001	1.118
Married	−0.330 (0.118)***	0.005	0.719	−0.270 (0.119)**	0.023	0.763	−0.268 (0.119)**	0.024	0.765
Income satisfaction	0.059 (0.036)*	0.098	1.061	0.005 (0.037)	0.897	1.005	0.003 (0.037)	0.940	1.003
Theist	0.049 (0.119)	0.681	1.050	−0.369 (0.140)***	0.008	0.691	−0.368 (0.140)***	0.009	0.692
Male	−0.176 (0.114)	0.124	0.839	−0.106 (0.116)	0.359	0.899	−0.102 (0.116)	0.378	0.903
Time-dependent migration status									
Period 2 × east–west movers	–	–	–	–	–	–	−1.037 (0.511)**	0.043	0.354
Period 2 × west stayers	–	–	–	–	–	–	−0.465 (0.281)*	0.097	0.628
Constant	−2.467 (0.462)***	<0.001	0.085	−3.115 (0.480)***	<0.001	0.044	−3.328 (0.496)***	<0.001	0.036

Note *$p < 0.10$; **$p < 0.05$; ***$p < 0.01$; () Standard Error in parenthesis models are significant improvements over the null model ($p < 0.001$). When evaluating Pseudo R^2 values (e.g., Model 2: McFadden's $R^2 = 0.042$) and receiver operating characteristics (ROC) curves (e.g., Model 2: area under ROC curve = 0.655), we find the goodness of our predictions to be rather poor. This poorness, however, is a well-known phenomenon and a consequence of both, the latent and multifactorial nature of post-materialist values as well as the latter's operationalization via Inglehart's (1977) four-item ranking scale (Braithwaite et al., 1996).

Model 1 and Model 2 are proportional odds models, assuming that the difference in log odds between respondents with different covariates is constant over time. This consistency corresponds to a constant ratio of the odds over different time intervals, here period 1 and period 2. We are first going to discuss the results for our focal variable, migration status, with the means of Model 2 and Model 3 before we briefly discuss the results for the control variables with Model 1. In Model 2, the logit coefficient for the group of East–West Movers is estimated as 0.654 (p-value = 0.009), corresponding to an odds ratio of exp(0.654) = 1.924 (Table 1). This result implies that the odds of a transition to post-materialism for East–West Movers in any given period–given that transition has not already occurred are 1.924 times the odds of East Stayers, controlling for the other covariates. This result directly refers to our hypothesis. We, therefore, find supporting evidence, that migration from East to West Germany after the fall of the Berlin Wall is indeed associated with an accelerated shift towards post-materialist values on an individual level.

Interestingly, the odds of a transition to post-materialism for West Stayers are 2.677 ($p < 0.001$) times higher than for East Stayers. No statistically significant difference is found between East–West Movers and West Stayers. In Model 3, we relax the proportional odds assumption by allowing the effect of the migration dummies to vary with the period. Here, we observe that East–West Movers have 3.139 ($p = 0.001$) times higher odds of transiting to post-materialism than East Stayers for period 1 (Table 1). Given that the transition has not occurred until the beginning of period 2, however, there is no such effect for period 2 (odds ratio = 3.139 * 0.354 = 1.111, $p = 0.784$). Therefore, Model 3 implies that our hypothesis is supported for period 1 but not for period 2. This result also complies with the descriptive findings of Fig. 1.

Concerning the control variables, see Model 1, we mainly find the anticipated directional effects. Although showing the anticipated directional effect, income satisfaction is only marginally significant in Model 1 and even non-significant in Model 2 and Model 3. As a proxy for perceived individual wealth and material security, it should be strongly associated with the transition to post-materialism from a theoretical perspective. Interestingly, being theist is negatively associated with a transition to post-materialism, which might result from religion, often embracing traditional values that attach great importance to respect for authority (Inglehart, 2008).

5 Discussion

Our results are the first longitudinal evidence for an accelerated shift towards post-materialism associated with migration from East to West Germany. The duration until a transition to post-materialism is shortened for East–West Movers compared to East Stayers. Thus, as envisaged, we find the confrontation with more available social capital and related social norms to result in leaps in post-materialism on an individual level. Consequently, drastic changes in living conditions can be assumed to result in an alteration of an individual's value orientation. As no lifelong longitudinal observation of post-materialism in Germany is available, we cannot altogether exclude the possibility that both groups already had a different chance of becoming post-materialists before migration. A deeper understanding of the nature of value transition after migration can be gained by reconciling the results from the event-history analysis with the proportions of post-materialism over time, depicted in Fig. 1.

Comparing West Stayers with East Stayers, Fig. 1 uncovers a parallel development of the proportions of post-materialists, though on different absolute levels. For both groups, the development of proportions follows a U-shape. Whether the decline in period 1 is directly associated with the abolition of the inner-German border or with other changes remains unclear. There exists no longitudinal data on post-materialism for East Stayers before 1996 or for West Stayers between 1986 and 1996. However, this observation is in line with Inglehart and Welzel's (2005) notion of the non-inevitability and non-linearity of post-materialism. The late 1990s and early 2000s in Germany were characterized by low economic growth, high unemployment rates, and political insecurity. Only in the late 2000s did Germany start to strengthen its economic position within the European Community (Storm & Naastepad, 2015). Besides the found differences in proportions, Model 2 and Model 3 suggest that, also, the time-to-transition depends on the migration status. In other words, not only absolute differences in post-materialism but also its rate of adoption is a function of migration status. These findings support the idea of unique paths towards post-materialism, depending on a society's culture (Inglehart & Welzel, 2005). It underlines the position that traditional values have an enduring influence and the value gap between East and West Germany is, therefore, unlikely to vanish. Given a faster rate of adoption, the value gap between East and West Germany should become even more substantial. However, we found differences in the proportions of post-materialists to be constant over time; a phenomenon also observed by other authors (Scheuer, 2016; van Deth, 2001). This constancy implies that West Stayers are more likely to fall back into non-post-materialism (origin state) after having adopted post-materialistic values.

Comparing East–West Movers with East Stayers, Model 3 indicates an accelerated transition to post-materialism for East–West Movers in period 1, which is mirrored by an increasing difference in proportions of post-materialists between the groups (see Fig. 1). Given a transition has not occurred until the beginning of period 2, there is no accelerated transition for any of the two groups. Our data suggest a convergence of the proportions of post-materialists. Thus, analogous to West Stayers, East–West Movers are more likely to fall back into non-post-materialism (origin state). The proportion of post-materialists among East–West Movers decreased in the second interval. A high proportion of East German non-post-materialists entering the East–West Mover group in period 2 can partly explain this decline. Still, the number of East–West Movers reverting towards materialism exceeds the number of East–West Movers becoming post-materialists in period 2. In this respect, post-materialism among East Germans after the fall of the Berlin Wall appears to behave similarly to the development of Schwartz's personal values observed for Ingrian Finnish migrants two years after migration (Lönnqvist et al., 2013).

At the outset, we summarized the ongoing discussion on the degree to which the current conditions of an individual shape the personal value structure. Our findings support both positions: The degree to which post-materialist values are adopted does react to radical changes in living conditions. Over time, however, the value orientation seems to revert. A survival data analysis allowing for competing events and multiple failure-times could provide a more profound understanding of this presumed rebound trend.

Summarizing, one can say that value change is not entirely ruled out by socialization and stratification. The level of post-materialism is likely to increase after migration to an economically more developed region with presumably higher social capital. Unlike the higher chance of becoming a post-materialist caused by growing up in societies with high levels of agency, this impact seems not to be enduring. More detailed, there is a specific time interval associated with higher odds of becoming a post-materialist. Besides, there seems to be a rebound trend after reaching post-materialism within this period. Thus, the development towards post-materialism is path-dependent on an individual level but can be changed for a limited time through migration. These findings may bring the focus of studies on value change and social capital back from the macro- to the micro-perspective. Future studies should shed light on the factors influencing the duration of an increased relative chance for value change after migration.

Generally, the results are in line with the notion of post-materialism not only reinforcing but also resulting from social capital. The consistently lower scores for cohesion found in East Germany (Unzicker, 2017) seem to have an enduring impact on the value-structure of its citizens. As this result shows, even with enhancing living standards, additional inclusive steps are necessary to promote a sense of community in societies.

References

Abramson, P., & Inglehart, R. (1995). *Value change in global perspective.* University of Michigan Press.

Allison, P. (1982). Discrete time methods for the analysis of event histories. In S. Leinhardt (Ed.), *Jossey-Bass management series. Jossey-Bass social and behavioral science series. Sociological methodology 1982* (pp. 61–97). San Francisco: Jossey-Bass Publ.

Braithwaite, V., Makkai, T., & Pittelkow, Y. (1996). Inglehart's materialism-postmaterialism concept: Clarifying the dimensionality debate through Rokeach's model of social values. *Journal of Applied Psychology, 26*(17), 1536–1555.

Clarke, H. D., & Dutt, N. (1991). Measuring value change in western industrialized societies: The impact of unemployment. *The American Political Science Review, 85*(3), 905–920.

Clarke, H. D., Dutt, N., & Rapkin, J. (1997). Conversations in context: The (mis)measurement of value change in advanced industrial societies. *Political Behavior, 19*(1), 19–39.

Cleves, M. A., Gould, W., & Marchenko, Y. V. (2016). *An introduction to survival analysis using stata* (Revised 3rd edition). College Station, Texas: Stata Press.

Dalton, R. J. (2006). Citizen politics. Public opinion and political parties in advanced industrial democracies. CQ Press.

Dalton, R. J., & Welzel, C. (2014). From allegiant to assertive citizens. In: Dalton, R.,& Welzel C. (Eds.), The Civic Culture Transformed: From Allegiant to Assertive Citizens (pp. 282–306). Cambridge University Press.

Delhey, J. (2010). From materialist to post-materialist happiness? national affluence and determinants of life satisfaction in cross-national perspective. *Social Indicators Research, 97*(1), 65–84.

Diener, E. (2000). Subjective well-being. The science of happiness and a proposal for a national index. *American Psychologist, 55*(1).

Duch, R. M., & Taylor, M. A. (1993). Postmaterialism and the economic condition. *American Journal of Political Science, 37*(3), 747–779.

Duch, R. M., & Taylor, M. A. (1994). A reply to Abramson and Inglehart's 'education, security, and postmaterialism.' *American Journal of Political Science, 38*(3), 815–824.

Ferraro, K. F., & Shippee, T. P. (2009). Aging and cumulative inequality: how does inequality get under the skin? *The Gerontologist, 49*(3), 333–343.

Flanagan, S. C., & Lee, A.-R. (2000). Value change and democratic reform in Japan and Korea. *Comparative Political Studies, 33*(5), 626–659.

Frijters, P., Haisken-DeNew, J. P., & Shields, M. A. (2004). Investigating the patterns and determinants of life satisfaction in Germany following reunification. *The Journal of Human Resources, 39*(3), 649–674.

Frommert, D., & Himmelreicher, R. K. (2010). Angleichung oder zunehmende Ungleichheit? Alterseinkünfte in den alten und den neuen Bundesländern. In P. Krause & I. Ostner (Eds.), *Leben in Ost-und Westdeutschland: Eine sozialwissenschaftliche Bilanz der deutschen Einheit 1990–2010* (pp. 351–372). Campus.

Gouveia, V. V., Vione, K. C., Milfont, T. L., & Fischer, R. (2015). Patterns of value change during the life span: Some evidence from a functional approach to values. *Personality and Social Psychology Bulletin, 41*(9), 1276–1290.

Guisinger, S., & Blatt, S. J. (1994). Individuality and relatedness: Evolution of a fundamental dialectic. *American Psychologist, 49*(2), 104–111.

Haerpfer, C., Kizilova, K. (2014). Chapter 7. Support for political system in post-communist Europe and post-Soviet Eurasia. In: Dalton, R. J., & Welzel, C. (Eds.), The civic culture transformed (pp. 158–190). Cambridge University Press.

Hall, J., & Ludwig, U. (1994). *East Germany's transitional economy, 37*(5), 26–32.

Inglehart, R. (1977). *The silent revolution: Changing values and political styles among western publics.* Princeton.

Inglehart, R. (1997). *Modernization and postmodernization; cultural, economic, and political change in 43 societies*. Princeton University Press.
Inglehart, R. (2008). Changing values among western publics from 1970 to 2006. *West European, 31*(1–2), 130–146.
Inglehart, R., & Welzel, C. (2005). *Modernization, cultural change, and democracy—the human development sequence*. Cambridge University Press.
Jenkins, S. P. (2005). *Advanced methods for the analysis of complex event history data: Survival analysis*. Essex: University of Essex. Retrieved from http://www.iser.essex.ac.uk/survival-analysis
Johnson, M. K. (2001). Job values in the young adult transition: Change and stability with age. *Social Psychology Quarterly, 64*(4), 297–317.
Kielmansegg, P. G. (2000). *Nach der Katastrophe: Eine Geschichte des geteilten Deutschland*. Siedler Verlag.
Kilburn, H. W. (2009). Personal values and public opinion. *Social Science Qarterly, 90*(4), 868–885.
Kluckhohn, C. (1951). Value and value orientation in the theory of action. In T. Parsons & E. A. Shils (Eds.), *Toward a general theory of action* (pp. 388–433). Harvard University Press.
Kumpmann, I., Gühne, M., & Buscher, H. (2012). Old age poverty—Causes and a projection for 2023. *Journal of Economics and Statistics, 232*(1), 61–83.
Lenhart, O. (2018). More than just the adoption of western capitalism? Time use changes in east Germany following reunification. *Journal of Labor Research, 39*(3), 306–328.
Lönnqvist, J.-E., Jasinskaja-Lahti, I., & Verkasalo, M. (2013). Rebound effect in personal values: Ingrian finnish migrants' values two years after migration. *Journal of Cross-Cultural Psychology, 44*(7), 1122–1126.
Maercker, A., Zhang, X. C., Gao, Z., Kochetkov, Y., Lu, S., Sang, Z., Yang, S., Schneider, S., Margraf, J. (2015). Personal value orientations as mediated predictors of mental health: A three-culture study of Chinese, Russian, and German university students. *International Journal of Clinical and Health Psychology, 15*, 8–17.
Maslow, A. H. (1987). *Motivation and personality* (3rd ed.). Harper and Row.
Masoom, M. R., & Sarker, M. M. (2018). The effect of materialistic value-orientation on religiosity in Bangladesh: An empirical investigation. *Religions, 9*(1), 1–14.
McAdamy, D. P. (1997). *The stories we live by: Personal myths and the making of self*. The Guilford Press.
McCullagh, P., & Nelder, J. A. (1999). *Generalized linear models* (2. ed., [Nachdr.]). *Monographs on statistics and applied probability* (Vol. 37). London: Chapman & Hall.
Mishler, W., & Rose, R. (2007). Generation, age, and time: The dynamics of political learning during Russia's transformation. *American Journal of Political Science, 51*(4), 822–834.
Motel-Klingebiel, A., Simonson, J., & Tesch-Römer, C. (2010). Alter und Altern in Ost und West: Zur Entwicklung der Lebensqualität alternder und alter Menschen seit der Vereinigung. In P. Krause & I. Ostner (Eds.), *Leben in Ost-und Westdeutschland: Eine sozialwissenschaftliche Bilanz der deutschen Einheit 1990–2010* (pp. 387–409). Campus.
Nový, M., Smith, M., & Katrňák, T. (2017). Inglehart's scarcity hypothesis revisited: Is postmaterialism a macro- or micro-level phenomenon around the world? *International Sociology, 32*(6), 1–24.
Pacheco, G., & Owen, B. (2014). Moving through the political participation hierarchy: A focus on personal values. *Applied Economics, 47*(3), 222–238.
Pallas, A. M. (2000). The effects of schooling on individual lives. In M. T. Hallinan (Ed.), *Handbook of the sociology of education* (pp. 499–525). Springer.
Pavlović, Z. (2009). Is there a sociodemographic model of acceptance of postmaterialist values? The case of Serbia. *Sociologija, 51*(2), 177–188.
Pepper, M., Jackson, T., & Uzzell, D. (2009). An examination of the values that motivate socially conscious and frugal consumer behaviors. *International Journal of Consumer Studies, 33*(2), 126–136.

Prince-Gibson, E., & Schwartz, S. H. [Shalom] (1998). Value priorities and gender. *Social Psychology Quarterly, 61*(1), 49–67.
Putnam, R. D. (1993). *Making democracy work: Civic traditions in modern Italy*. Princeton University Press.
Rabe-Hesketh, S., & Skrondal, A. (2012). *Categorical responses, counts, and survival. Multilevel and longitudinal modeling using stata:/Sophia Rabe-Hesketh (University of California, Berkeley, Institute of Education, University of London); Anders Skrondal (Norwegian Institute of Public Health)* (Vol. 2, 3rd ed.) College Station, Texas: StataCorp LP.
Rokeach, M. (1968). *Beliefs, attitudes and values: A theory of organization and change*. Jossey-Bass.
Sagiv, L. (2002). Vocational interests and basic values. *Journal of Career Assessment, 10*(2), 233–257.
Sapiro, V. (2004). Not your parents' political socialization: Introduction for a new generation. *Annual Review of Political Science, 7*(1), 1–23.
Scheuer, A. (2016). Werte und Einstellungen. In Statistisches Bundesamt (Ed.), *Datenreport 2016: Ein Sozialbericht für die Bundesrepublik Deutschland* (pp. 417–432). Bonn: Bundeszentrale für politische Bildung.
Schwartz, S.H., & Rubel, T. (2005). Sex differences in value priorities: Cross-cultural and multimethod studies. *Journal of Personality and Social Psychology, 89*(6), 1010–1028.
Schwartz, S. H. [Shalom]. (2007). Value orientations: Measurement, antecedents and consequences across nations. In R. Jowell, C. Roberts, R. Fitzgerald, & E. Gillian (Eds.), *Measuring attitudes cross-nationally: Lessons from the European social survey* (pp. 161–193). London: Sage.
Sortheix, F. M., & Lönnqvist, J.-E. (2014). Personal value priorities and life satisfaction in Europe: The moderating role of socioeconomic development. *Journal of Cross-Cultural Psychology, 45*(2), 282–299.
Storm, S., & Naastepad, C. W. M. (2015). Crisis and recovery in the German economy: The real lessons. *Structural Change and Economic Dynamics, 32*(1), 11–24.
Tooby, J., & Cosmides, L. (2005). Evolutionary psychology: Conceptual foundations. In D. M. Buss (Ed.), *The handbook of evolutionary psychology* (pp. 5–67). Wiley.
Tormos, R. (2012). Postmaterialist values and adult political learning: Intra-cohort value change in Western Europe. *Revista Espanola De Investigaciones Sociológicas, 140*(1), 201–228.
Trommsdorff, G. (1999). Social change and individual development in East German: A methodological critique. In R. K. Silbereisen & A. Eye von (Eds.), *Growing up in times of social change* (pp. 171–202). Berlin: Walter de Gruyter.
Unzicker, K. (2017). Social cohesion in Germany 2017. Retrieved from https://www.bertelsmann-stiftung.de/fileadmin/files/user_upload/LW_Abstract_Social_Cohesion_in_Germany_2017.pdf
Uslaner, E. M. (2001). Volunteering and social capital: How trust and religion shape civic participation in the United States. In P. Dekker & E. M. Uslaner (Eds.), *Social capital and participation in everyday life* (pp. 104–117). Routledge.
Uslaner, E. M. (2001b, September). *Trust as a moral value*. University of Exeter. Social Capital: Interdisciplinary Perspectives, Exeter.
Uslaner, E. M. (2002). *The moral foundations of trust*. Cambridge University Press.
Van Deth, J. W. (2001). Wertewandel im internationalen Vergleich. Ein deutscher Sonderweg? *Aus Politik und Zeitgeschichte, 51*(B29), 23–30.
Vogel, N., Gerstorf, D., Ram, N., Goebel, J., & Wagner, G. G. (2017). *Terminal Decline in Well-Being Differs between Residents in East Germany and West Germany, 41*(1), 115–126.
Welzel, C., & Inglehart, R. (2010). Agency, values and well-being: A human development model. *Social Indicators Research: An International and Interdisciplinary Journal for Quality-of-Life Measurement, 97*(1), 43–63.

Eric Holdack is a Ph.D. student at the marketing chair of HHL Leipzig Graduate School of Management. His current research interests focus especially on the digitization of employee and customer experiences. He is also interested in urban modernization and value change. He is an active lecturer with a professional background in project management and digital marketing.

Rico Bornschein is a Ph.D. student in the field of Marketing at HHL Leipzig Graduate School of Management. He earned a bachelor's degree in Economics and Business and a master's degree in Management—both with distinction. His current research focusses on birth cohort differences in work-related attitudes, such as work values and work centricity. Particularly, he deals with disentangling cohort from simultaneous action effects, that is, age or period effects.

Silko Pfeil is an assistant professor at the marketing chair of HHL Leipzig Graduate School of Management. His dissertation deals with the topic of value orientation and job choice behaviour of millennial candidates. His current research interests focus especially on the digitization of employer branding. He is an active lecturer at several universities and offers courses on marketing, market research, HR management, employer branding, strategic management and applied statistics.

The Impact of Economic Insecurity on Social Capital and Well-Being: An Analysis Across Different Cohorts in Europe

Tim Reeskens and Leen Vandecasteele

1 Introduction

Taken place more than ten years ago, studies on the social impact of the Great Recession, initiated by the collapse of Lehman Brothers in 2008, are accumulating. In an overview article, Redbird and Grusky (2016) for instance review its socioeconomic impact on social inequality, employment, health, well-being, demographic behaviour (Dooley et al., 1996; Stuckler et al., 2015). More importantly, however, they pinpoint the lack of research into the potential of recessions to drive larger social change, manifesting itself in changes in social and political attitudes. In terms of attitudinal outcomes, economics shocks have shown to alter political attitudes (for a review, see Margalit, 2019), with demonstrated peaks in demands for welfare state intervention when encountering hardship (see also Margalit, 2013). Even though these findings show how difficult the Great Recession has been to cope with, evidence about the extent that it has affected distinct values, attitudes and well-being differently are scarce and rather scattered. This is surprising, precisely because of the unique context that the Great Recession has shaped for testing the assumptions of one of the most influential theories on social change.

Indeed, modernization theory (Inglehart, 1977, 1997) predicts that economic downturns have social consequences, in the sense that particularly young people

T. Reeskens (✉)
Department of Sociology, Tilburg University, Tilburg, Netherlands
e-mail: t.reeskens@uvt.nl

L. Vandecasteele
Institute for Social Sciences - Lifecourse and Inequality Research Centre, University of Lausanne, Lausanne, Switzerland

LIVES Centre, Swiss Centre of Expertise in Life Course Research, Lausanne, Switzerland

L. Vandecasteele
e-mail: leen.vandecasteele@unil.ch

A. Almakaeva et al. (eds.), *Social Capital and Subjective Well-Being*, Societies and Political Orders in Transition,
https://doi.org/10.1007/978-3-030-75813-4_5

in their formative years will prioritize material over postmaterial values when experiencing harsh economic circumstances. In more general terms, Inglehart (1977, 1997) argued that, as economic development progressed, industrial societies gradually moved towards self-expression values like tolerance and autonomy with generational change: younger cohorts, exposed to optimal economic life-conditions in their formative years, replace older cohorts that were more exposed to severe economic conditions. Because of the slow replacement of older more «traditional» or «conservative» cohorts by younger more «progressive» cohorts, this shift is referred to as the «Silent Revolution» (Inglehart, 1977). In this context, it is important to note that youth and early adulthood are formative life stages wherein the influence of the societal context on a generation is expected to be greater. Put differently, the influence of material prosperity on value properties, or alternatively a major event like the economic crisis in which scarcity dominates, differs across cohorts depending on what life stage they are in (Elder, 1974).

Research on the influence of the Great Recession on the social outcomes of young people exists, demonstrating that while human values dispositions are unaffected, more sociotropic social and political attitudes have shifted (Reeskens & Vandecasteele, 2017). However, a formal test whether different cohorts react differently to the economic crisis in terms of social and political attitudes and preferences, as well as value priorities, is to our knowledge not undertaken yet. In this chapter, we will empirically examine to what extent human values, social attitudes and well-being are affected by the recent economic crisis, making use of longitudinal data for 24 European countries that have been hit to varying extents by the Great Recession. Our main expectation is that the social attitudes of younger age groups are more strongly affected by the economic crisis of 2008, because economic shocks earlier in the life course have worse scarring effects (scarcity and socialization), while we expect less or no impact among the older cohorts. Human values, on the other hand are more stable personality traits that have been socialized in early childhood and are not expected to change drastically in response to an economic crisis or across age groups.

We employ a fixed effects pseudo-panel analysis of the 2008–2016 waves of the European Social Survey to detect whether changes over time in the socio-demographic group's exposure to poverty and changes in national-level prosperity—both useful indicators for measuring the exposure to the Great Recession in a pseudo-panel design—affect individual dispositions to varying degrees according to the cohort they belong to. Unique for this set-up is that we can test whether the findings hold for over-time changes in the country-level economic situation (GDP/capita), as well as changes in the economic situation of the person's socio-demographic group.

2 Theory and Hypotheses

In modernization theory (Inglehart, 1997), one crucial mechanism is the *scarcity hypothesis*, positing that periods of economic downturns result in an emphasis of materialistic values; embracing materialism in times of scarcity would particularly hold for those in their most formative years, also known as the *socialization hypothesis*. The aim of our contribution is to subject these two hypotheses to an empirical test by studying how the Great Recession, initiated by the collapse of Lehman Brothers in 2008, impacts people differently depending on their life stage. While economic downturns have been shown to have adverse effects on people's life chances, it has often been argued that big societal events such as an economic recession have differential effects on people's futures depending on their life stage (Elder, 1974). This in turn, can lead to generational clashes, not only in labour market chances and well-being but also in attitudes and values.

The empirical test into the differential impact of economic hardship caused by the Great Recession on different age cohorts requires distinguishing between the outcomes studied. First, we consider whether *human values* are affected by economic hardship. Here, we follow Schwartz (1992, p. 4), relying on earlier insights (Schwartz & Bilsky, 1987), who defines values as «concepts or beliefs [that] pertain to desirable end states or behaviors [and that] transcend specific situations, guide selection or evaluation of behaviour and events, and are ordered by relative importance». Emphasizing that values transcend specific situations implies that they are relatively stable over the lifespan (Rokeach & Ball-Rokeach, 1989), while they result from socialization at a young age (Hooghe & Wilkenfeld, 2008). In a more strict test, Inglehart (1985, p. 110) showed the stability of value priorities at the aggregate, yet at the individual level more variation is present. In a recent study on the question whether the Great Recession has influenced value priorities of young people, Reeskens and Vandecasteele (2017) have shown that exposure to economic hardship did not change the value priorities of young adults. In line with these outcomes, we can expect that across all cohorts of our study, the Great Recession will not affect human values.

By contrast, an attitude is defined as «a disposition to respond favourably or unfavourably to an object, person, institution or event» (Ajzen, 2005, p. 3). Attitudes are more situational (Converse, 1964) and therefore open to be influenced by everyday experiences. Research on attitude stability fuels this idea, as stability is particularly low among young adults (Alwin & Krosnick, 1991). Nevertheless, we do not expect that all attitudes are equally affected by the economic crisis. Particularly for the more sociotropic evaluations, or attitude objects which are closely linked to the Great Recession (e.g. evaluations of politics and the economy), we can expect that they are affected by exposure to economic hardship. Hobolt (2014, p. 56) combined Eurobarometer data showing that across Europe, trust in national political institutions declined from 40% in 2007 to 30% in 2013, which is supplemented with national findings of some European countries (e.g. O'Sullivan et al., 2014). Further, because of relatively low value stability among younger cohorts, we expect that particularly young people see their sociotropic attitudes shift, something that was also diagnosed in a study on the influence of the Great Recession on political and social attitudes across Europe (Reeskens & Vandecasteele, 2017).

However, in light of Inglehart's theory of value change (1997), we are interested in attitudes that are more distal and not necessarily a direct reflection of the economic conditions of the country. Previous research found that exposed to material prosperity, people in their formative years are more likely to express self-expression values, and this has been linked to the development that advanced industrialized societies have grown increasingly tolerant towards LGBTQ and more tolerant towards immigrants (Inglehart & Baker, 2000). The experience of the Great Recession would, if modernization theory holds, therefore hinder the shift towards societal tolerance that was witnessed during the last few decades. Recent research is lukewarm about this this idea. On the one hand, Inglehart (2018) has updated his own theory by arguing that not necessarily objective economic conditions but also economic insecurity, which is a rather subjective perception, influences self-expression values like tolerance and autonomy. Second, reflecting on the success of the populist surge across industrialized societies, Norris and Inglehart (2019) also discuss the Silent Revolution in reverse. Exposed to the increasing progressive values of the younger cohorts, the elderly have taken a more conservative turn. Even though our study focuses on the influence of economic conditions and therefore will put these updates not to a formal test, our longitudinal test is nevertheless able to detect over-time stability or change in the elderly cohorts. Yet, given the focus of the economic crisis and derived from modernization theory, we expect that particularly young age cohorts will express less progressive attitudes when exposed to economic downturns, while older age cohorts see their attitudes not affected. Further, we expect this impact to be weaker compared to attitudes that are proximal to the economic crisis.

Last but not least, in line with recent findings of health downturns in response to the economic crisis, we also consider subjective well-being (cf. Tausig & Fenwick, 1999). Previous research on the expectation between economic resources and well-being has shown a positive albeit non-linear relationship, because particularly the lower income groups see stronger increases in their well-being influenced by economic prosperity (see Clark et al., 2008; Diener & Oishi, 2000). Important for our study is that income losses have stronger scarring effects than income gains (Wolbring et al., 2013). Summarized, this allows us to hypothesize that the experience of economic hardship lowers well-being, with two underlying mechanisms (see Diener & Biswas-Diener, 2002). On the one hand, material resources allow for covering basic needs; as these needs are covered, individuals see their happiness increase and devote resources to other ways to increase happiness (Ferrer-i-Carbonell, 2005). On the other hand, well-being has been shown to depend upon relative positions and comparison either with other people or with the past (Clark et al., 2008; Easterlin, 1995; Ferrer-i-Carbonell, 2005). Because the change in economic hardship following a recession reminds people of their better times in the past, happiness is expected to thwart. Combined, we propose that exposure to the economic crisis lower well-being; we do not expect that different cohorts are affected differently.

3 Data and Methods

We use bi-annual data for 24 OECD countries from the 2008–2016 releases of the European Social Survey (ESS Rounds 4–8). The 2008 wave was specifically selected as baseline as the fall of Lehman Brothers in September 2008 is considered to have initiated the Great Recession. Since economic growth figures in most European countries were still positive in 2008 (see Eurostat, 2015), the consequences of the economic crisis were not visible until after 2008. We focus on the labour active population in 2008, as these are arguably more affected by the economic recession. Although the youngest cohort is not anymore in their formative years, we still expect that the youngest cohort is more vulnerable for scarring effects of the Great Recession. The selected sample includes people aged 25–64 in 2008 and were followed until 2016 where they were aged 33–72. The countries included are: Belgium, Bulgaria, Switzerland, Cyprus, Czech Republic, Germany, Denmark, Estonia, Spain, Finland, France, UK, Greece, Croatia, Hungary, Ireland, Lithuania, Netherlands, Norway, Poland, Portugal, Sweden, Slovenia, Slovakia.

3.1 Research Design and Sample Selection

This study uses a pseudo-panel design investigate over-time changes in human values, well-being indicators and social attitudes. In the absence of individual-level longitudinal data, a pseudo-panel design allows for an assessment of changes in socio-demographic groups on the basis of repeated cross-sectional data (Deaton, 1985; Meier Jaeger, 2013). This method is useful for the questions of interest in this study as no comprehensive cross-national panel data at the individual level covers the social attitude questions. Initially groups are defined on the basis of a number of non-time-varying characteristics—in this case country, gender and educational level. These groups are then matched over the cross-sectional releases of the ESS survey. All respondents aged 25–64 (in 2008) were divided in groups according to country (24 countries), birth cohort (born 1974–1983/1964–1973/1954–1963/1944–1953), gender (Male/Female) and educational level (Lower secondary and below/Upper secondary and Post-secondary non tertiary/Tertiary). For instance, one group could be «female, cohort 1974–1983, tertiary educated in Belgium», while another group would be «male, cohort 1954–1963, upper secondary education in France». These groups were constructed in five ESS waves (2008, 2010, 2012, 2014 and 2016). Not all countries participated in all ESS waves, and we also exclude groups in years wherein they comprised less than 30 respondents. We end up with 1723 group observations and Table 3 in Appendix shows the number of groups per country and wave.

3.2 Dependent Variables

The dependent variables are time-varying socio-demographic group averages (mean) of the Schwartz' human values inventory (self-transcendence, conservation, self-enhancement, hedonism, openness-to-change), a well-selected set of political and social attitudes that either reflect sociotropic orientations towards society (social trust, political trust, satisfaction with the economy), or are good proxies for postmaterialism (attitudes towards migrants and attitudes towards gay people); last but not least, we also consider subjective well-being.

The construction of the human values is based on the ESS Human Values Scale (see Davidov et al., 2008). The 21 items on which basis the human values are created, can be found in Appendix Table 4. The response scales—ranging from «not like me at all» (code '1') to «very much like me» (6)—are reversed if necessary to ensure the same direction of interpretation. In line with recommendations (Schwartz, 2003), we controlled for acquiescence in response behaviour by subtracting the average across all 21 items from the specific item, making that each item measures the relative value priority. The five second-order values are distinguished, namely self-transcendence (mean of «universalism» and «benevolence»), conservation (mean of «security», «conformity», and «tradition»), self-enhancement (mean of «power» and «achievement»), hedonism, and openness-to-change (mean of «self-direction» and «stimulation»). For more information on how to handle the human values based on the ESS, see Schwartz (2003).

Second, we examine social attitudes with respect to social trust, political institutions, the economy, migrants and gay people. Social trust is measured using three items measuring whether (a) most people can be trusted or whether you cannot be too careful at all, (b) most people try to be fair or try to take advantage of you, and (c) most people are helpful or are mostly looking out for themselves. The response scales range from 0 to 10, with a higher score indicating more trusting opinions. For political trust, we measure trust in representational institutions, i.e. (a) trust in the country's parliament, (b) politicians and (c) political parties. Responses range from «no trust at all» (0) to «complete trust» (10). Furthermore, satisfaction with the economy is investigated, which in the ESS is questioned by «On the whole how satisfied are you with the present state of the economy in [country]?», with responses from «extremely dissatisfied» (0) to «extremely satisfied» (10). Attitudes towards migrants are measured on the basis of three items: «Immigrants make country worse or better place to live», «Immigration is bad or good for the country's economy» and «Country's cultural life undermined or enriched by immigrants» with a response scale ranging from 0 to 10 with higher values denoting more positive attitudes towards migrants. Attitudes towards gay people are measured on the basis of the question whether people agree or disagree with the statement «gays and lesbians free to live life as they wish» on a 5-item response scale.

Finally, we examine «subjective well-being», which is the average of life satisfaction and happiness. Life satisfaction is measured by the item «All things considered, how satisfied are you with your life as a whole nowadays?» ranging from «extremely dissatisfied» (0) to «extremely satisfied» (10) while «happiness» is measuring by «Taking all things together, how happy would you say you are?» ranging from «extremely unhappy» (0) to «extremely happy» (10). Descriptive details of the dependent variables are given in Appendix Table 5.

3.3 Explanatory Variables

The fixed-effects models will show cohort-specific effects of over-time changes in the country's GDP/capita as well as the % of socio-demographic group members belonging to the lowest income quintile on the dependent variables. In this study, we examine the effect of changes in one variable of the socio-demographic group: changes in the group-specific percentage of group members belonging to the lowest income quintile. Additionally, the effect of one country level variable is assessed, changes in GDP/capita. We use the Eurostat indicator for real GDP/capita, which measures real expenditure per capita adjusted for price-level differences across the countries. The explanatory variables are measured bi-annually between 2008 and 2016. Importantly, the effect of these variables is assessed across four birth cohorts: born 1974–1983, born 1964–1973, born 1954–1963 and born 1944–1953. The largest concern for the validity of a pseudo-panel analysis is when the composition of the socio-demographic groups varies over time on characteristics that are relevant for the dependent variables but which are not used for composing the groups. To control for the possibility that the socio-demographic groups differ in age composition over the different waves, the analysis controls for the mean age in the socio-demographic group at any particular wave. Table 4 shows descriptive statistics for all variables used in the analysis.

3.4 Analytical Technique

We use fixed effects regression estimation to examine within-group change in both explanatory and dependent variables (Wooldridge, 2002). The Models for the effects of socio-demographic groups (1) and the effects of country characteristics (2) look as follows:

$$Y_{gct} = \alpha + Cohort * x_{gct}\beta 1 + q_{gc} + \varepsilon_{gct} \tag{1}$$

$$Y_{gct} = \alpha + Cohort * z_{ct}\beta 2 + q_{gc} + \varepsilon_{gct} \tag{2}$$

The dependent variable Y_{gct} is the group-average on our dependent variables in the socio-demographic group g (i = 1,…, N) in country c (c = 1,…, 24) at time t (t = 2008, 2010, 2012, 2014, 2016). x_{gct} is the explanatory group variable, percentage in lowest income quintile, which varies across the socio-demographic groups and time-points. z_{ct} refers to the country characteristic (GDP/capita) that varies across countries and over time. q_{gc} stands for time-constant individual characteristics and ε_{gct} indicates the residual error term. We run separate models with fixed-effects estimation and interaction terms to examine cohort-specific effects of change in (1) the explanatory group-variables x_{gct} and (2) change in country variables z_{ct} on group changes in the Y_{gct}, i.e. the human values, social attitudes and well-being.

By examining strictly over time variation, a main advantage of this design is that it controls for omitted time-constant characteristics of groups that affect both the explanatory variables as well as the human values, social attitudes or well-being indicators. This could for instance be norms in the socio-demographic group affecting both people's value orientation as well as the group's socio-economic position, or the cultural and institutional characteristics of the welfare regime the country belongs to.

4 Results

Table 1 presents the results of the fixed effects analysis of the pseudo-panel displaying the outcomes of the Schwartz human values. The analysis shows interaction effects between birth cohort and over-time changes in the percentage of the socio-demographic group belonging to the lowest income quintile and changes in GDP/capita on over-time changes in the pseudo-group means of the dependent variables. This analysis is presented over the cohort categories in order to assess whether the change in economic circumstances has a stronger effect on younger cohorts.

The results for human values show that significant effects remain limited to a few of the human values. An increase in the group's share belonging to the lowest income quintile decreases conservation and increases the openness to change. This is surprising, because it could be expected that when confronted with sudden economic shocks, people fall back to more traditional value priorities, including conservation values and hence opposing openness to change. This finding is further evidenced by the GDP/capita effect, as a decrease in GDP/capita reduces the conservation score, while it also increases the hedonism score. Overall, effects are small and do not change much across cohorts, except for the effect of GDP/capita change on conservation that is non-existent in the oldest cohort.

In Table 2, the results for the social attitude and well-being variables are presented. It shows that an increase in the percentage of group-members belonging to the lowest income quintile reduces political trust, satisfaction with the economy and subjective well-being for all cohorts, but this effect is stronger for the youngest cohort. Similarly, the effect on social trust varies by cohort as it's only negative for the youngest cohort. Only the attitudes towards migrants and gay people remain unaffected by changes in the percentage of group-members belonging to the lowest income quintile. Similar effects can be found for a decrease in GDP/capita which results in a reduction of social trust, political trust, satisfaction with the economy and subjective well-being, while it renders more negative attitudes towards migrants and gay people. Overall, these effects don't differ by cohort.

Table 1 Fixed effects pseudo-panel-regression of human values regressed on birth cohort interacted with time-varying percentage in lowest income quintile in socio-demographic group and country's GDP/capita (2008–2016)

	Self-transcendence	Conservation	Self-enhancement	Hedonism	Openness to change
% in lowest income quintile in socio-demographic group	0.0002 (0.0007)	−0.0019** (0.0006)	0.0001 (0.0009)	0.0006 (0.0011)	0.0020** (0.0007)
x cohort 1964–1973	−0.0004 (0.0010)	0.0009 (0.0010)	0.0002 (0.0014)	−0.0003 (0.0017)	−0.0007 (0.0011)
x cohort 1954–1963	−0.0005 (0.0009)	0.0016 (0.0009)	0.0002 (0.0013)	0.0002 (0.0016)	−0.0020 (0.0011)
x cohort 1944–1953	−0.0022* (0.0009)	0.0014 (0.0008)	0.0015 (0.0012)	0.0018 (0.0015)	−0.0014 0.0010
GDP/capita	−0.000005 + (0.000002)	0.000005* (0.000002)	−0.000006 + (0.000003)	0.000010* (0.000004)	−0.000001 (0.000003)
x cohort 1964–1973	0.000003 (0.000003)	−0.000004 (0.000003)	0.000002 (0.000005)	−0.000007 (0.000005)	0.000004 (0.000004)
x cohort 1954–1963	0.000003 (0.000003)	−0.000004 (0.000003)	0.000002 (0.000005)	−0.000008 (0.000006)	0.000005 (0.000004)
x cohort 1944–1953	−0.000002 (0.000003)	−0.000007* (0.000003)	0.000006 (0.000005)	−0.000002 (0.000006)	0.000007 + (0.000004)

$+ p < 0.10$; $^{*}p < 0.05$; $^{**}p < 0.01$; $^{***}p < 0.001$. Controlled for age composition in group. Standard errors in parenthesis

5 Conclusion

From different angles, research findings indicate that the Great Recession has shown adverse socioeconomic outcomes and affected those experiencing hardship in various ways. However, a systematic test on an extensive set of value properties has not taken place. Because countries have been hit by the recession in varying degrees, describing the aftermath of the recession requires a cross-national panel design. In the absence of such design, we have constructed a cross-national pseudo-panel where we model socio-demographic groups composed on the basis of the time-invariant characteristics country, cohort, gender and educational level. Focusing on the labor active population—25–64 years old—from the onset of the Great Recession until 2016, when this group was 33–72, we have tested whether the changing economic context—GDP per capita—as well as he changing economic composition of the socio-demographic group—percentage of respondents in the lowest income decile—relates to changes in group averages in human values, relevant political and social attitudes, as well as subjective well-being.

The results of our study mostly confirm our initial expectations. First and foremost, we can confirm that economic conditions have an influence on social and political attitudes, while on the opposite, the influence on the Schwartz human values is inconsistent and rather small in terms of effect size. Second, the effects are particularly

Table 2 Fixed effects pseudo-panel-regression of social attitudes and well-being regressed on birth cohort interacted with time-varying percentage in lowest income quintile in socio-demographic group and country's GDP/capita (2008–2016)

	Social trust	Political trust	Satisf. with the economy	Attitudes tow. migrants	Attitudes towards gay people	Subjective well-being
% in lowest income quintile in socio-demographic group	−0.0039 + (0.0022)	−0.0189*** (0.0037)	−0.0262*** (0.0055)	−0.0044 (0.0029)	−0.0007 (0.0013)	−0.0146*** (0.0023)
x cohort 1964–1973	−0.0013 (0.0033)	0.0032 (0.0056)	−0.0033 (0.0083)	−0.0013 (0.0044)	0.0028 (0.0020)	−0.0053 (0.0035)
x cohort 1954–1963	−0.0010 (0.0031)	0.0049 (0.0052)	0.0090 (0.0078)	−0.0030 (0.0041)	0.0000 (0.0019)	0.0031 (0.0033)
x cohort 1944–1953	−0.0011 (0.0029)	0.0178*** (0.0049)	0.0256*** (0.0073)	−0.0057 0.0038	0.0022 (0.0018)	0.0094** (0.0030)
GDP/capita	0.000017* (0.000008)	0.000090*** (0.000013)	0.00014*** (0.000014)	0.000028** (0.000010)	0.000010* (0.000005)	0.000028*** (0.000006)
x cohort 1964–1973	−0.000003 (0.000011)	−0.000014 (0.000018)	0.000002 (0.000018)	0.000010 (0.000014)	−0.000008 (0.000007)	0.000003 (0.000008)
x cohort 1954–1963	−0.000012 (0.000011)	−0.000011 (0.000018)	−0.000003 (0.000018)	0.000009 (0.000014)	0.0000001 (0.000007)	0.000015 + (0.000008)
x cohort 1944–1953	−0.000005 (0.000011)	−0.000014 (0.000019)	0.000015 (0.000019)	0.000013 (0.000015)	−0.000003 (0.000007)	−0.000005 (0.000009)

$^{*}p < 0.05$; $^{**}p < 0.01$; $^{***}p < 0.001$. Controlled for age composition in group. Standard errors in parenthesis pronounced among the youngest age cohorts. Our results show that over the course of eight years, when exposed with economic hardship, the youngest cohort is more negative about politics, the state of the economy, their political representatives, and their subjective well-being. Interestingly, attitudes towards gays and towards immigrants, which are proxies for evaluating modernization theory, are unaffected by the composition of the poorest quintile; yet, in a poorer economy (expressed in lower levels of GDP per capita), younger groups become more negative towards immigrants and towards gays and lesbians.

The findings pose us with two interpretations, namely one optimistic and one pessimistic interpretation. The optimistic one indicates that if young people's attitudes most proximal towards the economy are affected, these opinions can bounce back as soon as the economy veers up. In the end, young people are quite resilient towards adverse experiences (Schoon & Mortimer, 2017), meaning that the Great Recession might be a little wrinkle in the course of the Fourth Industrial Revolution.

The more negative interpretation is that in the absence of more data points, our findings provide tentative confirmation for modernization theory in the presence of the Great Recession, in the sense that young people, confronted with economic hardship, will take a more conservative turn. Such interpretation would align to some initial findings of the European Values Study (Muis et al., 2019), where it is shown that the youngest age cohorts are becoming sexually less permissive. However, more research needs to be conducted about the long-run implications, and particular in terms of social change, our initial findings might indicate that economic downturns might influence the social course of societies.

One liability in that respect is that we have focused on objective economic conditions. As Inglehart (2018) has recently underscored, economic insecurities will take a more prominent position with the turn towards the «Artificial Intelligence Society». Subjective perceptions of the economy, and their influence on various political and social outcomes, which would form a good test for the Thomas theorem (see Merton, 1995), has not been part of our study. Yet, it is without any doubt that it will matter a lot. Also, to compensate for the experiences of deprivation, across Europe there is variation in welfare traditions. Although welfare states not only redistribute material resources but also immaterial properties (see Paskov, 2016; van Ingen & van der Meer, 2011), it is expected that they cushion the impact of the Great Recession on values, attitudes and well-being, too. We have refrained from testing this given the complex empirical set-up of such design. Last but not least, a pseudo-panel data study is not undisputed; however, it is the best available option given the fact that real longitudinal data on social attitudes do, at this point, not exist yet for a comparative sample of countries.

Finally, looking at the other end of the age distribution, our findings also question the dominant turn that the Silent Revolution has taken in recent years, with an emphasis to the «Silent Revolution in Reverse» (Norris & Inglehart, 2019). While the argument goes that older age cohorts, confronted with the social change towards increasing self-expression values, have become also quite persistent in articulating more traditional values. Although our study has not tested this assumption, our study finds that the conditions that have characterized the first decade of the twenty-first century has been particularly relevant for the younger age cohorts.

Acknowledgements The authors thank Sophia Degen for excellent student assistance.

Appendix

See Tables 3, 4, and 5.

Table 3 Number of groups per country and ESS wave

Country	2008	2010	2012	2014	2016	Total
Belgium (BE)	0	20	21	20	21	102
Bulgaria (BG)	17	21	20	0	0	58
Switzerland (CH)	17	11	13	14	13	68
Cyprus (CY)	14	10	12	0	0	36
Czech Republic (CZ)	9	9	10	11	14	53
Germany (DE)	17	17	17	16	16	83
Denmark (DK)	16	19	18	15	0	68

(continued)

Table 3 (continued)

Country	2008	2010	2012	2014	2016	Total
Estonia (EE)	17	14	16	15	16	78
Spain (ES)	20	19	18	20	19	96
Finland (FI)	19	18	19	18	19	93
France (FR)	21	15	16	17	15	84
United Kingdom (GB)	17	23	24	23	23	110
Greece (GR)	19	22	0	0	0	41
Croatia (HR)	13	11	0	0	0	24
Hungary (HU)	13	11	13	11	10	58
Ireland (IE)	18	21	21	20	22	102
Lithuania (LT)	0	13	15	15	15	58
Netherlands (NL)	22	23	22	23	20	110
Norway (NO)	16	17	16	17	16	82
Poland (PL)	12	18	19	19	18	86
Portugal (PT)	15	13	14	11	10	63
Sweden (SE)	18	15	16	15	15	79
Slovenia (SI)	12	12	10	10	11	55
Slovakia (SK)	12	13	11	0	0	36
Total	374	385	361	310	293	1723

Table 4 ESS human values scale to measure Schwartz human values

Second order value	Human value	Item in ESS (variable name)
Self-transcendence	Benevolence	Important to help people and care for others well-being (iphlppl)
		Important to be loyal to friends and devote to people close (iplylfr)
	Universalism	Important that people are treated equally and have equal opportunities (ipeqopt)
		Important to understand different people (ipudrst)
		Important to care for nature and environment (impenv)
Conservation	Security	Important to live in secure and safe surroundings (impsafe)
		Important that government is strong and ensures safety (ipstrgv)
	Conformity	Important to do what is told and follow rules (ipfrule)
		Important to behave properly (ipbhprp)
	Tradition	Important to be humble and modest, not draw attention (ipmodst)
		Important to follow traditions and customs (imptrad)

(continued)

Table 4 (continued)

Second order value	Human value	Item in ESS (variable name)
Self-enhancement	Achievement	Important to show abilities and be admired (ipshabt)
		Important to be successful and that people recognize achievements (ipsuces)
	Power	Important to be rich, have money and expensive things (imprich)
		Important to get respect from others (iprspot)
Hedonism	Hedonism	Important to have a good time (ipgdtim)
		Important to seek fun and things that give pleasure (impfun)
Openness-to-change	Self-direction	Important to think new ideas and being creative (ipcrtiv)
		Important to make own decisions and be free (impfree)
	Stimulation	Important to try new and different things in life (impdiff)
		Important to seek adventures and have an exciting life (ipadvnt)

Table 5 Descriptives of the socio-demographic group variables of interest (2008–2016)

Variable	N	Scale range	Mean/prop	Std. dev
Cohort born 1974–1983	440		25.54	
Cohort born 1964–1973	433		25.13	
Cohort born 1954–1963	431		25.01	
Cohort born 1944–1953	419		24.32	
Male	812		47.13	
Female	911		52.87	
Low educated	370		21.47	
Mid educated	794		46.08	
High educated	559		32.44	
Percentage in lowest income quintile	1652	0–88	15.91	14.3
Self-transcendence	1723	−0.14–1.24	0.67	0.22
Conservation	1723	−0.65–1.1	0.08	0.27
Self-enhancement	1723	−1.7–0.35	−0.68	0.32
Hedonism	1723	−1.68–0.6	−0.25	0.39
Openness-to-change	1723	−1.29–0.49	−0.13	0.23
Social trust	1723	2.67–7.69	5.32	0.99
Political trust	1723	1.1–6.69	3.82	1.24
Satisfaction with economy	1723	0.87–8.66	4.39	1.59
Attitude towards migrants	1723	2.2–7.97	5.31	0.99
Attitude towards gay people	1723	1.05–4.11	2.05	0.59
Subjective well-being	1723	3.02–8.94	7.14	0.89

References

Ajzen, I. (2005). *Attitudes, personality and behavior* (2nd ed.). Open University Press.

Alwin, D. F., & Krosnick, J. A. (1991). Aging, cohorts, and the stability of sociopolitical orientations over the life span. *American Journal of Sociology, 97*(1), 169–195.

Clark, A. E., Frijters, P., & Shields, M. A. (2008). Relative income, happiness, and utility. An explanation for the Easterlin paradox and other puzzles. *Journal of Economic Literature, 46*(1), 95–144.

Converse, P. (1964). The nature of belief systems of mass sublics. In D. E. Apter (Ed.), *Ideology and discontent* (pp. 206–261). Free Press.

Davidov, E., Schmidt, P., & Schwartz, S. H. (2008). Bringing values back: In the adequacy of the European social survey to measure values in 20 countries. *Public Opinion Quarterly, 72*(3), 420–445.

Deaton, A. (1985). Panel data from time series of cross-sections. *Journal of Econometrics, 30*(1–2), 109–126.

Diener, E., & Biswas-Diener, R. (2002). Will money increase subjective well-being? A literature review and guide to needed research. *Social Indicators Research, 57*(2), 119–169.

Diener, E., & Oishi, S. (2000). Money and happiness: income and subjective well-being across nations. In E. Diener & E. Suh (Eds.), *Culture and subjective well-being* (pp. 185–218). MIT Press.

Dooley, D., Fielding, J., & Levi, L. (1996). Health and unemployment. *Annual Review of Public Health, 17*, 449–465.

Easterlin, R. A. (1995). Will raising the incomes of all increase the happiness of all? *Journal of Economic Behavior & Organization, 27*(1), 35–48.

Elder, G. H. (1974). *Children of the great depression: Social change in life experiences.* University of Chicago Press.

Ferrer-i-Carbonell, A. (2005). Income and well-being: An empirical analysis of the comparison income effect. *Journal of Public Economics, 89*(5–6), 997–1019.

Hobolt, S. B. (2014). Public attitudes towards the Euro crisis. In O. Cramme & S. B. Hobolt (Eds.), *Democratic politics in a European Union under stress* (pp. 48–66). Oxford University Press.

Hooghe, M., & Wilkenfeld, B. (2008). The stability of political attitudes and behaviors across adolescence and early adulthood: A comparison of survey data on adolescents and young adults in eight countries. *Journal of Youth and Adolescence, 37*(2), 155–167.

Inglehart, R. (1977). *The silent revolution: Changing values and political styles in advanced industrial society.* Princeton University Press.

Inglehart, R. (1985). Aggregate stability and individual-level flux in mass belief systems. The level of analysis paradox. *American Political Science Review, 79*(1), 97–116.

Inglehart, R. (1997). *Modernization and post-modernization. Cultural, economic, and political changes in 43 societies.* Princeton University Press.

Inglehart, R. (2018). *Cultural evolution: People's motivations are changing, and reshaping the world.* Cambridge University Press.

Inglehart, R., & Baker, W. E. (2000). Modernization, cultural change, and the persistence of traditional values. *American Sociological Review, 65*(1), 19–51.

Margalit, Y. (2013). Explaining social policy preferences: Evidence from the great recession. *American Political Science Review, 107*(1), 80–103.

Margalit, Y. (2019). Political responses to economic shocks. *Annual Review of Political Science, 22*, 277–295.

Meier Jaeger, M. (2013). The effect of macroeconomic and social conditions on the demand for redistribution: A pseudo panel approach. *Journal of European Social Policy, 23*(2), 149–163.

Merton, R. K. (1995). The Thomas theorem and the Matthew effect. *Social Forces, 74*(2), 379–422.

Muis, Q., Sieben, I., Reeskens, T., & Halman, L. (2019). Seksueel-ethische permissiviteit: Trends in Nederland 1981–2017. *Mens & Maatschappij, 94*(4), 429–458.

Norris, P., & Inglehart, R. (2019). *Cultural backlash: Trump, brexit, and authoritarian populism*. Cambridge University Press.

O'Sullivan, S., Healy, A. E., & Breen, M. J. (2014). Political legitimacy in ireland during economic crisis: Insights from the European social survey. *Irish Political Studies, 29*(4), 547–572.

Paskov, M. (2016). Is solidarity less important and less functional in egalitarian contexts? *Acta Sociologica, 59*(1), 3–18.

Redbird, B., & Grusky, D. B. (2016). Distributional effects of the great recession: Where has all the sociology gone? *Annual Review of Sociology, 42*, 185–215.

Reeskens, T., & Vandecasteele, L. (2017). Hard times and European youth. The effect of Economic insecurity on human values, social attitudes and well-being. *International Journal of Psychology, 52*(1), 19–27.

Rokeach, M., & Ball-Rokeach, S. J. (1989). Stability and change in American value priorities, 1968–1981. *American Psychologist, 44*(5), 775–784.

Schoon, I., & Mortimer, J. (2017). Youth and the great recession: Are values, achievement orientation and outlook to the future affected? *International Journal of Psychology, 52*(1), 1–8.

Schwartz, S. H. (1992). Universals in the content and structure of values: Theoretical advances and empirical tests in 20 countries. *Advances in Experimental Social Psychology, 25*(1), 1–65.

Schwartz, S. H. (2003). A proposal for measuring value orientations across Nations. Chapter 7 in the ESS questionnaire development report. London: City University. http://www.europeansocialsurvey.org

Schwartz, S. H., & Bilsky, W. (1987). Toward a psychological structure of human values. *Journal of Personality and Social Psychology, 53*(3), 550–562.

Stuckler, D., Reeves, A., Karanikolos, M., & McKee, M. (2015). The health effects of the global financial crisis: Can we reconcile the differing views? A network analysis of literature across disciplines. *Health Economics, Policy and Law, 10*(1), 83–99.

Tausig, M., & Fenwick, R. (1999). Recession and well-being. *Journal of Health and Social Behavior, 40*(1), 1–16.

Van Ingen, E., & van der Meer, T. (2011). Welfare state expenditure and inequalities in voluntary association participation. *Journal of European Social Policy, 21*(4), 302–322.

Wolbring, T., Keuschnigg, M., & Negele, E. (2013). Needs, comparisons, and adaptation: The importance of relative income for life satisfaction. *European Sociological Review, 29*(1), 96–104.

Wooldridge, J. M. (2002). Econometric Aaalysis of cross section and panel data. Cambridge: MIT Press.

Tim Reeskens is an Associate Professor at the Department of Sociology at Tilburg University. His research interests lie in the social consequences of immigration and diversity, with a particular focus on social capital and social trust, national identity and support for welfare redistribution. Tim is the program director for the Netherlands of the European Values Study.

Leen Vandecasteele is an Associate Professor at the Life Course and Inequality Centre of the University of Lausanne. Her research is in the areas of inequality, poverty and social policy in the life course. She is associated with the national centre of competence on vulnerability in the life course (LIVES).

Rainbows in Latin America: Public Opinion and Societal Attitudes Towards Homosexuality

David Sulmont and Kiara Castaman

1 Introduction

Over the last decades, the issues around sexual rights and the struggle against the discrimination of lesbian, gays, bisexual, transgender, and intersex people (LGBTI) have increasingly become an important feature of social debate and political mobilization in many countries around the globe. Social movements in several countries have been raising awareness of the discrimination and social injustices suffered by LGBTI and have been advocating for the expansion of their civil rights. Most governments have decriminalized homosexuality, and the most progressive ones have recognized same-sex marriages or allowed the change of gender on identification documents. Likewise, public opinion attitudes have shifted towards higher levels of recognition and support of the LGBTI community and their rights (International Lesbian, Gay, Bisexual, Trans and Intersex Association et al., 2017; Pew Research Center, 2013a).

Latin America has not been an exception to those social, cultural and political changes. Since 2007, countries in the region have introduced legislation to protect sexual and civil rights of LGBTI individuals, including legislation that recognized same-sex partnerships rights (Mexico, Ecuador, Chile, Argentina, Colombia, Brazil, and Uruguay). In countries without such legislation, LGTBI social movements have encountered increasing support in their attempt to promote social and political changes. The advances mentioned above are happening in a region characterized by deep traditional values and Catholic roots but, which since the end of the XX century, has also experienced substantial structural changes: rapid economic development; the consolidation of democratic institutions; and the expansion of secular and democratic values.

D. Sulmont (✉) · K. Castaman
Department of Social Sciences, Pontificia Universidad Católica del Perú, Lima, Peru
e-mail: sulmont@pucp.pe

A. Almakaeva et al. (eds.), *Social Capital and Subjective Well-Being*, Societies and Political Orders in Transition,
https://doi.org/10.1007/978-3-030-75813-4_6

This contribution aims at discussing and analyzing how societal attitudes in Latin America have changed towards the recognition of sexual diversities and the support of LGBTI rights. Moreover, is going to address to what extent those changes reflect more profound cultural and generational shifts related to socioeconomic and cultural modernization processes. How are public opinion changes toward homosexuality related to economic modernization, political democratization, and progressive legislation in the region? Those are some the research questions we will try to answer in this work.

To explore this subject, we will analyze public opinion data from two comparative projects: the World Values Survey (Inglehart et al., 2020) and the Latin American Public Opinion Project (LAPOP) of the University of Vanderbilt (2021),[1] which have included in their consecutive surveys (from 1996 to 2017) questions about acceptance towards homosexuality and the advancement of LGBTI rights.

In the upcoming section, we present some of the legislative advances that several Latin American countries have been implementing regarding LGBTI rights and the political challenges that gender equality is still facing in the region. Later, we introduce some of the explanations to the changes in public opinion towards homosexuality and LGBTI, according to the literature on those issues.

In the empirical section of this contribution, we start by describing the data on Latin American public opinion that we used for our analysis, its scope and the variables available to measure attitudes towards homosexuality and LGBTI in the region. We show how those attitudes vary across countries and over time, and how these societal attitudes are associated with economic development and political democratization. Then, we will analyze the specific weight of individual factors (age, gender, education, religion, and traditional values) on the attitudes towards homosexuality.

This contribution shows that, as in other regions of the world (see for example: Andersen & Fetner, 2008a; Halman & van Ingen, 2015; Manalastas et al., 2017; Pew Research Center, 2013a; van den Akker et al., 2013), Latin American public opinion attitudes have changed towards a wider acceptance of homosexuality and the LGBTI community. Indeed, those changes are related to economic and political modernization and the cultural transformations accompanying those processes. However, we also point out that negative attitudes towards homosexuality and LGBTI rights are still widespread in the region, representing a political challenge for the advancement of a progressive social agenda on these matters. We also discuss the necessity of taking a more nuanced approach in the analysis of the relationship between religiosity, religious values, and attitudes towards homosexuality, in a region characterized by a predominantly Christian and Catholic population.

[1] We thank the Latin American Public Opinion Project (LAPOP) and its major supporters (the United States Agency for International Development, the Inter-American Development Bank, and Vanderbilt University) for making the data available.

2 LGBTI Rights in Latin America: Advances and Challenges

Over the last years, several Latin American countries have been strengthening the protection and recognition of LGBTI rights. These advances started with the decriminalization of homosexuality, currently widely expanded in the region. The following legislative changes had been oriented to anti-discrimination laws, employment protection or the ban of conversion therapies for the LGBTI. More recently, the legislation shift has driven the expansion of LGBTI civil rights to a more progressive path. In some countries of the region, individuals can change their name and/or gender identity on official documents (Argentina, Bolivia, Colombia, Ecuador and Uruguay). In others, same-sex civil unions or marriages are now permitted, and in a few other countries, same-sex couples are allowed to joint adoption (International Lesbian, Gay, Bisexual, Trans and Intersex Association et al., 2017).

Table 1 shows the year of legal recognition of some same-sex couples' rights in Latin America: legal recognition of same-sex partnership, same-sex marriage and adoption by same-sex couples.[2]

However, Latin American also presents some contradictory features in the advancement of LGBTI people's rights. The International LGBTI Association recognizes that despite the normative improvements, LGTBI are victims of high levels of violence in the region (International Lesbian, Gay, Bisexual, Trans and Intersex Association et al., 2017, pp. 158–162). This violence affects the LGBTI people even in countries with substantial normative advances on the protection and recognition of their civil rights. For example, in Argentina, 103 hate crimes based on sexual orientation were committed in 2017. In Brazil, the death reports of lesbians, gays,

Table 1 Progressive legislation in Latin America: year of legal recognition of same-sex couples' rights

Country	Same-sex partnership	Same-sex marriage	Adoption
Argentina		2010	2010
Brazil	2011	2013	2010
Chile	2015		
Colombia	2011	2016	2015
Ecuador	2014		
Mexico[a]	2007	2009	
Uruguay	2008	2013	2013

[a] At a subnational level

Table: Authors; *Source* International LGBTI Association et al. (2017)

[2] Mexico has not approved national legislation in those matters, but some subnational entities, notably Mexico City, have recognized same-sex partnership since 2007 and same-sex marriage since 2009 (International Lesbian, Gay, Bisexual, Trans and Intersex Association et al., 2017, pp. 68–70).

bisexuals, and transsexuals has increased by 30% from 2016 to 2017 (Mott et al., 2017). Unfortunately, this situation is common around the region and ruthless acts such rapes, tortures, stabbings, and murders are some of the hate crimes LGBTI community suffers, as each countries' police reports confirm.

Nevertheless, physical attacks are not the only expression neither the most common one of the LGBTI rejection in Latin American societies. Numerous faith-based civil organizations[3] set out a politically conservative and ultra-conservative agenda, which includes intolerant discourses against the LGBTI community. In many countries, those groups are able to organize political campaigns and massive demonstrations in order to prevent or protest against the advancement of civil rights for LGBTI people. Generally, this kind of anti-LGBTI activism is part of larger campaigns whose purpose is to block the development of sexual and reproductive rights (abortion, sexual education in schools, sexual health programs, etc.) and the promotion of gender equality rights.

In most cases, those campaigns have the explicit participation and support of church authorities (Catholic and/or Evangelical), some of them linked with transnational conservative groups which promote an anti-LGBTI agenda. According to Corrales (2015b, p. 54), faith-based groups and religious actors are the most important veto players in the LGBTI politics around Latin America.

The spread of the negative attitudes towards the LGBTI community (so-called homonegativity) in the political sphere is quite common in the region, therefore, it is essential to understand how this homonegativity is distributed and which predictors are related to it in Latin America.

3 Predictors of Attitudes Towards LGBTI

A long history of prejudice has marked attitudes towards LGBTI people all over the globe. Hence, many scholars and activists have been analyzing which predictors are more linked to the support or rejection of this historically discriminated group.

The most commons are found to result from societal factors related to the modernization processes. The economic growth, the consolidation of democracy, and the secularization process have been found aligned with a declining level of homosexuality prejudice all around the world (Andersen & Fetner, 2008a, b; Corrales, 2015a, b; Inglehart & Welzel, 2005).

Consistently with Inglehart's modernization theory (Inglehart 1997; Inglehart & Welzel, 2005), we assume that economic prosperity increases the capabilities that enable people to raise their free choices. The expansion of the capabilities shifts

[3] "CitizenGo" in several countries; "Movimiento Vida y Familia" (Ecuador, Colombia, Mexico, Paraguay); "Con mis Hijos no te Metas" and "Coordinadora Pro-Familia" (Peru); "Red por la Vida y la Familia" (Bolivia); "Padres Objetores de Chile" and "El Observatorio Legislativo Cristiano" (Chile); "Comisión Nacional de Pastoral de Familia y de Vida" (Costa Rica); "ProFamilia" (Dominican Republic); "Familia, Desarrollo y Población" (Guatemala); "La Alianza Panameña por la Vida y la Familia" (Panama); "Movimiento Pro Vida" (Honduras, El Salvador); among others.

people's preferences from materialist concerns to postmaterialist ones, which emphasize on self-expression and lead people to demand and defend their freedom of choice. The emphasis on self-expression, supported by the existence of democratic institutions, set the bases that allow people from any economic position or way of living to exert their free choices. This results in higher levels of social tolerance among citizens.

Tolerance can be understood as an engagement with practices or beliefs that are different from or conflicting with one's own beliefs or attitudes (Schirmer et al., 2012). It can be considered as a way of valuing or celebrating the difference by treating others equitably despite the differences. This can be taken as an opposition to discrimination or prejudice (Wise & Driskell, 2017). Tolerance is essential for the functioning of the civic society in democracies (Coleman, 1988; Putnam, 1996; Stevenson, 1988).

Increasing tolerance reduces prejudice and discrimination towards groups that had been recognized as minorities (such as LGTBI people), and whose rights have been historically vulnerable (Djupe & Calfano, 2012; Jones, 2006; Lee, 2014; Parekh et al., 2018; Schirmer et al., 2012; Stevenson, 1988). Hence, it is possible to argue that tolerance can foster social cohesion, and in that sense, being one of the core elements of democratic political culture (OECD, 2014). It is important to understand that tolerance is only relevant in a pluralistic context where disagreement and dislike are a possibility. Also, tolerance foster the openness to the diversity of opinions, behaviors, identities, beliefs, among other characteristics of the diverse people who coexist within the same social group (Sullivan & Transue, 1999).

By recognizing differences, people are more likely to build familiarity and trust with others (Lee, 2014), and thus, the composition of a person's social network can be broadened to include a variety of "beings" (Baliamoune-Lutz, 2011; Bureekul & Thananithichot, 2012; Cigler & Joslyn, 2002; Hooghe et al., 2010). Tolerance facilitates the expansion and diversification of social networks and organizations, key components of "social capital" in contemporary societies (Putnam, 1996, p. 66). In that sense, acceptance of LGBTI people and the expansion of their civic, political and social rights, can be also related with increased levels of social capital in contemporary pluralistic and secularized societies.

Nevertheless, as the LGBTI population remains a largely disadvantaged group, authors had also explored the effects of individual-level variables as predictors of the attitudes that diminish homosexuality prejudice. Since cultural change takes effect over time, younger and single individuals tend to be less prejudiced than older cohorts. Hence, there is empirical evidence that correlates attitudes of support for the LGBTI people with age and marital status (Andersen & Fetner, 2008b; Flores, 2014; Pew Research Center, 2013b; Slootmaeckers & Lievens, 2014; Smith et al., 2014; van den Akker et al., 2013).

Additionally, the rising of educational attainment increases the exposure to a diversity of ideas and realities, encouraging people to be more open-minded (Andersen & Fetner, 2008b; Collier et al., 2015; Decco, 2014; Ellison & Musick, 1993; Hicks & Lee, 2006). On the other hand, researchers have shown that opposition to LGBTI rights had been concentrated in men, what bear out gender as a variable to take into account (Herek, 2002; Hooghe et al., 2010; Whitley & Aegisdóttir, 2000).

Even though religiosity is generally associated with conservative values and negative attitudes towards LGBTI (Pew Research Center, 2013a; b), some authors argue that in Latin America religion and religiosity are not necessarily incompatible with more secular and progressive values or attitudes (Corrales, 2015a; Romero, 2013, 2016). By the end of the 1960s, the discussions around the II Vatican Council led the Latin American Catholic Church and its grass root movements to get more involved in causes that promoted progressive civil, social and political rights. The "Liberation Theology" in Latin America advocated for further involvement of the Catholic Church, clergy, and laity, with that kind of causes. Notwithstanding Pope John Paul II's (1978–2005) promotion of a conservative turn in the Latin American Catholic Church, a commitment with progressive causes and values (political freedom, social and human rights) continued to be important in many sectors of the Catholic Church and its laity. From the 1980s onwards, the proliferation of protestants Christian Evangelical churches contributed to enhancing the religious diversity and pluralism in the region. In that sense, conservative versions of Catholicism and Christian religion ended up coexisting with more progressive ones, more open or supportive of secularized values and principles.

Some authors have discussed the effects that LGBTI civil rights legal recognition might have on public opinion (Flores & Barclay, 2016). If changes in the status quo can cause polarized responses, the authors point up the importance of analyzing possible mass opinion backlash, which is understood as an adverse reaction to public policy initiatives most of the time aligned to the benefit of disadvantaged groups. "Policy backlash" towards the LGBTI rights have mostly been studied in the U.S and Canada (Andersen & Fetner, 2008b; Bishin et al., 2016; Flores & Barclay, 2016; Kazyak & Stange, 2018; Redman, 2018), in their analysis, the authors have found little evidence supporting backlash theories, concluding that instead of that, progressive legislation tends to enhance consensus and legitimacy of LGBTI rights.

Our analysis will consider the factors identified by the literature mentioned above, both at an aggregate level (economic development, political liberties and progressive legislation), and at individual level (gender, age, education, marital status, religion, interpersonal trust and postmaterialist values).

4 Attitudes Towards Homosexuality in Latin America

4.1 Data and Dependent Variables

As we mentioned before, we use two different data sources for the analysis of public opinion and societal attitudes towards homosexuality in the region: The World Values Survey (WVS) and the Latin American Public Opinion Project (LAPOP). As we can see in Table 2, those data sets have different coverage across time and countries.

Table 2 Countries and years covered by WVS & LAPOP surveys

Country	WVS				LAPOP						
	1994/98	1999/04	2005/09	2010/14	2004	2006	2008	2010	2012	2014	2016/17
Argentina	1995	1999	2006	2013			X	X	X	X	2017
Bolivia					X	X	X	X	X	X	2017
Brazil			2006	2014		2007	X	X	X	X	2017
Chile	1996	2000	2006	2011		X	X	X	X	X	2017
Colombia	1997/98		2005	2012	X	X	X	X	X	X	2016
Costa Rica					X	X	X	X	X	X	2016
Dominican Rep	1996				X	X	X	X	X	X	2016
Ecuador				2013	X	X	X	X	X	X	2016
El Salvador		1999	2004		X	X	X	X	X	X	2016
Guatemala					X	X	X	X	X	X	2017
Honduras					X	X	X	X	X	X	2016
Mexico	1995/96	2000	2005	2012	X	X	X	X	X	X	2017
Nicaragua					X	X	X	X	X	X	2016
Panama					X	X	X	X	X	X	2017
Paraguay						X	X	X	X	X	2016
Peru	1996	2001	2006	2012		X	X	X	X	X	2017
Uruguay	1996		2006	2011		2007	X	X	X	X	2017
Venezuela	1996	2000				2007	X	X	X	X	2016

WVS covers a more extensive period with survey waves every five years. The first wave (1981–1983) included only two Latin American countries, Argentina and Mexico, but Wave 6 (2010–2014) expanded its sample up to 8 countries. For our analysis, we will use the data from Wave 3 (1994–1998) thru Wave 6, which allow us to analyze changes in the long run over a period of 15–18 years depending on the country. WVS sample size for each country/wave varies mostly around 1200–1500 respondents.

LAPOP, coordinated by Vanderbilt University, covers most of the region's countries in the seven biennial surveys it has run between 2004 and 2017. Although the time frame is narrower than the WVS, LAPOP offers a broader geographical coverage, allowing more inter-case comparisons. The average sample size of the LAPOP surveys is around 1500–1700 cases.

As dependent variables, we will use the questions about attitudes towards homosexuality on both projects. The WVS questionnaire considers two questions:

- Please tell me for each of the following actions whether you think it can always be justified, never be justified, or something in between, using this card (1 = "Never justifiable"; 10 = "Always justifiable"): Homosexuality
- On this list are various groups of people. Could you please mention any that you would not like to have as neighbors? Homosexuals

The LAPOP questionnaire includes the following questions:

- Thinking of homosexuals, how strongly do you approve or disapprove of such people being permitted to run for public office? (1 = "Strongly disapprove"; 10 = "Strongly approve").
- How strongly do you approve or disapprove of same-sex couples having the right to marry? (1 = "Strongly disapprove"; 10 = "Strongly approve") (Note: This question was first included in the 2010 wave).

4.2 Attitudes Across Countries and Years

Figure 1 shows the mean of the justification of homosexuality variable by country for the last available wave of the WVS in Latin American countries (2010–2014).

As we can see, three countries (Chile, Argentina and Uruguay) have a mean greater than 5, which indicates that favorable opinions towards homosexuality tend to be more frequent than negative ones. Ecuador, Colombia and Peru show the lower levels of justification of homosexuality among the Latin American countries of the WVS.

For the same countries and WVS wave, Fig. 2 shows the proportion of people who mention that they would not like to have homosexuals as neighbors. As in the previous variable, Colombia, Peru and Ecuador are the countries where homonegativity is more frequent (more than a third of respondents would not like homosexuals as neighbors). On the other side, Uruguay, Argentina and Brazil are the countries where rejection of homosexuals as neighbors is the lowest.

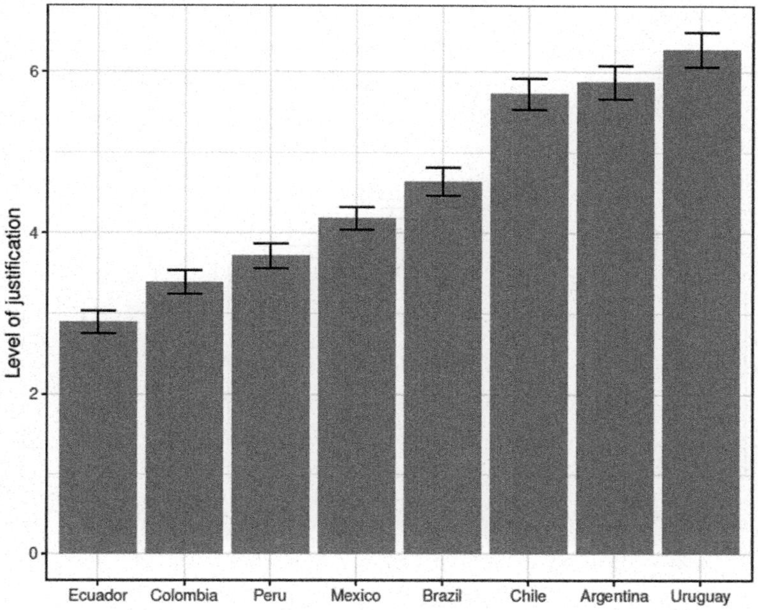

Fig. 1 WVS 2010–2014: homosexuality is justifiable, by country (Mean and 95% confidence interval)

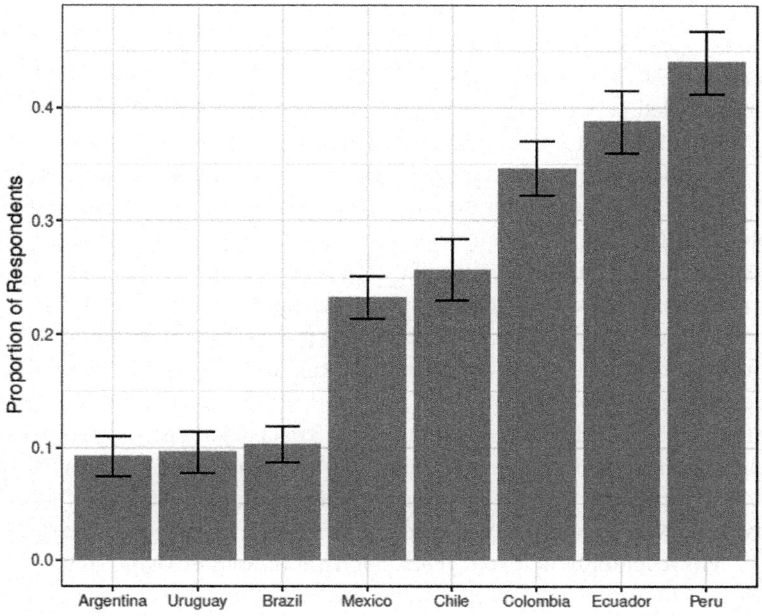

Fig. 2 WVS 2010–2014: proportion of respondents that do not want homosexuals as neighbors, by country (Proportion and 95% confidence interval)

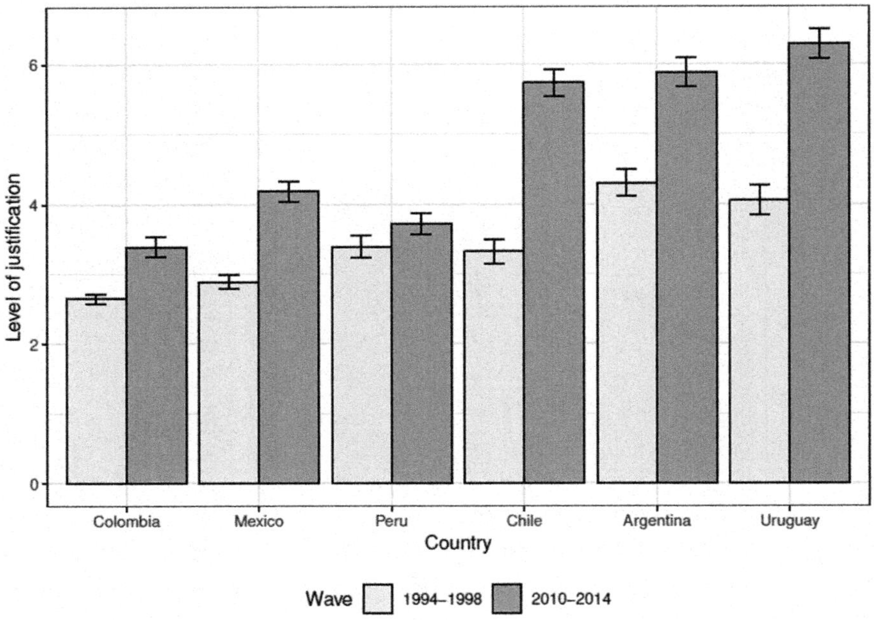

Fig. 3 WVS: homosexuality is justifiable, changes between 1994 and 2014 by country and wave (Mean and 95% confidence interval)

Figures 3 and 4 show the WVS indicators in the six countries which were part of both the 1994–98 and the 2010–14 waves, which allows us to compare changes over an extended period. As we can see, changes were more radical in Argentina, Chile, and Uruguay. In those countries, by the mid-1990s, the mean value of the justification question indicates that the most prevalent attitudes were intolerant ones (mean < 5); 15 or 18 years later they show the opposite situation (mean > 5).

Colombia, Mexico, and Peru have also experienced positive changes but in a lesser extent, and their levels still indicate a prevalence of homonegativity, which could mean that in those countries, cultural change leading towards more open-minded attitudes take place in a slower pace. It is striking to note that in Colombia, regarding some attitudes (rejection of homosexual neighbors) the change over time has been in the negative direction.

LAPOP data presents similar patterns to WVS data results, although over a shorter time lapse and for a wider sample of countries. As we can see in Fig. 5, between 2004 and 2016/17, in Latin America[4] approval of homosexuals' right to run for office has increased, as well as approval of same-couples' right to marry between 2010 and 2016/17. However, only in recent years, approval of homosexuals' rights to run for office has mean values indicating a slight predominance of more tolerant attitudes

[4] Figure 5 shows the mean approval level of all the countries included in each wave's sample. To calculate the regional mean each country mean has the same weight.

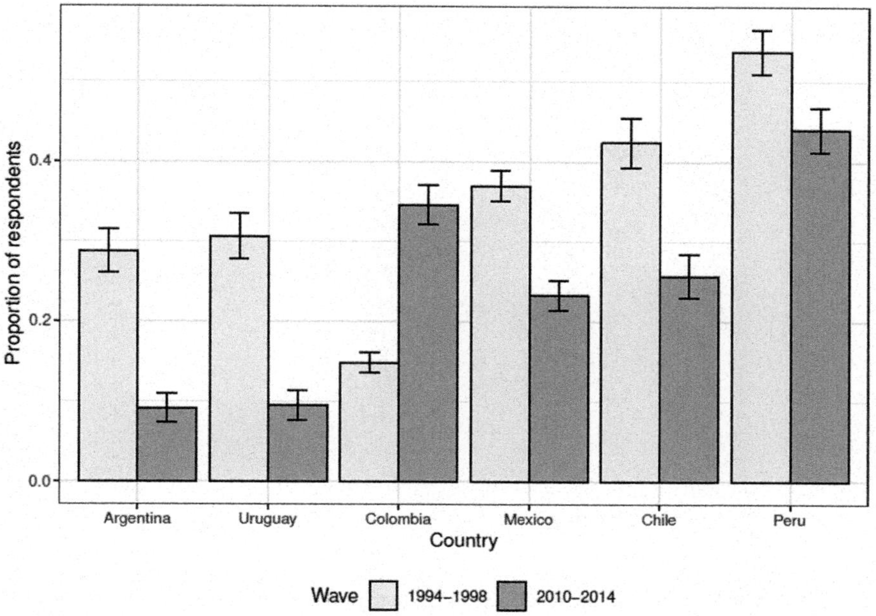

Fig. 4 WVS: don't want homosexuals as neighbors, changes between 1994 and 2014 by country and wave (Proportion and 95% confidence interval)

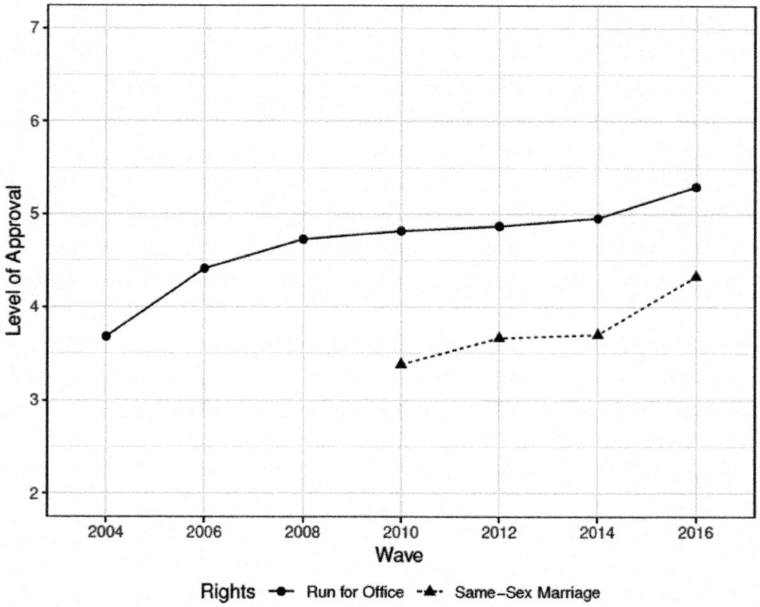

Fig. 5 LAPOP 2004–2016: approval for homosexuals' rights, by type of right and survey wave

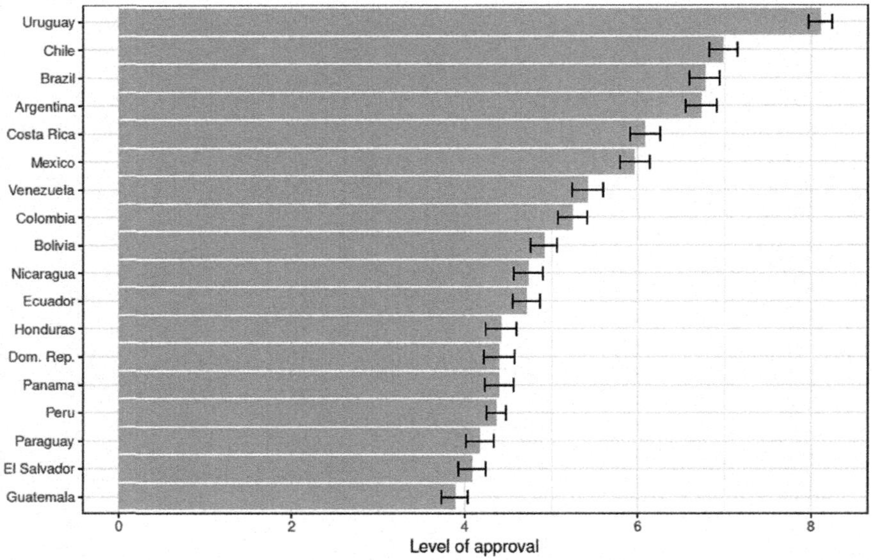

Fig. 6 LAPOP 2016: approval of homosexuals' right to run for office, by country (Mean and 95% confidence interval)

(mean > 5). On the other side, same-sex marriage still encounters a majoritarian opposition in the region.

Figures 6 and 7 show the mean values of LAPOP indicators distribution across countries for the last available wave of this survey (2016/17). As expected, the most tolerant countries are the ones already identified using WVS data: Uruguay, Argentina, Brazil, and Chile. At the bottom of the distribution, among the most intolerant cases, we find mostly some Central American countries: El Salvador, Guatemala, Honduras, Panama. Paraguay and the Dominican Republic also share that position. Andean countries (Colombia, Ecuador, Peru, and Bolivia) are in a middle position, but closer to the group of intolerant countries than the more tolerant ones.

As the results show, countries that have implemented progressive legislation (see Table 1) usually present more favorable attitudes towards homosexuals. That could be a sign that instead of provoking a public opinion backlash, the adoption of favorable legislation towards LGBTI might accompany or enhance open-minded attitudes among the public.

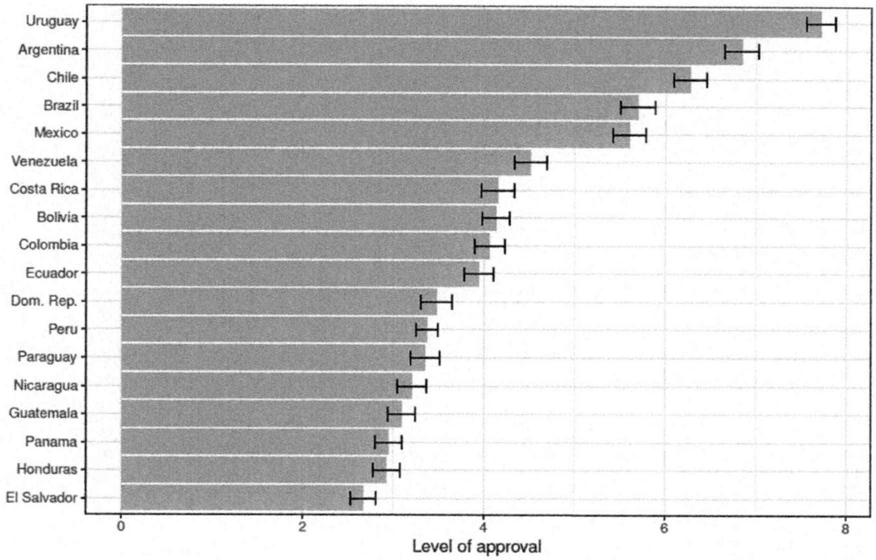

Fig. 7 LAPOP 2016: approval of same-sex couples' right to marry, by country (Mean and 95% confidence interval)

5 Economic Development, Democratization and Attitudes Towards Homosexuality

Modernization theory proposes a positive relationship between economic development, democratization and cultural change towards more progressive values. Figure 8 shows the relationship, at country level, between per capita GDP (in US$), political freedom and the level of approval of homosexuals' rights measured by LAPOP 2016/17 survey wave. Figures for per capita GDP correspond to 2016 (World Bank, 2021). Political Freedom Index was calculated using data from the 2016 "Freedom in the World" report elaborated by Freedom House (2021).[5]

As we can see, countries with higher economic development or higher political and civil liberties levels tend to have higher approval levels of homosexuals and same-sex couples' rights. Table 3 shows the correlation coefficients for those variables, in the table we have included the correlations calculated with data from the 2006 and 2010 LAPOP survey waves. Correlations between economic development and attitudes towards homosexuality are quite important and have remained almost at the same level in 2006 and 2016. Political freedom is correlated, at lower levels, with the dependent variables in 2016 but not in 2006 and 2010.

[5] In order to calculate the "Freedom Index", we reversed the original values of Freedom House's "Political Rights" (PR) and "Civil Liberties" (CL) indexes, and then added them into a single index with a theoretical 0–12 range. In its original form, lower PR or CL values indicate higher levels of freedom (Freedom House, 2018).

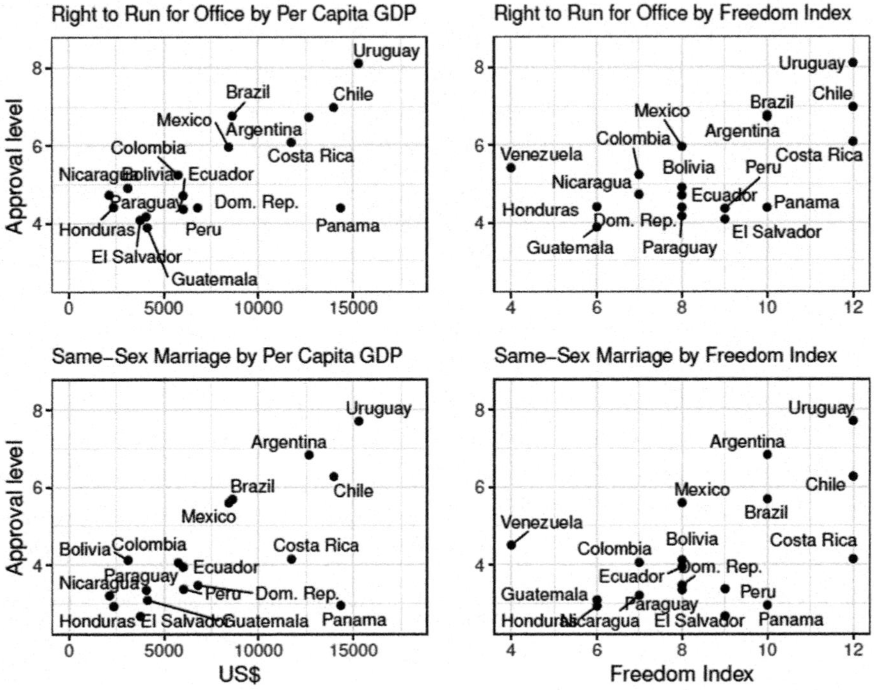

Fig. 8 LAPOP 2016/17: homosexuals' rights, economic development and political freedoms

Table 3 Correlations (Pearson's r) between attitudes towards homosexuals' rights, economic development and political freedom

Dependent variable	Year	Per capita GDP	Freedom index
Run for office	2006	0.724***	0.478
	2016	0.734***	0.612**
Same-sex marriage	2010	0.657**	0.433
	2016	0.695**	0.521*

Note *p < 0.05; **p < 0.01; ***p < 0.001

In general, those results are consistent with the hypotheses of Inglehart's modernization theory. Economic prosperity and political democratization establish the underlying conditions for cultural value changes over time and across societies, shifting preferences from materialist concerns to postmaterialist ones. That can foster the acceptance of diverse living styles and choices, which in this case, enhance acceptance of homosexuality and homosexuals and same couples' rights.

6 Individual Level Predictors and Attitudes Towards Homosexuality

In order to analyze the effect of individual predictors of attitudes towards homosexuality, we have run several multilevel regression models using data from our two sources. A multilevel model allows us to estimate the effect of the predictor variables on the independent variables when our cases are nested in "levels" or groups that also affect the outcome variable. In our case, the Level-1 of our analysis is the individual (each respondent), and Level-2 is each country-year of the survey. The following equation can represent our models (Finch et al., 2014, p. 31).

$$y_{ij} = \gamma_{00} + \gamma_{10}x_{1ij} + \gamma_{20}x_{2ij} + \cdots + \gamma_{n0}x_{nij} + u_{0j} + e_{ij}$$

where: i defines Level-1 (individuals); j defines Level-2 (country-year); γ_{00} is the constant or intercept; γ_{10} is the estimate for the effect for each x_n; u_j: is the Level-2 residual; and e_{ij}: is the Level-1 residual.

6.1 *LAPOP Models for Attitudes Towards Homosexuality*

The first sets of models are based on LAPOP data from 2010 to 2017. In this case, we estimated two Multilevel Linear Models (MLM), one for each of LAPOP's dependent variables: approval of homosexuals' right to run for office and approval for same-sex couples' right to marry.

For each model we included the following dependent variables for Level-1 (individuals):

- Gender, as a dichotomous dummy variable, where Male = 0; and Female = 1.
- Age
- Marital status as a dichotomous dummy variable, where 1 = single/never married; and 0 = Other situations (married, living in couple, widowed, divorced).
- Education: Years of formal education.
- Religious denomination, as a polytomous dummy variable with four categories: 0 = Catholic; 1 = Other Christian (protestants, evangelical and others)[6]; 2 = Other religion; 4 = None. The contrast category is Catholic. Figure 9 shows the distribution of this variable by country in the 2016/17 LAPOP survey wave. Besides Uruguay, which is the most secularized country in our sample, more than 50% of respondents in Latin America belongs to a Christian religion, mostly Catholic. Evangelical Christians are an important group, mainly in Central America and Brazil.

[6] According to LAPOP 2014 wave, among "Other Christians", 57% were evangelicals and 38% other protestant denominations.

- Importance of religion, based on the question "Could you please tell me how important is religion in your life?" with values: 0 = Not at all important; 1 = Not very important; 2 = Rather important; 3 = Very important.
- Progressive legislation: a dichotomous dummy variable indicating if the country has approved progressive legislation (see Table 1) before the survey year: 1 = Yes; 0 = No.

Level 2 is each country-year, our models will estimate a constant or intercept which represents a base value (holding all the other variables equal to 0) for our dependent variable for each country-year, as a way of considering the specific particularities of a Latin American society (for example the level of economic development or political freedoms) at a given year and their effects in the dependent variables.

Table 4 shows the results of the MLM. Coefficients have been estimated using the maximum likelihood method. As we can see, results are consistent with the findings of the literature on this subject: acceptance of homosexuals and same-sex couples' rights is higher among women than among men; it increases in the younger age groups, among single people, and in individuals with higher educational attainment.

People who consider religion more important in their lives tend to disapprove homosexuals' rights, confirming that more religious people have negative attitudes towards homosexuals. However, not all religions hold the same level of homonegativity, Catholics and other non-Christian believers tend to be less intolerant towards homosexuals than other Christians (mostly Evangelical).

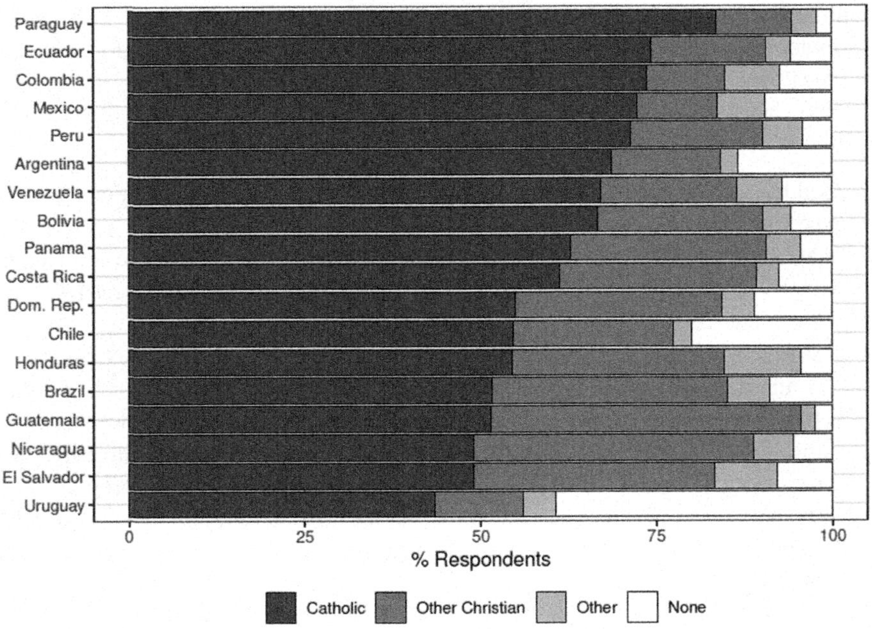

Fig. 9 LAPOP 2016/17: religious denomination by country (% of respondents)

Table 4 LAPOP 2010–2017: multilevel lineal models for approval of homosexuals' rights

	Dependent variables	
	Run for office (1)	Same-sex marriage (2)
Gender = Female	0.425*** (0.019)	0.632*** (0.019)
Age	−0.009*** (0.001)	0–0.024*** (0.001)
Education	0.132*** (0.002)	0.067*** (0.002)
Relig.: other christian versus catholic	−0.841*** (0.024)	−0.970*** (0.024)
Relig.: other versus catholics	−0.081 (0.069)	−0.074 (0.067)
Relig.: none versus catholics	0.201*** (0.037)	0.117*** (0.037)
Importance of religion	−0.226*** (0.013)	−0.404*** (0.013)
Progressive legislation	1.627*** (0.237)	2.195*** (0.216)
Constant	4.116*** (0.133)	4.269*** (0.125)
Observations	109,981	95,549
Log likelihood	−280,386.50	−238,771.40
Akaike inf. crit	560,797.00	477,566.90
Bayesian inf. crit	560,912.20	477.680.50

Note Standard errors in parentheses
*p < 0.05; **p < 0.01; ***p < 0.001

Finally, in LAPOP models we can see that individuals in countries that had approved progressive legislation before the surveyed year show much higher levels of approval for homosexuals and same-sex couples' rights.

6.2 *WVS Models for Attitudes Towards Homosexuality*

Using WVS data from waves 3 thru 6, we estimated four different multilevel models. The first two consider justification of homosexuality as the dependent variable and are Multilevel Linear Models (MLM). The last ones are Multilevel Generalized Linear Models (MGLM) for a dichotomous outcome variable (Finch et al., 2014, pp. 141–144), since they consider whether respondents reject (1) or not (0) homosexuals as neighbors as the dependent variable and the coefficients are based on logistic binomial regressions.

Our WVS models share many of the Level-1 (individual) independent variables that we used in LAPOP models: Gender, age, marital status, religious denomination (considering "Catholic" as the control category) and progressive legislation. In the case of education, WVS measures "level of education", with values from 0 = "None", thru 8 = "Complete University".

Instead of "importance of religion", we used the following question about the "importance of God":

> How important is God in your life? Please use this scale to indicate your answer, where 10 means "very important" and 1 means "not at all important".

WVS models include three other variables which are not measured in LAPOP. The first one is the Postmaterialist scale based on the 12 values index (Inglehart, 1997, 355). The second is the question about interpersonal trust, which can be considered as an indicator for "social capital". The wording of this question is:

> Generally speaking, would you say that A) most people can be trusted or that B) you need to be very careful in dealing with people?

Table 5 shows the results for the variables of importance of God (mean), interpersonal trust (% of people who answer that "most people can be trusted") and postmaterialism (12 index scale) for the six countries of the WVS that where surveyed both in the 1994–1998 and 2010–2014 waves. As we can see, in both waves the importance of God was quite high, whit the relative exception of Uruguay. Despite economic and political development, besides Argentina, interpersonal trust has declined in our sample of countries. The same can be said (although in at a lesser level) about postmaterialism.

The third variable considered in our WVS models is a question about the "Meaning of Religion" (MR) which was only included in the WVS general questionnaire in Wave 6. The question wording is:

> With which one of the following statements do you agree most? The basic meaning of religion is: A) To follow religious norms and ceremonies; or B) To do good to other people.

Table 5 WVS 1994–2014: importance of God (mean), interpersonal trust (%) and postmaterialism (mean), by country and wave

Country/wave	Importante of God		Interpersonal trust		Postmaterialism	
	1994–1998	2010–2014	1994–1998	2010–2014	1994–1998	2010–2014
Argentina	8.4	7.2	17.6	23.2	2.7	2.1
Chile	8.7	8.2	21.4	12.8	2.5	2.5
Colombia	9.6	9.6	10.8	4.1	n.a	2.3
Mexico	7.9	9.4	31.2	12.4	2.3	2.3
Peru	9.0	8.9	5.0	8.3	2.2	2.0
Uruguay	6.7	6.7	21.6	15.2	2.7	2.4
Mean	8.4	8.3	17.9	12.7	2.5	2.3

Table 6 WVS 2010–2014: meaning of religion, % of respondents by country

Country	Follow norms and ceremonies	Do good to other people
Argentina	16.5	83.5
Brazil	12.6	87.4
Chile	20.7	79.3
Colombia	12.5	87.5
Ecuador	16.7	83.3
Mexico	14.8	85.2
Peru	17.9	82.1
Uruguay	10.3	89.7
Mean	15.3	84.7

Table 6 shows the distribution of the answers to this question by country. As we can see, in most countries, more than 80% of respondents agree with the second choice.

The question was first introduced in the Peruvian WVS questionnaire during wave 2 in 1996 by Catalina Romero (1996). Its objective was to explore religious pluralism and the different meanings and attitudes towards Christian faith (Romero, 2013, pp. 147–148), particularly religious values which prioritize the respect to norms and authority over those which give more emphasis to solidarity. The underlying hypothesis is that inside the same religion we can find different values sets, which are not necessarily incompatible with secularization or the development of more tolerant attitudes in society. Therefore, after testing the results from Peruvian surveys, the WVS project decided to include this question (among others) into its general questionnaire in the 6th wave (2010–2014) to explore inter and intrareligious diversity around the world. In the models we present, the "Meaning of Religion" variable (MR) is also considered as an interactive dummy variable with religious denomination.

Table 7 shows the results of MLM and MGLM for the WVS data. For each dependent variable, the first model uses data from waves 3 thru 6, while the second model, which includes the MR variable uses only data from wave 6.

Our results confirm many of the findings we have already seen in the LAPOP models: positive attitudes towards homosexuality are more common among women, young people and individuals with higher educational attainment.

Interpersonal trust is positively associated with acceptance of homosexuality (in our models the "no trust" category—"you need to be very careful in dealing with people"—was coded as 1). Since interpersonal trust is an indicator of social capital, we could say that people with higher levels of social capital tend to show more tolerant and open attitudes toward different groups in society.

The relationship between postmaterialism and attitudes towards homosexuals is also consistent with the cultural modernization theory, people with more postmaterialist values tend to be less intolerant towards homosexuals.

Table 7 WVS: multilevel models for justification of homosexuality and for homosexuals as neighbors

	Dependent variables			
	Justifiable homosexuality MLM		No homosexual neighbors MGLM	
	Waves 2–6	Wave 6	Waves 2–6	Wave 6
Gender = Female	0.463*** (0.035)	0.512*** (0.063)	−0.324*** (0.027)	−0.288*** (0.051)
Age	−0.020*** (0.001)	−0.019*** (0.002)	0.010*** (0.001)	0.011*** (0.002)
Single/never married	0.060 (0.043)	0.048 (0.078)	−0.009 (0.033)	0.035 (0.064)
Education	0.154*** (0.008)	0.135*** (0.015)	−0.072*** (0.006)	−0.068*** (0.012)
Relig.: other christian versus catholic	−0.835*** (0.058)	−0.573* (0.238)	0.120* (0.044)	0.077 (0.178)
Relig.: other versus catholics	−0.422*** (0.094)	−0.813* (0.379)	0.160* (0.075)	0.492 (0.277)
Relig.: none versus catholics	0.186*** (0.047)	0.477* (0.208)	0.011 (0.037)	−0.291 (0.176)
MR: good to other people versus norms		0.284* (0.112)		−0.388*** (0.085)
Interpersonal trust = No	−0.114*** (0.009)	−0.132*** (0.018)	0.048*** (0.007)	0.012 (0.016)
Importance of God	−0.167*** (0.048)	−0.285** (0.104)	0.253*** (0.039)	0.020 (0.089)
Postmaterialist index (12 items)	0.214*** (0.015)	0.169*** (0.028)	−0.141*** (0.012)	−0.051* (0.023)
Progressive legislation	1.117* (0.556)	0.749 (0.846)	−1.163*** (0.346)	−1.173** (0.446)
Relig.: other christian versus catholic * MR		−0.355 (0.261)		0.261 (0.199)
Relig: other versus catholic * MR		0.274 (0.402)		0.039 (0.301)
Relig.: none versus catholic * MR		−0.423 (0.221)		0.401* (0.188)
Constant	4.396*** (0.269)	4.908*** (0.715)	−0.888*** (0.175)	−0.366 (0.411)
Observations	27,891	8,783	30,406	9,151
Log likelihood	−68,627.68	−21,819.77	−17,365.21	−4,743.88
Akaike inf. crit	137,283.40	43,675.54	34,756.41	9,521.76
Bayesian inf. crit	137,398.70	43,802.99	34,864.60	9,642.83

Note Standard error in parentheses
*p < 0.05; **p < 0.01; ***p < 0.001

However, as we saw in Table 5, the levels of interpersonal trust and postmaterialism have declined or remained quite unchanged in our sample of Latin American countries between 1994–2014, while the acceptance of homosexuality has increased in the same countries and the same period. This could mean that other macro-level phenomena, such as economic development, democratization, secularization, generational change and increased levels of education, might have more important effects on the acceptance of LGBTI people and their rights.

Homonegativity is associated with religiosity, considering the importance of God as an indicator of this dimension. Nevertheless, as we saw in LAPOP models, people from different religious denomination tend to have different levels of acceptance of homosexuality: Catholics are more open-minded towards homosexuality than Christians from other denominations (mostly evangelicals) and then people from other religions.

An interesting finding is that people who belong to a religious denomination and agree with religious meanings oriented towards solidarity tend to have more positive attitudes towards homosexuality than those who associate religion with the respect of norms and ceremonies. Those results support the argument proposed by Romero (2013, 151–152): an operational definition which associates religion and religiosity with traditional values is insufficient to understand the relationship between religion and cultural change. It is also vital to consider intra-religion differences and religious change: some religious values and faith inspired attitudes are compatible with the support of self-expression and postmaterialist values, which can also foster acceptance of human diversity and, in this case, of homosexuality.

Finally, as we have also seen in the LAPOP models, people from countries that had approved progressive legislation tend to express less rejection of homosexuals as neighbors. This supports the idea that legislation that aims to expand and protect the LGBTI rights does not provoke a "backlash" in the Latin American public's attitudes, but instead might accompany or support social consensus on those matters.

7 Conclusions

Our results show that over the last 20 years in Latin America there have been positive changes in public opinion towards homosexuality and LGBTI. Those changes are related to socioeconomic development and democratization, but they are also driven by generational cultural changes: younger and more educated generations, socialized in contexts of better economic conditions and democratic political institutions, develop more open-minded values and attitudes towards different ways of life.

These changes are similar than those observed in studies on other countries and regions that have analyzed longitudinal tends, such as in the USA (Flores, 2014; Hicks & Lee, 2006) and Europe (Halman & van Ingen, 2015; van den Akker et al., 2013).

Those changes are not homogeneous, some Latin American countries have experienced more radical value and attitude shifts than others, the pace or rhythm of the cultural change is also associated with the different levels of socioeconomic and political development, richer and politically freer countries tend to experience more rapid changes. Concerning political dynamics, the approval of progressive legislation towards LGBTI rights seems to foster or enhance cultural changes in public opinion.

Despite a positive evolution, homonegativity levels are still significantly high in the region, in most countries most of the population hold intolerant or negative attitudes toward LGBTI, as measured by our dependent variables. Using data from the WVS, Manalastas et al. (2017) have also observed important homonegativity attitudes and heterogeneous patterns in the acceptance of homosexuality in South East Asian countries, attributing those differences on the particular religious characteristics of those countries, pointing out on the differences between Muslim, Christian and Buddhist countries.

In many Latin America countries, conservative and faith-oriented groups can politically mobilize those prevalent anti-LGBTI attitudes to block the advancement of progressive legislation or government programs, not only concerning LGBTI rights but also gender equality and reproductive and sexual rights.

As in other regions of the world, religiosity is correlated with negative attitudes towards homosexuality, that is why some conservative Church authorities (Catholic and Evangelical) and faith-based organizations can still enjoy political leverage and become the most crucial veto players in LGBTI and gender politics.

However, it is essential to consider more nuanced relationships between religion and secular and progressive values. Over the last decades, religious pluralism has increased in the region, and Latin America has diverse religious traditions and ways to experience and conceive Christian and, particularly, Catholic faith. Some of them are not incompatible with secularization and postmaterialist values. Some meanings of religion emphasize solidarity instead of following norms (which are traditionally enforced by religious authorities), and those meanings can be associated with favorable attitudes towards homosexuality. It is important to consider those nuances since most of the Latin American countries are still profoundly Catholic societies. LGBTI activists might find sympathetic ears and even allies among Christians and Catholics in their countries, widening their support base for their political mobilization.

It is also important to consider that not always positive public opinion attitudes precede progressive legislative changes. As we can see in the cases of Colombia, Ecuador, Mexico and—at some extent—Brazil, before the adoption of progressive legislation the majority of the population held rather negative attitudes towards homosexuality (some still do). Thus, political mobilization and taking advantage of the structure of political opportunities opened for LGBTI social movements in each country is a key factor in advancing LGBTI civil rights in the region. Once progressive legislation is adopted, it can enhance positive attitudes towards homosexuality and LBGTI, normalizing their status as full citizens of their respective societies.

References

Andersen, R., & Fetner, T. (2008a). Cohort differences in tolerance of homosexuality: Attitudinal change in Canada and the United States, 1981–2000. *Public Opinion Quarterly, 72*(2), 311–330. https://doi.org/10.1093/poq/nfn017

Andersen, R., & Fetner, T. (2008b). Economic inequality and intolerance: Attitudes toward homosexuality in 35 democracies. *American Journal of Political Science, 52*(4), 942–958.

Baliamoune-Lutz, M. (2011). Trust-based social capital, institutions, and development. *The Journal of Socio-Economics, 40*(4), 335–346. https://doi.org/10.1016/j.socec.2010.12.004

Bishin, B. G., Hayes, T. J., Incantalupo, M. B., & Smith, C. A. (2016). Opinion backlash and public attitudes: Are political advances in gay rights counterproductive? Opinion backlash and public attitudes. *American Journal of Political Science, 60*(3), 625–648. https://doi.org/10.1111/ajps.12181

Bureekul, T., & Thananithichot, S. (2012). Trust and social cohesion, the key to reconcile Thailand's future. *The International Journal of Social Quality, 2*(2), 81–97. https://doi.org/10.3167/IJSQ.2012.020206

Cigler, A., & Joslyn, M. R. (2002). The extensiveness of group membership and social capital: The impact on political tolerance attitudes. *Political Research Quarterly, 55*(1), 7–25. https://doi.org/10.1177/106591290205500101

Coleman, J. (1988). Social capital in the creation of human capital. *American Journal of Sociology, 94*(1988), S95-120.

Collier, K. L., Horn, S. S., Bos, H. M. W., & Sandfort, T. G. M. (2015). Attitudes toward lesbians and gays among American and Dutch adolescents. *The Journal of Sex Research, 52*(2), 140–150. https://doi.org/10.1080/00224499.2013.858306

Corrales, J. (2015a). The politics of LGBT rights in Latin America and the Caribbean: Research agendas. *European Review of Latin American and Caribbean Studies/revista Europea De Estudios Latinoamericanos y Del Caribe, 100*, 53–62.

Corrales, J. (2015b). *LGBT rights and representation in Latin America and the Caribbean: The influence of structure, movements, institutions, and culture*. LGBT Representation and Rights Initiative at the University of North Carolina at Chapel Hill. https://globalstudies.unc.edu/files/2015/04/LGBT_Report_LatAm_v8-copy.pdf

Decco, E. (2014). *Changing attitudes toward homosexuality in the United States from 1977 to 2012* [MSc]. Brigham Young University.

Djupe, P. A., & Calfano, B. R. (2012). American Muslim investment in civil society: Political discussion, disagreement, and tolerance. *Political Research Quarterly, 65*(3), 516–528. https://doi.org/10.1177/1065912911401417

Ellison, C. G., & Musick, M. A. (1993). Southern intolerance: A fundamentalist effect? *Social Forces, 72*(2), 379–398. https://doi.org/10.1093/sf/72.2.379

Finch, W. H., Bolin, J. E., & Kellet, K. (2014). *Multilevel modeling using R*. CRC Press. http://www.crcnetbase.com/isbn/9781466515864

Flores, A. R. (2014). *National trends in public opinion on LGBT rights in the United States*. The Williams Institute UCLA. https://escholarship.org/uc/item/72t8q7pg

Flores, A. R., & Barclay, S. (2016). Backlash, consensus, legitimacy, or polarization: The effect of same-sex marriage policy on mass attitudes. *Political Research Quarterly, 69*(1), 43–56. https://doi.org/10.1177/1065912915621175

Freedom House. (2021). *Freedom in the world*. Freedom House. https://freedomhouse.org/report/freedom-world

Halman, L., & van Ingen, E. (2015). Secularization and changing moral views: European trends in church attendance and views on homosexuality, divorce, abortion, and Euthanasia. *European Sociological Review, 31*(5), 616–627. https://doi.org/10.1093/esr/jcv064

Herek, G. M. (2002). Heterosexuals' attitudes toward bisexual men and women in the United States. *Journal of Sex Research, 39*(4), 264–274. https://doi.org/10.1080/00224490209552150

Hicks, G. R., & Lee, T.-T. (2006). Public attitudes toward gays and lesbians: Trends and predictors. *Journal of Homosexuality, 51*(2), 57–77. https://doi.org/10.1300/J082v51n02_04

Hooghe, M., Claes, E., Harell, A., Quintelier, E., & Dejaeghere, Y. (2010). Anti-gay sentiment among adolescents in Belgium and Canada: A comparative investigation into the role of gender and religion. *Journal of Homosexuality, 57*(3), 384–400. https://doi.org/10.1080/00918360903543071

Inglehart, R. (1997). *Modernization and postmodernization: Cultural, economic, and political change in 43 societies.* Princeton University Press.

Inglehart, R., & Welzel, C. (2005). *Modernization, cultural change, and democracy: The human development sequence.* Cambridge University Press.

Inglehart, R., Haerpfer, C., Moreno, A., Welzel, C., Kizilova, K., Diez-Medrado, J., Lagos, M., Norris, P., Ponarin, E., & Puranen, B. (2020). *World values survey: All rounds—Country-pooled datafile.* JD Systems Institute & WVSA Secretariat. http://www.worldvaluessurvey.org/WVSDocumentationWVL.jsp

International Lesbian, Gay, Bisexual, Trans and Intersex Association, Carroll, A., & Mendos, R. (2017). *State sponsored homophobia 2017: A world survey of sexual orientation laws: Criminalisation, protection and recognition* (No. 12). ILGA. https://ilga.org/downloads/2017/ILGA_State_Sponsored_Homophobia_2017_WEB.pdf

Jones, P. (2006). Toleration, recognition and identity*. *Journal of Political Philosophy, 14*(2), 123–143. https://doi.org/10.1111/j.1467-9760.2006.00246.x

Kazyak, E., & Stange, M. (2018). Backlash or a positive response? Public opinion of LGB issues after *Obergefell v. Hodges*. *Journal of Homosexuality*, 1–25. https://doi.org/10.1080/00918369.2017.1423216

Latin American Public Opinion Project. (2021). *The Americas barometer.* http://www.LapopSurveys.org

Lee, F. L. F. (2014). "Tolerated one way but not the other": Levels and determinants of social and political tolerance in Hong Kong. *Social Indicators Research, 118*(2), 711–727. https://doi.org/10.1007/s11205-013-0433-5

Manalastas, E. J., Ojanen, T. T., Torre, B. A., Ratanashevorn, R., Chee Hong, B. C., Kumarezan, V., & Veeramuthu, V. (2017). Homonegativity in Southeast Asia: Attitudes toward lesbians and gay men in Indonesia, Malaysia, the Philippines, Singapore, Thailand, and Vietnam. *Asia-Pacific Social Science Review, 17*(1), 25–33.

Mott, L., Michels, E., & Paulinho. (2017). *Mortes violentas de LGBT no Brasil: Relatório 2017.* Grupo Gay da Bahia. https://homofobiamata.files.wordpress.com/2017/12/relatorio-2081.pdf

OECD. (2014). Society at a glance 2014: OECD social indicators. *OECD.* https://doi.org/10.1787/soc_glance-2014-en

Parekh, R., Maleku, A., Fields, N., Adorno, G., Schuman, D., & Felderhoff, B. (2018). Pathways to age-friendly communities in diverse urban neighborhoods: Do social capital and social cohesion matter? *Journal of Gerontological Social Work, 61*(5), 492–512. https://doi.org/10.1080/01634372.2018.1454564

Pew Research Center. (2013a). *The global divide on homosexuality.* http://www.pewglobal.org/2013/06/04/the-global-divide-on-homosexuality/

Pew Research Center. (2013b). *The global divide on homosexuality.* http://www.pewglobal.org/2013/06/04/the-global-divide-on-homosexuality/

Putnam, R. D. (1996). The strange disappearance of civic America. (Cover Story). *The American Prospect, 24,* 34.

Redman, S. M. (2018). Effects of same-sex legislation on attitudes toward homosexuality. *Political Research Quarterly*, 106591291775307. https://doi.org/10.1177/1065912917753077

Romero, C. (1996). *World values survey—Wave 3, questionnaire Peru.* http://www.worldvaluessurvey.org/WVSDocumentationWV3.jsp

Romero, C. (2013). Las Creencias Religiosas y el Cambio Cultural: Evidencia de Perú. In A. Moreno & M. Carballo (Eds.), *El Cambio de Valores en América Latina. Hallazgos de la Encuesta Mundial de Valores* (pp. 127–152). Centro de Estudios Sociales y de Opini6n Pública.

Romero, C. (2016). El Perú, País de Diversidad Religiosa. In C. Romero (Ed.), *Diversidad Religiosa en el Perú: Miradas Múltiples* (pp. 13–40). Centro de Estudios y Publicaciones; Pontificia Universidad Católica del Perú.

Schirmer, W., Weidenstedt, L., & Reich, W. (2012). From tolerance to respect in inter-ethnic contexts. *Journal of Ethnic and Migration Studies, 38*(7), 1049–1065. https://doi.org/10.1080/1369183X.2012.681448

Slootmaeckers, K., & Lievens, J. (2014). Cultural capital and attitudes toward homosexuals: Exploring the relation between lifestyles and homonegativity. *Journal of Homosexuality, 61*(7), 962–979. https://doi.org/10.1080/00918369.2014.870848

Smith, T. W., Son, J., & Kim, J. (2014). *Public attitudes towards homosexuality and gay rights across time and countries*. NORC—University of Chicago; The Williams Institute—UCLA. https://williamsinstitute.law.ucla.edu/wp-content/uploads/public-attitudes-nov-2014.pdf

Stevenson, M. (Ed.). (1988). Promoting tolerance for homosexuality: An evaluation of intervention strategies. *Journal of Sex Research, 25*(Nov 88), 500–511.

Sullivan, J. L., & Transue, J. E. (1999). The psychological underpinnings of democracy: A selective review of research on political tolerance, interpersonal trust, and social capital. *Annual Review of Psychology*, 625.

van den Akker, H., van der Ploeg, R., & Scheepers, P. (2013). Disapproval of homosexuality: Comparative research on individual and national determinants of disapproval of homosexuality in 20 European countries. *International Journal of Public Opinion Research, 25*(1), 64–86. https://doi.org/10.1093/ijpor/edr058

Whitley, B. E., Jr., & Aegisdóttir, S. (2000). The gender belief system, authoritarianism, social dominance orientation, and heterosexuals' attitudes toward lesbians and gay men. *Sex Roles, 42*(11/12), 947–967.

Wise, J., & Driskell, R. (2017). Tolerance within community: Does social capital affect tolerance? *Social Indicators Research, 134*(2), 607–629. https://doi.org/10.1007/s11205-016-1449-4

World Bank. (2021). *World dataBank*. http://databank.worldbank.org

David Sulmont got Ph.D. in Political Science and Government from the Pontificia Universidad Católica del Perú (PUCP) and M.A. in Sociology from the Ecole des Hautes Etudes en Sciences Sociales de Paris. He is a full professor at the Social Sciences Department of the PUCP, where he teaches political sociology and research methods, and does research on public opinion, electoral behaviour and ethnic and racial studies in Latin America. He's a collaborator of the Comparative Study of Electoral Systems (CSES) in charge of the Peruvian Electoral Study at the PUCP since 2006.

Kiara Castaman got M.A. in Poverty and Development from the University of Sussex, United Kingdom and B.A. in Sociology from the Pontificia Universidad Católica del Perú (PUCP). She has worked in project Monitoring and Evaluation focusing on community development and child protection. She is currently a research consultant at the International Initiative for Impact Evaluation (3ie), collaborating with the Synthesis and Meta-Analysis office in London.

Antecedents of Religious Tolerance in Southeast Asia

Sotheeswari Somasundram, Muzafar Shah Habibullah, Murali Sambasivan, and Ratneswary Rasiah

1 Introduction

Globalization has changed the landscapes of many nations, making it a norm for communities with different ethnicities, cultures and religions to be present within the same environment. The emerging trends require individuals with different views, religious inclinations and way of life to coexist within the same society. The social dynamics at play in these instances highlight the importance of trust and tolerance within the community for a harmonious existence. Tolerance and trust, illustrations of social capital, play a vital role in bridging divisive social cleavages (Norris & Davis, 2007). Studies indicate that social capital has the capacity to cope with societal changes (Hanna et al., 2009) by shifting communities' inclinations away from individualistic mindsets to supporting collective outcomes (Putnam, 1995a).

Given the importance of social capital in a diverse society, the focus of the present study is to gain insights on the role of tolerance, specifically religious tolerance, in social capital formation. In order to facilitate discussions on religious tolerance, we will first elaborate on a related concept of social capital, trust. In order to establish the role of trust in religion, the present study adopts the essence of trust from

S. Somasundram (✉) · R. Rasiah
Taylor's University, Selangor, Malaysia
e-mail: sotheeswari.somasundram@taylors.edu.my

R. Rasiah
e-mail: ratneswary.rasiah@taylors.edu.my

M. S. Habibullah
Putra Business School, University Putra Malaysia, Seri Kembangan, Malaysia
e-mail: muzafar@putrabs.edu.my

M. Sambasivan
Thiagarajar School of Management, Madurai, India
e-mail: director@tsm.ac.in

A. Almakaeva et al. (eds.), *Social Capital and Subjective Well-Being*,
Societies and Political Orders in Transition,
https://doi.org/10.1007/978-3-030-75813-4_7

social capital literatures to draw parallels to Adam Smith's capital value of reputation (Smith, 2007). Social capital as defined by Putnam (1995b) states that society pursues a shared objective through a social network which allows interaction based on norms and trust. In the social capital framework, trust is gained from the network by maintaining a degree of interaction and integration in the social environment (Beugelsdijk & van Schaik, 2005). This points towards the importance of reputational effect in the social network. Here parallels can be drawn between the reputational effects of social capital and Adam Smith's capital value of reputation. Anderson (1988), in making direct reference to Adam Smith's theory of capital value of reputation highlights that "religions produce and distribute moral information about individual members" (p. 1071) which provides prospective transactors the necessary information to gauge the risk involved in a given transaction. Thus the source of the moral information is individuals' attendance, interaction or membership with religious organization. Smith assumes that "man is naturally deceitful and unscrupulous and will quite willingly employ predatory practices so long as such practices are available to him" (Rosenberg, 1960, p. 558). In order to manage these tendencies, Adam Smith emphasized on the superiority of the price mechanism only in the presences of appropriate institutions (Rosenberg, 1960). In summary, Adam Smith's theory of capital value of reputation assumes that man's natural tendencies are towards insolence, however, religion provides an economic incentive to inculcate a self-monitoring system. Individuals aware of the economic costs of misbehavior will place great importance on not only maintaining but also enhancing the capital value of their reputation. Therefore religion provides the framework to neutralize deceitful tendencies, allowing for formation of trust enhancing behavior, a setting for social capital.

No religion in the world encourages its adherents to commit evil or be immoral, although an oft repeated cliché, but profoundly true. As such, religious intolerance should rightly be rejected by religious practitioners. Probing along these lines, can we rationalize that countries with higher level of religiosity should ideally record higher level of religious tolerance? Religiosity is defined as the level of religious commitment and captured through self-report of various practices such as frequency of practices, attendance and prayers (Association of Religion Data Archives, 2018). Although religiosity is a concept that is multidimensional in nature (Allport & Ross, 1967; Strabac & Listhaug, 2008; Yeung et al., 2009) but the current study focuses on two well-documented dimensions. Social religiosity which is a cornerstone in trust building for social capital formation; and individual religiosity which is on individual religious experiences (Okulicz-Kozaryn, 2010).

Social religiosity helps in building social capital through group dynamics and trust which provides support and scaffolding within the society (Helliwell & Putnam, 1995). However there is a downside to social religiosity which is excessive in-group trust (Portes, 2014). Individuals expressing religious intolerance might be mimicking group-level prejudice, and not necessarily expressing their own preference or belief. In-group trust might mandate support for group-level beliefs, and where members with different perspectives might not be viewed favorably or permitted to continue within the group (Hall et al., 2010). Thus, if an individual is a member of a group that propagates religious intolerance, one might be indirectly coerced to support the prejudicial views. In this case, the element of trust contributes towards increasing intolerance and negatively impacting social capital formation.

Individual religiosity akin to Allport and Ross (1967) intrinsic religious orientation focuses on following the religious prescriptions and said to 'live the religion' (Okulicz-Kozaryn, 2010, p. 156). If individuals follow and practice the teachings of one's religion, the incidences of religious intolerance are less likely to occur (Sedikides & Gebauer, 2010). Although some studies support the conclusion that intrinsic religious orientation contributes to tolerance (Greer et al., 2005; Hall et al., 2010) but there are counterclaims as well. Studies refuting this conclusion highlight a number of reasons for religious intolerance such as cognitively rigid ideologies (Johnson et al., 2011), uncertainty avoidances (Kossowska & Sekerdej, 2015) and perception that behaviors are inconsistent with their perceived traditional religious teachings (Rowatt et al., 2009). Thus, individual religiosity could negatively or positively impact religious tolerance, and on a broader perspective, influence the formation of social capital.

Given this setting, the present study investigates the impact of social religiosity and individual religiosity on religious tolerance among selected countries in Southeast Asia. The present study will focus on four Southeast Asian countries—Malaysia, Singapore, Thailand and Philippines. A comparative study among the different countries contributes as follows: (1) helps to compare the specific factors influencing religious tolerance among the countries in Southeast Asia, (2) helps to clarify the challenges faced and also provide a better understanding of the prevailing behaviors in these countries, and (3) assists the policy makers to understand the challenges and devise appropriate strategies to enhance tolerant behavior and prevent intolerance.

1.1 Religious Tolerance in Southeast Asia

Southeast Asia is home to three of the largest religions in the world. Indonesia, Malaysia and Brunei have a Muslim majority. Philippines houses a large Catholic population while Myanmar, Thailand, Cambodia and Laos have a significant Buddhist population (Pew Research Center, 2015). It is interesting to note that Southeast Asia is home to both the most as well as the least religiously diverse countries in the world.

A report on religious diversity by Pew Research Center (2014) ranked Malaysia, Brunei, Laos, Vietnam and Singapore as more diverse compared to the Philippines, Indonesia, Thailand, Cambodia and Myanmar. A pluralistic environment allows for assimilation through osmosis with societies having opportunities to familiarize themselves with other religions and in the process eliminating any negative stereotyping (Quinn, 2001). Religious plurality allows for a healthy interaction between the various religious practitioners promoting an attitude of religious understanding and tolerance. A proposition that can be supported using Myanmar, Thailand and Philippines. These countries have less diverse societies and face an increase in faith-based tensions. A correlation between religious diversity and religious tolerance among the

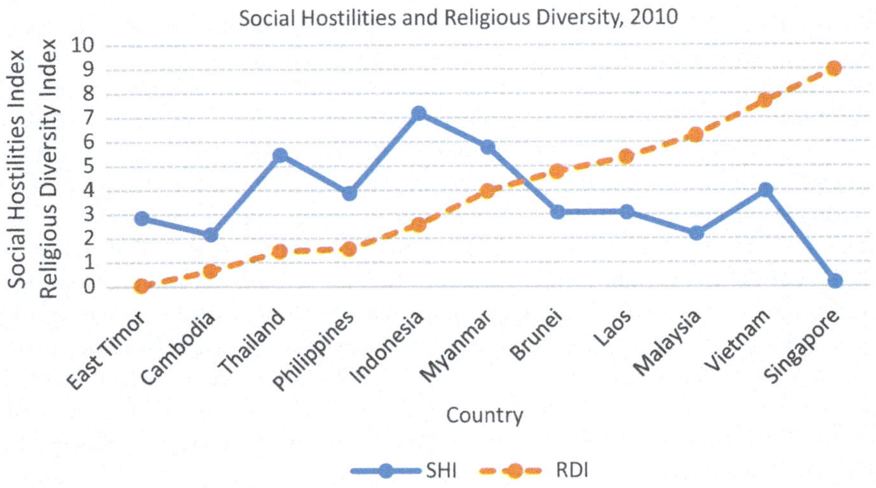

Fig. 1 Social hostilities and religious diversity in Southeast Asia, 2010. *Source* Pew Research Center (2016). Global Restrictions on Religion Data, Available at: http://www.pewresearch.org; Pew Research Centre (2014). Global Religious Diversity Data, Available at: http://www.pewresearch.org

Southeast Asian countries for 2010 highlights that countries with higher religious diversity record lower religious intolerance, further strengthening the conclusion that diversity has a positive impact on tolerance (see Fig. 1).

However is the proposition of religious tolerance in a diverse population cast in stone? Media reports claim that diverse populations are more intolerant. A report claims that religious tolerance prevailing in the Southeast Asian region is deceptive and cautions that the strength gained over the centuries through religious diversity may be eroded (Pilling, 2017). Another report highlights the rising religious intolerance in the region while stressing on the need to reject the politicization of religion (Bo & Wahid, 2016).

The prevalence of deceptive religious tolerance and rising intolerance are indeed strong claims. In order to verify this, the study looked at religious social oppression using the societal hostilities index (SHI) from 2007 to 2014 among the Southeast Asian countries (see Fig. 2). The scatter plots indicate high religious intolerance in Indonesia, Myanmar, Malaysia, Thailand and Vietnam. This indicates that close to forty five percent of countries in Southeast Asia are leaning towards intolerance. The preliminary analysis concurs with the claims by the media, justifying the need for further analysis.

This study focuses on four Southeast Asian countries—Malaysia, Thailand, Singapore and Philippines. The rational for choosing these countries was to ensure a fair representation of the three major religions in the Southeast Asian region. The countries identified represent different levels of economic growth and varying degrees of religious plurality in the region. Malaysia represents a developing economy with a

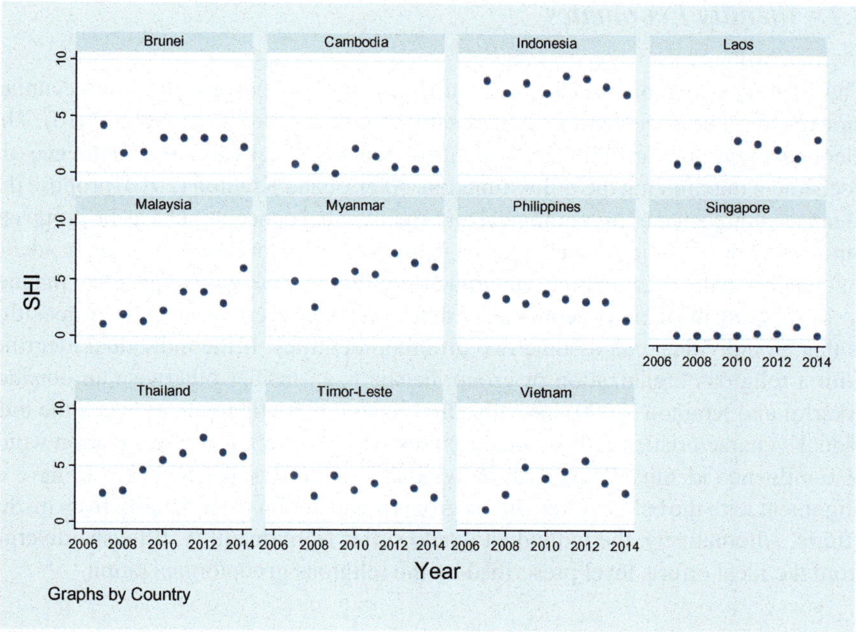

Fig. 2 Religious tolerance in Southeast Asia, 2007–2014. *Source* Pew Research Center (2016). Global Restrictions on Religion Data, Available at: http://www.pewresearch.org

pluralistic society housing a majority of Muslim population. Thailand and Philippines represent developing economies but with a less diverse religious population while housing a majority of Buddhist and Christian population, respectively. Singapore represents an advanced economy with a pluralistic society without a religious majority.

2 Theoretical Framework

The underpinning framework for our study is the proposition that decisions and behaviors are influenced by the need to maximize satisfaction or utility. Similarly, the decisions and behaviors around tolerance is also influenced by satisfaction. In order to support our analysis we utilize identity economics and the social comparison theory to explain the theoretical framework.

2.1 Identity Economics

The identity economics applies the utility function to capture the non-pecuniary motives that influence and maximizes satisfaction (Akerlof & Kranton, 2010). This theory explains how an individual's identity—a person's sense of self—influences the decision in maximizing the utility function. Akerlof and Kranton (2010) propose that identity is subjected to psychological and sociological concepts such as in-group and out-group within a social category. The identity of assuming one-self as an insider or an outsider in the organization can influence utility in a positive or negative manner.

In applying the identity economics framework to the present study, the proposition is that an individual can assume two different identities. If the individual identifies with a religious organization or group, he/she is an insider otherwise an outsider. Akerlof and Kranton (2000) have also highlighted that alignment between the individual's characteristics and the ideals expressed by the religious organization would also influence identity. Thus if an individual is an insider, he/she needs to have an alignment with the belief system of the group/organization to gain utility from his/her efforts. Alternatively, the individual would suffer from disutility, if he/she diverges from the ideal efforts level prescribed by the religious group/organization.

2.2 Social Comparison Theory

Festinger (1954) has proposed that a person's self-image (identity) is evaluated by comparing with those who are similar to themselves. Later studies in this area highlight that people make negative assessments of others to boost their own self-esteem (Fein & Spencer, 1997). In addition, although a downward evaluation is made against a target group but affiliation is sought with the favored group (Taylor & Lobel, 1989). Social comparison is argued to be the preferred approach for self-evaluations as it can result in gains of social and material benefits (Strickhouser & Zell, 2015) which would justify the affiliation one seeks with the favored group. However, a strong comparison reference is important, otherwise it can reduce the social comparison effects (Garcia et al., 2013).

Social comparison theory was employed as an explanatory framework for tolerance formation leading to utility maximization by Dima and Dima (2016). Their overarching argument, utility maximization decisions were influenced not only by one's gains but more so, the gains received in comparison to others within the society. In their framework, Dima and Dima (2016) emphasized on the significance of the perceived quality of social environment as it influences the comparison one makes with others within the society. The manner in which an individual perceives the quality of the social environment is influenced by group discrimination or behavioral predisposition where these views are supported with the realistic group conflict theory[1] and the strong reciprocity theory.[2] Dima and Dima (2016) elaborates that the level of tolerance and the predisposition towards tolerance or confrontation plays a crucial role in how one perceives the quality of the social environment. The level of tolerance differs significantly between individuals where according to Dima and Dima (2016) one might be tolerant to certain religious group but intolerant towards others or express preferences for certain behavior in public but intolerant in private life. Thus in their framework, the optimal level of tolerance is given as the level that would maximize individual utility.

Dima and Dima (2016) proposed that the explanatory power of their framework can be enhanced by incorporating subjective factors such as cultural biases, intergenerational transmitted behaviors, feeling of personal security among others. The present study incorporates two subjective factors; individual religiosity and social religiosity into Dima and Dima's (2016) framework. The rationale to include these two variables is supported by previous studies that justify the impact these variables have on predisposition for tolerance or confrontation. In the case of individual religiosity, studies highlight that individuals with intrinsic religiosity motives are less willing to engage in value judgment of others (Beck & Miller, 2000; Sedikides & Gebauer, 2010), indicating a predisposition towards tolerance rather than confrontation. On the other hand, social religiosity which is similar to Allport and Ross's (1967) extrinsic religiosity is associated with higher levels of intolerance (Batson, 2013) which to a large extent is motivated by the need for social acceptance and conformity (Hall et al., 2010).

The present study adopts the tolerance conceptual framework[3] by Dima and Dima (2016) which employs the social comparison theory as the overarching theoretical framework. Our contribution is the incorporation of two subjective factors; individual religiosity and social religiosity into the original framework. This framework will be applied to analyze the religious tolerance prevailing in four Southeast Asian countries.

[1] Theory proposes that group discrimination and prejudice are the outcomes of social groups being locked in the logic of zero-sum competition over material or symbolic resources (Dima & Dima, 2016, p. 443).

[2] "Strong reciprocity is the behavioral predisposition to cooperate conditionally on others' cooperation and to punish violations of cooperative norms even at a net cost to the punisher"(Dima & Dima, 2016, p. 443).

[3] For readers who are interested in the mathematical conceptual framework, please refer to Appendix 1.

3 Methodology

3.1 Model Specification

The baseline estimation model for our study from Dima and Dima (2016) is as shown below:

$$Tol_i = \beta_1 + \beta_2 g_i + \beta_3 g_i^2 + \beta_4 Gender_i + \beta_5 \log Age_i \\ + \beta_6 Education_i + \beta_7 Marital\ Status_i + \varepsilon_i \quad (1)$$

where Tol is religious tolerance for individual *i*, g_i is self-positioning in an income group, the square of g_i was included by Dima and Dima (2016) to capture the ∪-shape impact of income on tolerance. The remaining control variables are individuals' characteristics such gender, education, age and marital status. $\beta_i s$ are vector of estimated coefficients, and ε_i is the residual term.

The present study employs the hierarchical regression analysis estimation technique which is normally applied to assess theoretical assumptions and examine the impact of independent variables in a sequential manner (see for example, Petrocelli, 2003). The advantage of using this approach is that it allows us to determine relative importance of the additional variables introduced into the framework. The present study tests the control variables in Model 1, and incorporates the social religiosity and individual religiosity in Model 2. Social and individual religiosity are tested in the same model as both are different aspects of the same dimension, religiosity.

Thus, the extended model specification incorporating social religiosity and individual religiosity is expressed as:

$$Tol_i = \beta_1 + \beta_2 g_i + \beta_3 g_i^2 + \beta_4 Gender_i + \beta_5 \log Age_i \\ + \beta_6 Education_i + \beta_7 Marital\ Status_i \\ + \beta_8 SR_i + \beta_9 IR_i + \varepsilon_i \quad (2)$$

3.2 Variables and Sample

The dataset for this study is from the World Values Survey (WVS) 2010–2014 Wave 6. The control variables for this study are income (g_i), income square $\left(g_i^2\right)$, age, gender, education and marital status adapted from Dima and Dima (2016). The measures for social religiosity and individual religiosity are adopted from Okulicz-Kozaryn (2010). The WVS questions, descriptions and coding used in this study are shown in Table 1.

Table 1 World values survey questions and coding

WVS variable and question	Coding
Religious Tolerance (Tol_i)	
V41—on this list are various groups of people. Could you please mention any that you would not like to have as neighbors? People of a different religion	−1: Mentioned; 1: not mentioned; 0: non available/not answered
V154—please tell us if you strongly agree, agree, disagree, or strongly disagree with the following statements: the only acceptable religion is my religion	−2: Strongly agree; −1: agree; 1: disagree; 2: strongly disagree; 0: non available/not answered
V155—please tell us if you strongly agree, agree, disagree, or strongly disagree with the following statements: all religions should be taught in our public schools	2: Strongly agree; 1: agree; −1: disagree;−2: strongly disagree; 0: non available/not answered
V156—please tell us if you strongly agree, agree, disagree, or strongly disagree with the following statements: people who belong to different religions are probably just as moral as those who belong to mine	2: Strongly agree; 1: agree;−1: disagree;−2: strongly disagree; 0: non available/not answered
Social Religiosity (SR_i)	
V25—now I am going to read off a list of voluntary organizations. For each organization, could you tell me whether you are an active member, an inactive member or not a member of that type of organization? Church or religious organization	−1: Not a member; 1: inactive member; 2: active member; 0: non available/not answered
V145—apart from weddings and funerals, about how often do you attend religious services these days?	1: Never, 2: less often; 3: once a year; 4: only on special holidays; 5: once a month; 6: once a week; 7: more than once a week
Individual Religiosity (IR_i)	
V9—for each of the following, indicate how important it is in your life: religion	−2: Not at all important; −1: not very important; 1: rather important; 2 = very important; 0: non available/not answered
V147—independently of whether you attend religious services or not, would you say you are: a religious person	−2: Atheist; −1: not a religious person; 1: religious person; 0: non available/not answered
V148—do you believe in God?	−1: No; 1: yes; 0: non available/not answered
V152—how important is God in your life? Please use this scale to indicate. 10 means "very important" and 1 means "not at all important."	1: Not at all important; 10: very important; 0: non available/not answered

(continued)

Table 1 (continued)

WVS variable and question	Coding
Income Group (g_i)	
V239—on this card is an income scale on which 1 indicates the lowest income group and 10 the highest income group in your country. We would like to know in what group your household is	1: lower step; 2: second step; 3: third step; 4: fourth step; 5: fifth step; 6: sixth step; 7: seventh step; 8: eighth step; 9: ninth step; 10: tenth step; 0: non available/not answered
Gender	
V240—gender	1: Female; 0: otherwise
Age	
V242—this means you are ____ years old (write in age in two digits)	
Education	
V248—what is the highest educational level that you have attained?	−4: No formal education;−3: incomplete primary school; −2: complete primary school; −1: incomplete secondary school: technical/vocational type; 1: complete secondary school: technical/vocational type; 2: incomplete secondary school: university-preparatory type; 3: complete secondary school: university-preparatory type; 4: some university-level education, without degree; 5: university—level education, with degree
Marital Status	
V57—marital status	1: Single; 0: otherwise

Note Authors' compilation

The sample includes respondents from Malaysia (1250), Philippines (1170), Singapore (1429) and Thailand (946). The sample has a balanced proportion of male and female respondents, Malaysia has (51.2% male), Philippines (50% male), Singapore (44.5% male) and Thailand (52.8% male). The mean age of the respondents in Malaysia (39 years), Philippines (43 years), Singapore (43 years) and Thailand (46 years). The percentage of married respondents were higher in this sample with Malaysia having (68%), Philippines (69%), Singapore (62%) and Thailand (69%). The percentage of respondents having a university degrees in Malaysia (6%), Philippines (14%), Singapore (24%) and Thailand (15.4%).

Religious tolerance was measured using four questions from the World Values Survey (WVS) 2010–2014 Wave 6. The first question, V41, was on whether the respondents could mention people of other religion that they would not like to have as neighbors. This question recorded a higher percentage for respondents from Thailand (34%) and Malaysia (30%) indicating they did not like having neighbors from a different religion compared to Philippines (16%) and Singapore (11%). The second question, V154, on whether they agreed with the statement '*the only acceptable religion was my religion*' respondents from Malaysia (70.8%) strongly agreed or agreed with this statement, followed by Philippines (64.9%), Thailand (38.4%) and Singapore (25.9%). The third question, V155, higher percentage of respondents from Singapore (81%) strongly disagreed or disagreed that all religions should be taught in our public schools compared to Thailand (43.3%), Philippines (40.1) and Malaysia (35.6%). The final question of religious tolerance, V156, on whether '*people who belong to different religions are probably just as moral as those who belong to mine*', respondents from Thailand (81.1%) strongly agreed or agreed with this statement, followed by Malaysia (79.2%), Singapore (75.5%) and Philippines (73.2%).

Social religiosity was measured using four questions from the World Values Survey (WVS) 2010–2014 Wave 6. The first question, V25, on whether they are an active member, an inactive member or not a member of a church or religious organization, Philippines (35.9%) had the highest percentage of active members, followed by Singapore (28.4%), Thailand (14.8%) and Malaysia (14.7%). The second question, V145, on the frequency of attendance of religious services, Philippines (64.9%) recorded the highest frequency for once a week or more than once in a week, followed by Malaysia (52.4%), Singapore (35.7%) and Thailand (34%).

There were four items measuring individual religiosity. Firstly, V9, on how important religion was to the respondent. Religion was considered very important by respondents from Philippines (86.1%), Malaysia (85%), Thailand (58.5%) and Singapore (43.3%). The second item, V147, on whether the respondent is a religious person, the highest percentage of religious persons were from Philippines (81.2%), Singapore (59.1%), Malaysia (53.4%) and Thailand (35.9%). Third item, V148, on whether the respondents believed in God, Philippines (99.6%) recorded the highest percentage of believers, followed by Malaysia (98.9%), Singapore (84.3%) and Thailand (30%). The final item, V152, *'How important is God in your life'*, those who choose very important were from Philippines (83.4%), Malaysia (68.2%), Singapore (23.9%) and Thailand (6.9%).

4 Empirical Results

Hierarchical regression was performed to investigate the role of religiosity on religious tolerance, after controlling for income, education and other demographic factors. A diagnostic analysis was carried out to ensure no violation of normality, linearity, homoscedasticity and collinearity assumptions. The diagnostics flagged a concern on collinearity. The variance inflation factor (VIF) for income square and age were above the acceptable level, thus these control variables were removed. The subsequent diagnostic indicated that VIF was between 1.279 and 9.390 removing any concerns on multi-collinearity. The hierarchical regression results for the four countries are presented in Table 2. The first step of the hierarchical model (Model 1) included the control variables, income, education, gender and marital status these variables were statistically significant for all four countries. The second step of the

Table 2 Hierarchical regression analysis of predictors for religious tolerance

	Malaysia		Philippines		Thailand		Singapore	
	Model 1	Model 2	Model 1	Model 2	Model 1	Model 2	Model 1	Model 2
Income	0.431*** (11.406)	0.870*** (11.060)	0.305*** (8.121)	0.071 (1.354)	0.512*** (14.562)	0.353*** (7.160)	0.267*** (6.861)	0.078 (1.537)
Education	−0.037 (−1.295)	−0.052* (−1.869)	0.063** (2.068)	0.075** (2.514)	0.058** (2.220)	0.071*** (2.730)	0.158*** (5.182)	0.191*** (6.215)
Gender	−0.035 (−1.009)	−0.003 (−0.073)	0.099** (2.976)	−0.013 (−0.348)	0.125*** (4.276)	0.095*** (3.197)	0.134*** (3.643)	0.076** (2.040)
Marital status	0.044 (1.430)	0.053* (1.725)	0.048* (1.674)	0.017 (0.598)	−0.004 (−0.155)	−0.002 (−0.074)	0.116*** (3.552)	0.099*** (3.080)
Social religiosity		−0.227*** (−3.835)		0.018 (0.231)		−0.044 (−0.950)		0.093* (1.892)
Individual religiosity		−0.279*** (−2.947)		0.346*** (4.082)		0.240*** (4.550)		0.223*** (5.199)
R^2	0.178	0.206	0.183	0.211	0.409	0.420	0.229	0.261
ΔR^2	0.178	0.032	0.183	0.028	0.409	0.011	0.229	0.033
ΔF	67.264***	25.004***	65.108***	20.853***	246.683***	12.913***	69.785***	20.767***
Sample size	1250	1250	1170	1170	1429	1429	946	946

Note t-values in parentheses

*, **, *** denote significance at 10%, 5% and 1% respectively

hierarchical model (Model 2) included social religiosity and individual religiosity. Individual religosity was statistically significant for all four countries.

The results for Malaysia indicate that three of the control variables, income, education and marital status are significant in explaining religious tolerance. In addition, both social and individual religiosity significantly impact religious tolerance in Malaysia. Religiosity explains 3.2% of variance in religious tolerance. A one unit increase in social religiosity results in a 0.227 unit decrease in religious tolerance. Meanwhile, a one unit increase in individual religiosity results in 0.279 unit decrease in religious tolerance. The findings are intriguing as both social and individual religiosity contribute towards religious intolerance. However, the magnitude of impact of individual religiosity on religious intolerance is greater compared to social religiosity. In case of Philippines, for the control variable only education is significant in explaining religious tolerance. Individual religiosity significantly impacts religious tolerance in Philippines, while social religiosity does not impact religious tolerance. The introduction of the religiosity variables explain an additional 2.8% changes to religious tolerance, where the changes are solely from individual religiosity. It is also worth noting that individual religiosity has a positive impact on tolerance where a one unit increase in individual religiosity leads to a 0.346 units increase in religious tolerance.

The control variables impacting religious tolerance in Thailand are education, income and gender. For religiosity, individual and not social religiosity that impacts religious tolerance. This is similar to the case of Philippines. The incremental variance to religious tolerance explained by religiosity, or more specifically individual religiosity is 1.1%. Individual religiosity positively impacts religious tolerance where a one unit increase in individual religiosity increases religious tolerance by 0.240 units. In case of Singapore, marital status, education, gender and individual religiosity impact religious tolerance. The religiosity component, accounts for 3.3% of the changes in religious tolerance where a one unit increase in individual religiosity results in a 0.223 unit increase in religious tolerance.

5 Discussion and Conclusion

Individual religiosity impacts religious tolerance in all the four countries. In Malaysia, individual religiosity leads to religious intolerance. Malaysia differs significantly from Philippines, Thailand and Singapore, where in these countries individual religiosity enhances religious tolerance. Literature reports of mixed findings on the relationship between individual religiosity and tolerance (Farrell et al., 2018). Some studies show a positive relationship between individual religiosity (Beck & Miller, 2000; Ekici & Yucel, 2015; Lynch et al., 2017) and religious tolerance which is aligned to the results obtained for Philippines, Thailand and Singapore. Studies have also highlighted of individual religiosity leading to increased religious intolerance, as in the case of Malaysia. The motivation for this behavior includes among others uncertainty towards followers of other religion (Kossowska & Sekerdej, 2015), and selective intolerance towards persons perceived to exhibit behavior which are not consistent with some traditional religious teachings (Batson, 2013; Batson et al., 1993; Rowatt et al., 2009). Second aspect of religiosity, social religiosity, does not impact tolerance in Philippines, and Thailand but fuels religious intolerance in Malaysia. Studies justifying the impact of social religiosity on higher levels of intolerance highlight factors such as the need for social acceptance and conformity (Batson, 2013; Hall et al., 2010) and in-group cooperation which generates hostile attitudes towards out-groups (Lynch et al., 2017) as possible contributors. The subsequent discussion focuses on rationalizing the findings of why Malaysia significantly differs from the rest of her neighbors.

Malaysia has a higher religious diversity compared to Philippines and Thailand (Pew Research Center, 2014) but our findings indicate lower religious tolerance stemming from both individual and social religiosity. A finding which is of concern and alerts one to the caution raised earlier on the prevalence of a deceptive religious tolerance in a religiously pluralistic society (Bo & Wahid, 2016; Pilling, 2017). In order to decipher this phenomenon, an understanding of the ethno-religiosity of the country is essential. Malaysia was a colonial country under the British and was subjected to the divide and rule policy. The British segregated the three main ethnic groups—Malay (Muslims), Chinese (Buddhist and Christians) and Indian (Hindus and Christians)—by settlement and occupation (Abdul Ghani & Awang, 2017). Against this background of a divide and rule policy, the ethnic relations suffered from less interactions and economic disparities (Abdul Ghani & Awang, 2017). The ethnic-religiosity of the Malaysian society was aptly described by the country's longest serving Prime Minister in his book, the *Malay Dilemma* stating that a semblance of a harmonious society depicted not a lack, rather an absences of open display of conflicts (Mohamad, 1970).

Although acknowledging that the impetus for religious intolerance stemmed from colonial practices, however, it would be premature to attribute it purely to these policies. After all, Malaysia has been an independent nation for more than sixty years. A study by Talib and Gill (2012) highlights of the presence of two distinct communities in Malaysia. On one end of the spectrum, a highly tolerant society harmoniously coexisting with people of diverse beliefs. On the other end, a society with lower level of tolerance, agitated by differences, resulting in unwanted incidents. The ambiguity in religious tolerance in Malaysia is attributed to a lack of conscientious effort in pursuing this goal (Abdul Ghani & Awang, 2017). A point of contention is that domestic political conditions favored the existence of these religious and ethnic bubbles. The politicization of religion is seen as a zero sum game to cling to political power (Liow, 2015). It is claimed that religion is used as a divisive tool to magnify racial and ethnic differences to gain political mileage by allowing extreme right-wing ethno-nationalists and propagation of hateful and discriminatory speeches (Liow, 2015). Malaysia's religious tolerance has its genesis in history and is further compounded by politics but in the final analysis, it can be actualized by mutual respect and understanding which is crucial for a country housing a diverse and plural society. What is needed is the political will to give prominence to fostering religious tolerance. A change that appears feasible given that the previous ruling government has been ousted and the new government appears committed to pursuing a progressive role of tolerance.

Our findings on Thailand and Philippines have also raised some significant questions. How widely prevalent and pervasive is religious intolerance in countries experiencing faith-based tensions in Southeast Asia? Could these faith-based tensions be taken as an indication of rising religious intolerance? In the case of Thailand, reports indicate that religious intolerance might not be a contributing factor for the religious conflicts in the southern region of the country. The government of Thailand maintains that the religious conflicts are not fueled by religious intolerance but stems from dissatisfaction due to social and economic inequalities resulting from past development policies (International Panel of Parliamentarians for Freedom of Religion or Belief & Asia Centre, 2017). A claim that is supported by the findings of the present study where in Thailand and Philippines religiosity enhances religious tolerance.

In conclusion, the findings of this study has highlighted that religious intolerance is not a concern in countries that currently experience religious conflicts. However that is not the case for Malaysia, a country with a religiously diverse population and without any faith-based conflicts. This indicates that a façade of tolerance might guise the actual reality on the ground. And alternatively, incidents of faith-based conflicts might be wrongly perceived as an indication of rising religious intolerance within a society. However either way, it is important for the policymakers in Southeast Asia to be more vigilant and look into implementing policies that would promote religious tolerance in the region.

Appendix 1

The utility estimation from the decision making process was expressed in the function below

$$U^i : \propto_1 g_i^2 - \propto_2 g_i + \beta_1 s_i^2 - \beta_2 s_i + \chi_1 g_i^2 s_i^2 - \chi_2 g_i s_i + \delta_1 \psi_i^2 - \delta_2 \psi_1 \tag{3}$$

The self-positioning in an income group is denoted by g_i, while s_i is an evaluation of the quality of the social environment, the interaction term $g_i s_i$ expresses the synergy between comparison in income and the perceived quality of the social relationship while ψ_1 is a vector of other potential determinants of utility. The perceived quality of the social environment was expressed as:

$$s_i = w_1 tol^i - w_2 c^i \tag{4}$$

The perceived quality of social environment is expressed as influenced by degree of tolerance (tol^i) and the predisposition towards tolerance or confrontation (c^i).

Dima and Dima (2016) elaborates that Equation (4) captures the attitude of balance between tolerance and confrontation. Stating that an individual might be tolerant to one religious group but intolerant towards another or express preferences for certain behavior in public but intolerant in private life. Equation (4) was substituted in utility function (Equation 3). After having derived the new utility function, they proceeded to differentiate tolerance against utility to obtain the optimal level of tolerance that maximizes individual utility. Therefore, the optimal tolerance level was given as:

$$tol^{opt} = \frac{\beta_2 w_1 + \chi_2 g_i w_1 - 2w_1 w_2\left(\beta_1 c^i + \chi_1 g_i^2\right)}{2w_1^2 \beta_1\left(1 + w_1 w_2 c^i + \chi_1 g_i^2\right)} \quad (5)$$

In order to enhance the explanatory power of this framework, Dima and Dima (2016) suggested incorporating subjective factors (ϑ) into the framework. The present study incorporates two subjective factors; individual religiosity and social religiosity. The influence of these two subjective variables on predisposition towards tolerance and confrontation is expressed as follows:

$$c^i = c^i\left(\vartheta^i\right) \quad (6)$$

Taking into consideration the impact of these two variables, the optimal level of tolerance for the present study is re-written as:

$$tol^{opt} = \frac{\beta_2 w_1 + \chi_2 g_i w_1 - 2w_1 w_2\left(\beta_1 c^i\left(\vartheta^i\right) + \chi_1 g_i^2\right)}{2w_1^2 \beta_1\left(1 + w_1 w_2 c^i + \chi_1 g_i^2\right)} \quad (7)$$

Equation (7) shows the optimal level of tolerance which maximizes individual utility after the inclusion of the two subjective variables.

References

Abdul Ghani, R., & Awang, J. (2017). A review on writings on religious tolerance in Malaysia. *International Journal of Islamic Thought, 12*(1), 72–82. https://doi.org/10.24035/ijit.12.2017.007

Akerlof, G., & Kranton, R. (2000). Economics and Identity. *Quarterly Journal of Economics, 115*(3), 715–753. https://doi.org/10.1162/003355300554881

Akerlof, G., & Kranton, R. (2010). *Identity economics: How identities shape our work, wages, and well-being.* Princeton University Press.

Allport, G. W., & Ross, J. M. (1967). Personal religious orientation and prejudice. *Journal of Personality and Social Psychology, 5*(4), 432–443. https://doi.org/10.1037/h0021212

Anderson, G. M. (1988). Mr. Smith and the Preachers: The economics of religion in the wealth of nations. *Journal of Political Economy, 96*(5), 1066–1088. https://doi.org/10.1086/261576

Association of Religion Data Archives. (2018). Theories, concepts, and measurements|religiosity. Retrieved September 10, 2018, from http://wiki.thearda.com/tcm/concepts/religiosity/

Batson, C. D. (2013). Individual religion, tolerance, and universal compassion. In S. Clarke, R. Powell, & J. Savulescu (Eds.), *Religion, intolerance, and conflict: A scientific and conceptual investigation* (pp. 88–106). Oxford University Press.

Batson, C. D., Schoenrade, P., & Ventis, W. L. (1993). *Religion and the individual: A social-psychological perspective.* Oxford University Press.

Beck, R., & Miller, C. D. (2000). Religiosity and agency and communion: Their relationship to religious judgmentalism. *The Journal of Psychology, 134*(3), 315–324. https://doi.org/10.1080/00223980009600871

Beugelsdijk, S., & van Schaik, T. (2005). Social capital and growth in European regions: an empirical test. *European Journal of Political Economy, 21*(2), 301–324.https://doi.org/10.1016/j.ejpoleco.2004.07.004

Bo, C. M., & Wahid, A. (2016, September 27). Rejecting religious intolerance in Southeast Asia: Four steps to preserving the diversity that distinguishes this region. *The Wall Street Journal.* Retrieved from www.wsj.com/articles/rejecting-religious-intolerance-in-southeast-asia-1474992874

Dima, B., & Dima, ŞM. (2016). Income distribution and social tolerance. *Social Indicators Research, 128*(1), 439–466. https://doi.org/10.1007/s11205-015-1038-y

Ekici, T., & Yucel, D. (2015). What determines religious and racial prejudice in Europe? The effects of religiosity and trust. *Social Indicators Research, 122*(1), 105–133. https://doi.org/10.1007/s11205-014-0674-y

Farrell, J. E., Hook, J. N., Zhang, H., Mosher, D., Aten, J. D., Van Tongeren, D. R., & Davis, D. E. (2018). Religious attitudes and behaviors toward individuals who hold different religious beliefs and perspectives: An exploratory qualitative study. *Psychology of Religion and Spirituality, 10*(1), 63–71. https://doi.org/10.1037/rel0000143

Fein, S., & Spencer, S. J. (1997). Prejudice as self-image maintenance: Affirming the self through derogating others. *Journal of Personality and Social Psychology, 73*(1), 31–44. https://doi.org/10.1037//0022-3514.73.1.31

Festinger, L. (1954). A theory of social comparison processes. *Human Relations, 7*(2), 117–140. https://doi.org/10.1177/001872675400700202

Garcia, S. M., Tor, A., & Schiff, T. M. (2013). The psychology of competition. *Perspectives on Psychological Science, 8*(6), 634–650. https://doi.org/10.1177/1745691613504114

Greer, T., Berman, M., Varan, V., Bobrycki, L., & Watson, S. (2005). We are a religious people; we are a vengeful people. *Journal for the Scientific Study of Religion, 44*(1), 45–57. https://doi.org/10.1111/j.1468-5906.2005.00264.x

Hall, D. L., Matz, D. C., & Wood, W. (2010). Why don't we practice what we preach? A meta-analytic Review of religious racism. *Personality and Social Psychology Review, 14*(1), 126–139. https://doi.org/10.1177/1088868309352179

Hanna, K. S., Dale, A., & Ling, C. (2009). Social capital and quality of place: Reflections on growth and change in a small town. *Local Environment, 14*(1), 31–44. https://doi.org/10.1080/13549830802522434

Helliwell, J. F., & Putnam, R. D. (1995). Economic growth and social capital in Italy. *Eastern Economic Journal, 21*(3), 295–307.

International Panel of Parliamentarians for Freedom of Religion or Belief, & Asia Centre. (2017). *Country briefing on freedom of religion or belief in the universal periodic review process—Thailand.* Retrieved from http://ippforb.com/wp-content/uploads/2017/10/FORB-Thailand.pdf

Johnson, M. K., Rowatt, W. C., Barnard-Brak, L. M., Patock-Peckham, J. A., LaBouff, J. P., & Carlisle, R. D. (2011). A mediational analysis of the role of right-wing authoritarianism and religious fundamentalism in the religiosity–prejudice link. *Personality and Individual Differences, 50*(6), 851–856. https://doi.org/10.1016/j.paid.2011.01.010

Kossowska, M., & Sekerdej, M. (2015). Searching for certainty: Religious beliefs and intolerance toward value-violating groups. *Personality and Individual Differences, 83*, 72–76. https://doi.org/10.1016/j.paid.2015.03.053

Liow, J. C. (2015). Malaysia's ISIS conundrum. Retrieved August 1, 2018, from https://www.brookings.edu/opinions/malaysias-isis-conundrum/

Lynch, R., Palestis, B., & Trivers, R. (2017). Religious devotion and extrinsic religiosity affect in-group altruism and out-group hostility oppositely in Rural Jamaica. *Evolutionary Psychological Science, 3*(4), 335–344. https://doi.org/10.1007/s40806-017-0103-y

Mohamad, T. M. (1970). *The malay dilemma.* Times Books International.

Norris, P., & Davis, J. (2007). A continental divide? Social capital in the US and Europe. In *Measuring attitudes cross-nationally* (pp. 238–264) SAGE Publications, Ltd. https://doi.org/10.4135/9781849209458.n11

Okulicz-Kozaryn, A. (2010). Religiosity and life satisfaction across nations. *Mental Health, Religion & Culture, 13*(2), 155–169. https://doi.org/10.1080/13674670903273801

Petrocelli, J. V. (2003). Hierarchical multiple regression in counseling research: Common problems and possible remedies. *Measurement and Evaluation in Counseling and Development, 36*, 9–22. Retrieved from http://www.datapsyc.com/petrocelli_2003.pdf

Pew Research Center. (2014). Global Religious Diversity: Half of the Most Religiously Diverse Countries are in Asia-Pacific Region. Retrieved from http://www.pewresearch.org.

Pew Research Center. (2016). Global Restrictions on Religion 2007–2016 [Data file and code book]. Retrieved from http://www.pewresearch.org.

Pilling, D. (2017). Southeast Asia's religious tolerance is deceptive. *Financial Times.* Retrieved from https://www.ft.com/content/6128d792-9fea-11e4-aa89-00144feab7de

Portes, A. (2014). Downsides of social capital. *Proceedings of the National Academy of Sciences, 111*(52), 18407–18408. https://doi.org/10.1073/pnas.1421888112

Putnam, R. D. (1995a). Bowling alone: America's declining social capital. *Journal of Democracy, 6*(1), 65–78.https://doi.org/10.1353/jod.1995.0002

Putnam, R. D. (1995b). Tuning in, tuning out: The strange disappearance of social capital in America. *PS: Political Science & Politics, 28*(04), 664–683. https://doi.org/10.1017/S1049096500058856

Quinn, P. L. (2001). Religious diversity and religious toleration. *International Journal for Philosophy of Religion Issues in Contemporary Philosophy of Religion, 503*(1), 57–80. Retrieved from http://www.jstor.org/stable/40020983

Rosenberg, N. (1960). Some institutional aspects of the wealth of nations. *Journal of Political Economy, 68*(6), 557–570. https://doi.org/10.1086/258392

Rowatt, W. C., LaBouff, J., Johnson, M., Froese, P., & Tsang, J.-A. (2009). Associations among religiousness, social attitudes, and prejudice in a national random sample of American adults. *Psychology of Religion and Spirituality, 1*(1), 14–24. https://doi.org/10.1037/a0014989

Sedikides, C., & Gebauer, J. E. (2010). Religiosity as self-enhancement: A meta-analysis of the relation between socially desirable responding and religiosity. *Personality and Social Psychology Review, 14*(1), 17–36. https://doi.org/10.1177/1088868309351002

Smith, A. (2007). *Adam Smith. An inquiry into the nature and causes of the wealth of nations.* In R. H. Campbell & A. S. Skinner (Eds.), (Fourth). Oxford University Press. Retrieved from http://eet.pixel-online.org/files/etranslation/original/TheWealthofNations.pdf

Strabac, Z., & Listhaug, O. (2008). Anti-Muslim prejudice in Europe: A multilevel analysis of survey data from 30 countries. *Social Science Research, 37*(1), 268–286. https://doi.org/10.1016/j.ssresearch.2007.02.004

Strickhouser, J. E., & Zell, E. (2015). Self-evaluative effects of dimensional and social comparison. *JourNal of Experimental Social Psychology, 59*, 60–66. https://doi.org/10.1016/j.jesp.2015.03.001

Talib, A. T., & Gill, S. S. (2012). Socio-religious tolerance: Exploring the Malaysian experience. *Global Journal of Human-Social Science Research, 12*(8), 1–7.

Taylor, S. E., & Lobel, M. (1989). Social comparison activity under threat: Downward evaluation and upward contacts. *Psychological Review, 96*(4), 569–575. https://doi.org/10.1037//0033-295X.96.4.569

Yeung, J. W. K., Chan, Y.-C., & Lee, B. L. K. (2009). Youth religiosity and substance use: A meta-analysis from 1995 to 2007. *Psychological Reports, 105*(1), 255–266. https://doi.org/10.2466/PR0.105.1.255-266

Sotheeswari Somasundram is a senior lecturer with Taylor's Business School, Taylor's University. She has more than 20 years of experience in higher education, with extensive experience in curriculum design and new programme creation. Her research interests are in Economics of Religion, Urbanisation and Entrepreneurship Education.

Muzafar Shah Habibullah is a Professor at Putra Business School, Selangor, Malaysia. He holds a Ph.D. in Economics from the University of Southampton, United Kingdom. His specialization includes Applied Macroeconomics, Monetary Economics and Banking.

Murali Sambasivan has more than 20 years of teaching experience and 10 years of industry experience. His research interests are in the areas of Management Science, Operations Management, Supply Chain Management and other areas of management. He is currently working as a Professor and Director at Thiagarajar School of Management, Madurai, India. Prof Murali has published more than 120 articles in many international refereed journals such as International Journal of Production Economics, Journal of Cleaner Production, Technovation, Computers and Operations Research, International Journal of Physical Distribution and Logistics Management, International Journal of Project Management, International Journal of Medical Informatics, Journal of Biomedical Informatics and many more. He has supervised/co-supervised more than 60 Ph.D. and M.Sc. students.

Ratneswary Rasiah is an Associate Professor of Economics at Taylor's Business School, Taylor's University, where she has been attached for the last twenty one years. She has extensive teaching experience in the field of Economics, having taught numerous undergraduate and postgraduate modules. She received the Taylor's Education Group Chairman's Award for Excellence in Teaching for her immense contribution in the field of teaching and learning. Dr. Ratneswary also actively undertakes research and scholarly activities.

Social Capital as a Source of Subjective Well-Being

Formal and Informal Institutions as Drivers of Life Satisfaction in European Regions

Jesús Peiró-Palomino and Emili Tortosa-Ausina

1 Introduction

For several years the attention of economists has focused mostly on income and related issues. This tendency changed during the last decade, when citizen's well-being became a topic of increasing interest. In that regard, the appearance of new databases providing reliable data on variables such as happiness or life satisfaction spurred the number of empirical contributions. This chapter contributes to this literature by analysing the links between informal, formal institutions and life satisfaction for a wide sample of European regions.

Both types of institutions, whose importance has been highlighted in key contributions such as those by Douglass North, Joan Robinson or Daron Acemoglu (among others),[1] have been found to be positively associated to higher levels of life satisfaction, showing more intense effects than variables such as income or education. In these cases, significant associations hold only when relatively simple models are specified, which might suggest that they are mere transmission channels of other determinants (Helliwell, 2006; Helliwell et al., 2018). Today, the list of studies is extensive, although it is mostly confined to the country level.

Formal institutions are generally proxied by measures of quality of government. Frey and Stutzer (2000) linked government quality to higher levels of well-being,

[1] See, for instance, North (1986, 1989, 1991, 1994), or Robinson and Acemoglu (2012).

J. Peiró-Palomino (✉)
Department of Applied Economics II and INTECO, University of Valencia, Av dels Tarongers, 46022 Valencia, Spain
e-mail: jesus.peiro@uv.es

E. Tortosa-Ausina
Departament d'Economia, Universitat Jaume I and IIDL, Av Vicent Sos Baynat, 12071 Castelló de la Plana, Spain

A. Almakaeva et al. (eds.), *Social Capital and Subjective Well-Being*, Societies and Political Orders in Transition,
https://doi.org/10.1007/978-3-030-75813-4_8

suggesting as major mechanisms the existence of political outcomes more aligned to voters' preferences, as well as higher utility derived from increased political participation. Frey and Stutzer (2005) and Ott (2010) argued that people feel happier in good governance contexts. Similarly, Ott (2011) concluded that better government increases happiness and reduces happiness inequality. In addition to these direct effects, there may be important indirect effects too. For example, Helliwell et al. (2018) hold that high quality governments may increase the efficiency of companies, both private and public, and generate favorable conditions for progress. Moreover, a healthy institutional framework also benefits the relationships between government and citizens, and even relationships among citizens (Helliwell et al., 2018). Other authors such as Bjørnskov et al. (2010) provided results for different types of institutional quality, finding a preponderant impact of the quality of economic-judicial institutions on happiness in low-income countries, whereas middle- and high-income economies benefit more from improvements in political institutions. In this line, Orviska et al. (2014) found a positive effect from satisfaction with democracy to well-being.

Regarding informal institutions, these can be understood as social capital, a multifaceted concept encompassing a variety of elements (Bjørnskov, 2006). Social trust is the indicator for which more evidence is available, and its positive role in explaining subjective well-being is widely supported. In particular, Helliwell (2006) concluded that trustworthy environments foster people's contacts, which are, in addition, more successful. In this line, Bjørnskov (2008) concluded that in high trust areas people are more interactive, even with unknown fellows. Trust makes feel citizens safer, interactions are easier and more predictable, and this ultimately translates into a happier life. Considering data at the individual level, Han (2015) shows that individual social capital have a positive effect on happiness. At the country level, Kuroki et al. (2011) Tokuda et al. (2010) and Yamamura et al. (2015) provided additional empirical evidence on that regard for different geographical settings. For the European, context Portela et al. (2013) found that social networks, social trust and institutional trust are the social capital components showing a higher correlation with subjective well-being. More recently, Bartolini et al. (2017) suggested that the effect of trust on life satisfaction can be as powerful as that for income, but this association is only found for the medium term, whereas in the short run economic conditions generally dominate. Using individual level data, Neira et al. (2018) provide more refined results, showing that social capital improvements affect the most to the unhappiest people.

Whereas at the country level the number of studies is large, they are much more scant at the regional level due to data constrains. The main contribution of this chapter is the assessment of these linkages at the regional level, considering a wide sample of European regions. Formal institutions are proxied by a composite indicator of government quality, the European Quality of Government Index (EQI), available at the regional level. For informal institutions, i.e. social capital, we cover two dimensions with two indicators, social trust and perceived social network support. Results suggest a positive effect of both formal and informal institutions on self-reported levels of life satisfaction, although the impact is driven by the regional level of life satisfaction, i.e. a different effect is found for low and high levels of life satisfaction. These effects are robust to the inclusion of a wide set of regional control variables.

The chapter is structured as follows. After this introduction, in Sect. 2 we provide details on the sample and data used, as well as the corresponding sources, whereas Sects. 3 and 4 describe the methodology and discuss the results, respectively. Finally, Sect. 5 provides some concluding remarks.

2 Sample, Data and Sources

The sample comprises 166 European regions at NUTS1 and NUTS2 level of disaggregation, which is determined by the availability of data. The dependent variable of the analysis is self-reported life satisfaction, which lies between 0 (worst score) and 10 (best score). It is provided by the OECD Regional Well-being Dataset,[2] where figures are available only for years 2000 and 2014. However, figures for the 2014 dataset actually refer to the period 2006–2014, depending on the region. In any case, regional life satisfaction levels are expected to remain relatively stable is such a short period of time.

As independent variables, we measure formal institutions using the EQI index, an indicator of institutional quality at the regional level constructed by the Quality of Government Institute (QOG). It is a composite indicator based on three pillars: (i) corruption; (ii) impartiality; and (iii) quality. All the details on its construction can be found in the seminal papers (see Charron et al., 2014, 2015). Information is available for years 2010, 2013 and 2017, although for compatibility with the dependent variable we considered the average value of 2010 and 2013.

The informal institutions are proxied by two variables, namely the level of social trust and the perceived social network support, which represent two different dimensions of the more general concept social capital. As already commented, social trust is the most popular social capital indicator in the literature and information can be obtained from surveys. In particular, the question used to measure social trust reads as follows "Generally speaking, would you say that most people can be trusted, or that you can't be too careful in dealing with people?". The social trust indicator corresponds to the percentage of respondents that declared trusting others in each region. We used the most recent wave of the European Values Study (EVS) at the time of writing, corresponding to 2008. Using data from a previous year different to those for the dependent variable is not problematic in this case, as the specialised literature has considered trust as time-invariant, or at least remarkably stable in the short and medium run. At the country level, Bjørnskov (2007) reported high persistence in social trust levels across different waves of the World Values Survey (the macro survey providing country-level data). Following this strand of the literature, other authors have linked current trust levels to historical facts, thus showing that cultural features and personal beliefs are highly persistent over time. For instance,

[2] Available at https://www.oecdregionalwellbeing.org/.

Uslaner (2008) found a highly significant correlation between trust levels reported by descendants of immigrants to the USA and those in their ancestors' countries of origin. Similarly, Nunn and Wantchekon (2011) linked today's low trust levels in Africa to the transatlantic and Indian Ocean slave trade from a century ago. More recently, Geys and Qari (2017) concluded that individuals' social trust quickly returns to its long-run equilibrium level after violent unexpected events such as terrorist attacks.

The second indicator, perceived social network support, is measured as the percentage of people positively answering the question "Do you have relatives or friends you can count on?". Analogously to the dependent variable, the information is provided by the OECD Regional Well-being Dataset and it is labeled as 2014, although figures actually correspond to the period 2006–2014, depending on the region. Similarly to life satisfaction and trust, this variable is expected to be relatively stable too.

We also control for many other factors potentially explaining life satisfaction at the regional level, including income, education, the unemployment rate, safety levels, pollution, housing availability and broadband access. Other control variables are the dependency rate, the degree of urbanisation and the population density, all provided by the OECD Regional Database. Again, data labeled as 2014 correspond to earlier years, mostly to the period 2006–2014, which make them compatible with our variables of interest.[3] Table 1 reports all the variables together with a short description, their sources and some descriptive statistics.

Table 2 provides information by country for the main variables of interest. Regarding life satisfaction, Denmark, Finland and the Netherlands head the ranking, while Estonia, Greece and Portugal are at the bottom. Italy and Germany are the countries with the largest within-country disparities whereas the Nordic countries are the most homogenous. Focusing on government quality, Denmark, Finland and Sweden are in the top three and most of the Eastern European economies together with Italy and Greece show the worst performance. The largest within-country disparities are found in Italy, in line with the literature supporting the evidence of the great North-South divide in this country. Considering social trust, the pattern is fairly similar to that shown by government quality, with large disparities between the Nordic countries and the Netherlands, with the highest scores and the ex-soviet countries holding the worst social trust levels. Finally, the levels of social network support are generally high across the sample (in all countries the percentage is above 80%). Greece holds the lowest score (80.69%) in front of Ireland (96.60%), with the highest value. The largest within-country disparities for this variable are found in Germany and Italy, although in general this is the most evenly distributed indicator.

The above description reveals important inequalities across European economies. As a general tendency, the Nordic countries and the Netherlands score the best in terms of both types of institutions, and people report the highest levels of life satisfaction too. In contrast, those countries that were part of the soviet block together

[3] Detailed information for each variable and measurement year by country can be found at the user's guide of the dataset, freely available at the database website.

Table 1 Descriptive statistics

	Description (unit of measure)	Source	Mean	S.d.
Life satisfaction	Self-reported life satisfaction (0–10)	OECD Regional Well-being Dataset	6.57	0.65
Government quality	EQI index (-3 -3)	Quality of Government Institute	0.37	0.82
Social trust	People who report trust in others (%)	European Values Study	37.00	19.00
Social network	People who report having relatives or friends they can count on (%)	OECD Regional Well-being Dataset	91.61	4.13
Dependency rate	Population aged > 65 over total population 15–64 (%)	OECD Regional Well-being Dataset	27.30	5.58
Population density	Inhabitants per km^2	OECD Regional Well-being Dataset	346.28	846.64
Rural	Rurality index (1 totally urban, 5 totally rural)	OECD Regional Well-being Dataset	3.70	1.28
Education	Labour force with secondary education (%)	OECD Regional Well-being Dataset	78.45	12.46
Income	Disposable household income (US dollars)	OECD Regional Well-being Dataset	18,082	4,531
Unemployment	Unemployment rate 15–64 (%)	OECD Regional Well-being Dataset	10.71	6.30
Safety	Homicides per 100,000 inhabitants	OECD Regional Well-being Dataset	1.20	1.01
Pollution	Air pollution (level of PM2.5)	OECD Regional Well-being Dataset	11.86	4.08
Housing	Average number of rooms per inhabitant	OECD Regional Well-being Dataset	1.79	0.37
Broadband access	Population with broadband access (%)	OECD Regional Well-being Dataset	77.74	9.28

with Portugal and Greece show the worst levels of all the indicators and people declare lower satisfaction with life.

Figure 1 displays scatter plots for the basic relationships of interest. In all three cases a positive correlation is observed, similar in intensity. In particular, the Pearson's correlations are 0.80, 0.62 and 0.61 for government quality, social trust and social network, respectively. The densities in Fig. 2 support these arguments. For both the case of formal and the two indicators of informal institutions, life satisfaction is higher in those regions where these fundamentals are above the mean. Although this is merely a descriptive result, it provides the first insights on a positive association between institutions and life satisfaction in the European context.

Table 2 Life satisfaction and institutions by country

	# of regions	Life satisfaction		Government quality		Social trust		Social network support	
		Mean	S.d.	Mean	S.d.	Mean	S.d.	Mean	S.d.
Austria	9	7.300	0.122	1.065	0.167	36.833	14.189	92.978	1.547
Belgium	3	6.933	0.231	0.371	0.677	35.084	9.738	91.633	2.483
Czech Republic	8	6.450	0.214	−0.341	0.269	29.923	10.754	88.188	4.884
Germany	16	6.638	0.316	0.894	0.144	44.875	22.841	94.006	1.183
Denmark	5	7.600	0.100	1.648	0.113	76.043	0.000	96.160	1.115
Estonia	1	5.440	–	0.112	–	32.617	–	87.020	–
Spain	17	6.576	0.293	0.240	0.228	37.574	19.435	93.606	4.048
Finland	4	7.500	0.000	1.528	0.026	67.469	2.414	93.950	0.238
France	22	6.668	0.232	0.647	0.235	25.527	4.040	92.055	2.454
Greece	4	5.381	0.285	−0.790	0.231	18.502	5.428	80.692	1.174
Ireland	2	7.100	0.141	0.890	0.052	38.923	0.000	96.600	0.849
Italy	21	5.995	0.421	−0.646	0.918	32.170	13.908	88.576	4.367
Luxembourg	1	6.900	–	1.232	–	31.066	–	87.400	–
Netherlands	12	7.492	0.168	1.300	0.126	62.607	5.908	94.117	2.329
Poland	16	5.869	0.275	−0.529	0.165	27.408	9.085	90.613	2.176
Portugal	5	5.280	0.130	0.234	0.427	16.057	10.281	84.600	3.197
Sweden	3	7.406	0.082	1.418	0.089	71.683	2.146	92.111	0.908
Slovak Republic	4	6.150	0.238	−0.539	0.063	13.698	3.628	89.425	1.962
Slovenia	1	6.000	–	−0.006	–	24.204	–	91.950	–
United Kingdom	12	6.875	0.122	0.822	0.131	38.051	8.307	94.542	1.152

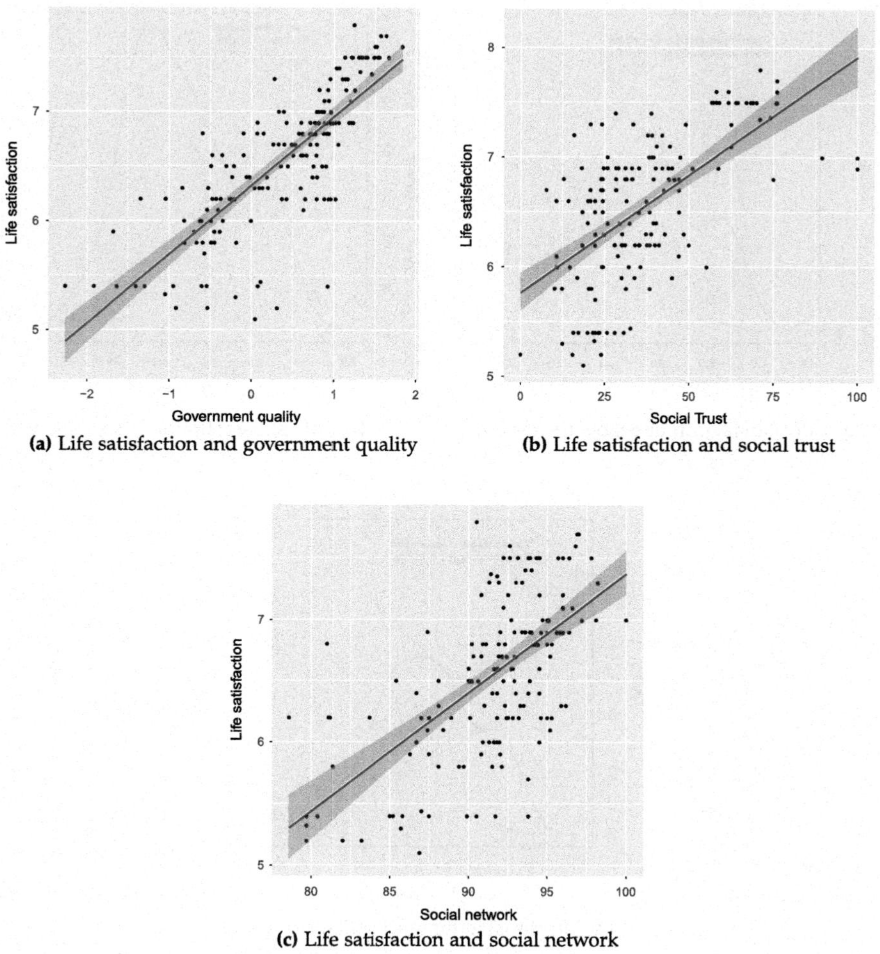

Fig. 1 Scatter plots for institutions and life satisfaction

3 Methodology

The empirical strategy relies on regression analysis. In particular, we run several Ordinary Least Squares (OLS) estimations using different model specifications. The most comprehensive model takes the form:

$$Y_i = \alpha + \beta X_i + \varepsilon_i \tag{1}$$

where i represents a region, Y stands for life satisfaction, X is a vector of the relevant variables, including our variables of interest and the control variables, α, β are parameters to be estimated and ε is the error term.

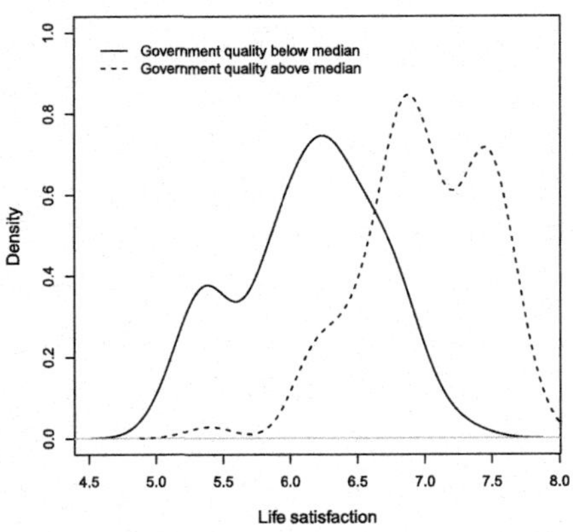

(a) Life satisfaction and government quality

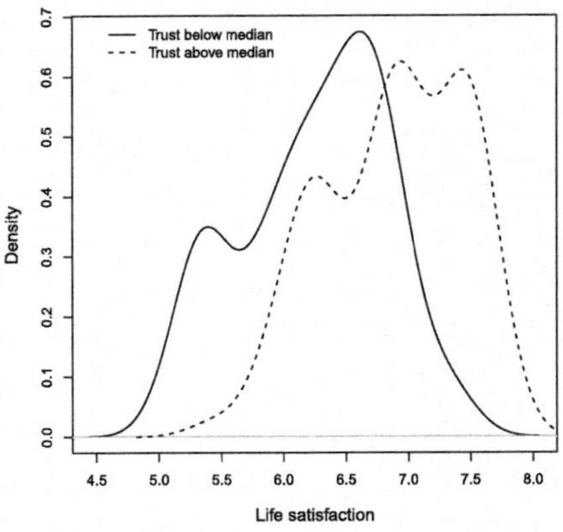

(b) Life satisfaction and social trust

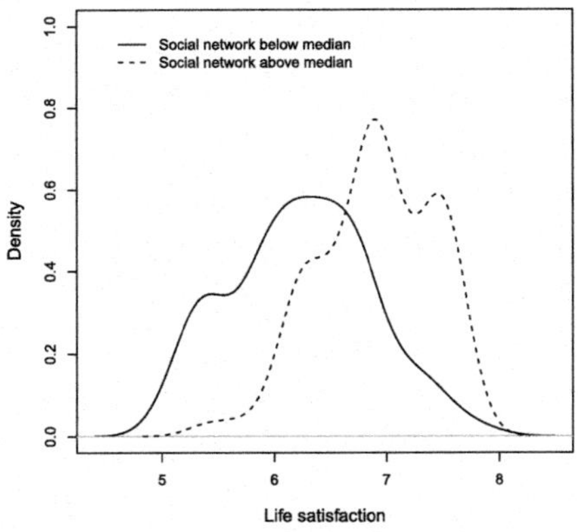

(c) Life satisfaction and social network

Fig. 2 Densities for institutions and life satisfaction

In addition, in order to assess whether the life satisfaction determinants are the same for people with low or high satisfaction with life, we also run quantile regression, providing estimates beyond the average effect yielded by OLS. Quantile regression was introduced by Koenker and Bassett (1978) and its application to different fields of economics has been common in recent years. It allows us to examine how the variable affect on the entire distribution of the dependent variable, namely life satisfaction. To do so, several quantiles (τ) are selected, providing different effects for each particular case and highlighting the existence of *heterogeneous effects* for low, medium and high levels of life satisfaction.

In line with Koenker and Bassett (1978), each β parameter can be estimated by minimizing the absolute sum of the residuals:

$$\min Q(\beta_q) = \sum_{i:y_i \geqslant x\prime_i \beta}^{N} \tau |y_i - x\prime_i \beta_\tau| + \sum_{i:y_i < x\prime_i \beta}^{N} (1-\tau)|y_i - x\prime_i \beta_\tau| \tag{2}$$

where τ, which lies within the [0, 1] interval, is a particular quantile.

The above function is not differentiable and it needs to be optimised with linear programming.[4] Each estimated $\hat{\beta}_\tau$ distributes asymptotically as $N \rightarrow (0, \Omega_\tau)$, where Ω_τ is the variance covariance matrix of $\hat{\beta}_\tau$ for a given τ.

4 Results

The results from OLS estimations are reported in Table 3. We estimated different models where variables are added sequentially. In all cases the dependent variable is life satisfaction. Model 1 only includes government quality (formal institutions). Model 2 considers the two indicators of informal institutions, while Model 3 accounts for all three indicators. Finally, the most comprehensive Model 4 adds to Model 3 all the control variables. For all the specifications we find a positive and significant coefficient for both formal and informal institutions. As expected, coefficients are lower when additional controls are included in the model.

Considering the control variables, a negative and significant sign is found for the rate of dependency, thus showing that younger populations are, on average, more satisfied with life. Living in rural areas, higher income levels and having access to internet are found to be positive for life satisfaction, while the rest of control variables are non-significant. Finally, Model 5 is a parsimonious model where only those significant variables are included. The results are in line with the previous models. All five models have substantial explanatory power (adjusted R^2 ranges from 54 to 76%) and are jointly significant.

Considering quantile regression estimations, Table 4 reports results for the main quantiles and for the parsimonious Model 5. These correspond to low levels of life satisfaction ($\tau = 0.1$) and high life satisfaction ($\tau = 0.9$), whereas the other quantiles correspond to intermediate levels. Detailed results for all the quantiles are displayed by Fig. 3, showing both the average impact from the OLS estimations and the impact for particular quantiles.

For all the variables we find that effects are not homogeneous across quantiles of life satisfaction. Focusing on formal institutions, the results show a crescent effect with a maximum level for those more satisfied with life. In places where life satisfaction is low (lower quantiles), increasing quality of government has a positive effect, although much lower.

[4] Additional explanations on quantile regression fall outside the aim of this chapter. See Koenker (2005) for further details.

Table 3 Institutions and life satisfaction, OLS estimations

	Dependent variable: life satisfaction				
Variables	Model 1	Model 2	Model 3	Model 4	Model 5
Intercept	6.333***	−0.297	2.798***	−2.432	−1.431
	(0.033)	(0.797)	(0.701)	(1.592)	(1.335)
Government quality	0.632***		0.434***	0.330***	0.298***
	(0.036)		(0.043)	(0.058)	(0.050)
Social trust		0.015***	0.007***	0.007***	0.007***
		(0.001)	(0.001)	(0.001)	(0.001)
Social network		0.068***	0.036***	0.028***	0.026***
		(0.008)	(0.007)	(0.007)	(0.007)
Dependency rate				−0.020***	−0.021***
				(0.006)	(0.005)
Population density				−1.20e−05	
				(3.55e−05)	
Rural				0.061**	0.056**
				(0.024)	(0.022)
Education				−0.001	
				(0.003)	
Income				0.506***	0.453***
				(0.152)	(0.133)
Unemployment				0.006	
				(0.006)	
Safety				0.045	
				(0.028)	
Pollution				0.009	
				(0.007)	
Housing				−0.005	
				(0.145)	
Broadband access				0.016***	0.014***
				(0.005)	(0.004)
N	166	166	166	166	166
Adjusted R^2	0.638	0.545	0.716	0.762	0.764
F-Statistic	292.80***	100.10***	140.20***	41.81***	77.66***

Robust standard errors are in parenthesis. *, ** and ***represent significance at 10%, 5%, and 1% significance levels, respectively

Table 4 Institutions and life satisfaction, quantile regressions for Model 5

	Dependent variable: Life satisfaction				
Variables	$\tau = 0.1$	$\tau = 0.25$	$\tau = 0.50$	$\tau = 0.75$	$\tau = 0.90$
Intercept	−2.714	−2.235	0.542	1.173	1.038
	(1.743)	(2.240)	(1.779)	(1.431)	(1.089)
Government quality	0.170**	0.252***	0.342***	0.376***	0.414***
	(0.065)	(0.090)	(0.059)	(0.053)	(0.062)
Social trust	0.009***	0.008***	0.008***	0.004**	0.002**
	(0.003)	(0.002)	(0.001)	(0.001)	(0.001)
Social network	0.028***	0.022*	0.014*	0.021**	0.030***
	(0.009)	(0.012)	(0.009)	(0.006)	(0.004)
Dependency rate	−0.039***	−0.019**	−0.017**	−0.013**	−0.020***
	(0.010)	(0.007)	(0.006)	(0.005)	(0.005)
Rural	0.061*	0.102***	0.047	0.022	0.025
	(0.036)	(0.035)	(0.032)	(0.021)	(0.016)
Income	0.562**	0.460**	0.330**	0.280*	0.290***
	(0.232)	(0.200)	(0.159)	(0.153)	(0.088)
Broadband access	0.014*	0.022***	0.017***	0.011**	0.006**
	(0.008)	(0.007)	(0.005)	(0.004)	(0.004)

Robust standard errors are in parenthesis. *, ** and *** represent significance at 10%, 5%, and 1% significance levels, respectively

Moving to the case of informal institutions, social trust exhibits a decreasing pattern across life satisfaction levels. This means that increases in social trust has the most prominent effect in those regions where life satisfaction is low. Finally, for the case of social networks, the other informal institutions indicator, we find relatively similar impacts across regions with different levels of life satisfaction (see Fig. 3).

Considering the rest of variables, the dependency rate is consistently negative in all cases. As expected, the greatest impact is found in places with the lowest life satisfaction. Living in a rural region only matters for those places with low levels of life satisfaction, whereas it becomes irrelevant once it increases sufficiently. Interestingly, income is especially important for places with low life satisfaction, finding a declining effect and showing that money becomes less important in regions with high life satisfaction. Finally, having broadband access shows a much more fuzzy trend, although in general the greatest impact is found again for low life satisfaction areas. These results suggest that material conditions together with social trust levels have a great effect for people with low life satisfaction, whereas in regions where life satisfaction is high the effect of having reliable formal institutions (high government quality) matters the most.

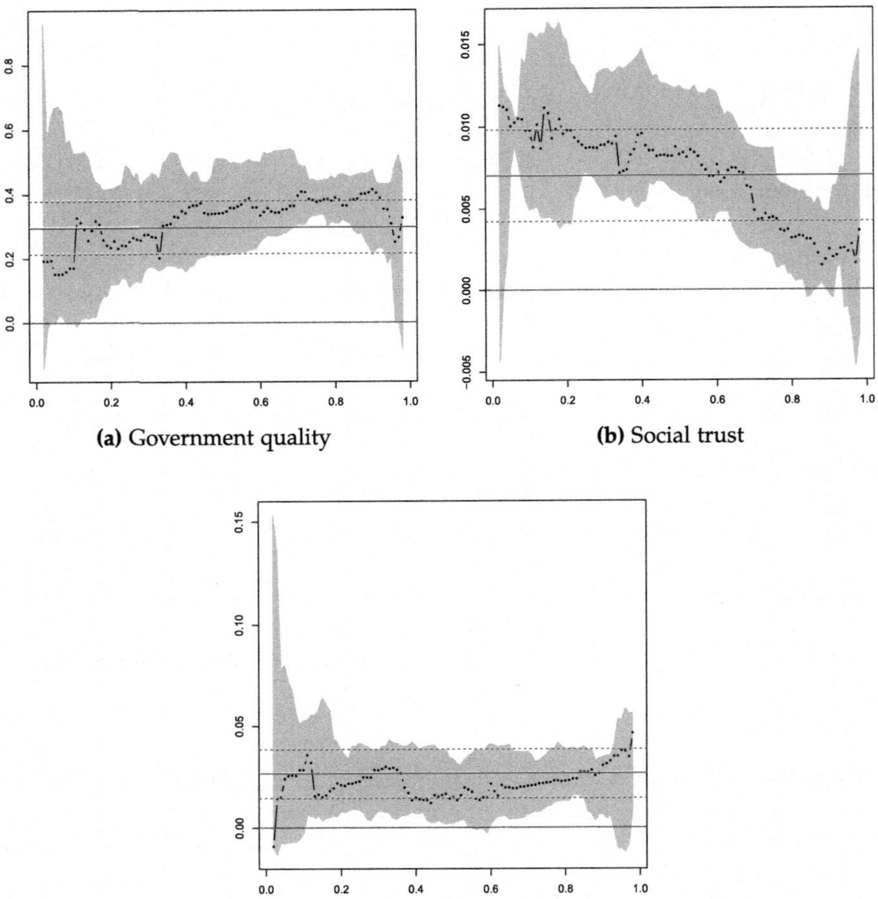

(a) Government quality

(b) Social trust

(c) Social network

Fig. 3 Quantile regressions, Model 5. Notes: Quantile estimates (black dotted line) are plotted as a function of the different quantiles of life satisfaction (from percentile 0 to 0.99), represented in the X axis. Low (high) quantiles represent regions where life satisfaction is low (high). The Y axis reports the impact of institutional variables on life satisfaction, which changes across life satisfaction levels. The red solid line corresponds to the OLS estimation (average effect, equivalent to all levels of life satisfaction). The dashed lines in red correspond to 90% confidence bands for the OLS estimation, whereas those for the quantile estimation are represented by the shaded area. In those areas where the confidence bands contain the zero, the estimated coefficient is non-significant

5 Conclusions

Over the last few years, the analysis of well-being has been gaining importance among economists and other social sciences researchers. Whereas the analysis of key economic variables such as per capita income and productivity still dominate the macroeconomic debate, the focus is now broader and also centred on related issues such as those covered in the present chapter—namely, well-being.

One of the reasons that has partly prevented more rapid advances on this related literature is the relative unavailability of databases on well-being for large samples of countries and years, as opposed to, for instance, per capita income—at least until recent times. However, the emergence of new databases providing information related to well-being variables such as life satisfaction and/or happiness has triggered an increase in the number of contributions in the field.

We have aimed to contribute in this field by analysing the links between informal, formal institutions and life satisfaction for a large sample of 166 European regions. For this, we used indicators of different nature to measure the quality of institutions: (i) the composite European Quality of Government Index (EQI), available for European regions and measuring the quality of formal institutions; and (ii) social trust and perceived social network support, to measure the quality of informal institutions. The geographical unit of analysis was also partly a contribution, given the relative scarcity of studies at the regional level.

In the available literature, mostly confined to the country level, the links between both types of institutions with life satisfaction have been found to be strong and positive. The effects have been generally found to be greater than those for income or education—for which only by specifying simple models it was possible to obtain relevant effects. Recent literature has suggested, though, the need for specifying more complex models which control for the existence of other determinants (Helliwell et al., 2018).

In our empirical strategy we have first considered a baseline model which was estimated via OLS. Additional controls were sequentially added, finding a robust positive association between our different indicators of institution quality (namely, government quality, social trust and social network) and our measure of well-being—life satisfaction. Regardless of the model considered, from the baseline model (model 1) to the most parsimonious one (model 5), the effects were always positive and strong. These robust results are in line with the available literature (see Neira et al., 2018; Rodríguez-Pose & von Berlepsch, 2014; Sarracino, 2010), suggesting that life satisfaction is not only motivated by economic factors—although we actually found a positive effect for income in our regressions.

Despite the importance of the results found, they reflect the average effect for the average region. However, results can vary remarkably across different quantiles of the conditional distribution of life satisfaction—i.e., results can differ for regions with either high or low life satisfaction levels. Results are also strong and significant for all the relevant regressors and *most* quantiles (τ). The most notable differences were found in the magnitudes of the estimated coefficients, which also varied depending on the quantile considered. For formal institutions the largest effects are found for high levels of life satisfaction. In spite of direct comparison with previous literature is not possible, a potential explanation is that people with low life satisfaction levels are more worried about getting the basic necessities covered. As the results show, the income dimension is more important for the unhappiest people. Oppositely, people which are already highly satisfied with life can improve happiness even more with other dimensions such as having a reliable formal institutional framework able to guarantee the welfare system.

In contrast, a different pattern is found for informal institutions. Regarding social trust, its effects are stronger for regions with low levels of life satisfaction. For social network support effects are similar across different levels of life satisfaction. These results are aligned to the recent findings by Neira et al. (2018), who reported similar evidence for informal institutions and life satisfaction but using individual-level data. It is likely that the very happy people are richer in terms of social capital than the unhappiest (Diener & Seligman, 2002). Therefore, further improvements of social capital have a more limited effect in increasing life satisfaction. Therefore, despite the results for quantile regression corroborate those found for OLS, results are more intricate than what average regressions based on the average effect might suggest. This calls for further research examining more closely the links between varying levels of life satisfaction and institutions, both formal and informal.

References

Bartolini, S., Mikucka, M., & Sarracino, F. (2017). Money, trust and happiness in transition countries: Evidence from time series. *Social Indicators Research, 130*(1), 87–106.

Bjørnskov, C. (2006). The multiple facets of social capital. *European Journal of Political Economy, 22*(1), 22–40.

Bjørnskov, C. (2007). Determinants of generalized trust: A cross-country comparison. *Public Choice, 130*(1–2), 1–21.

Bjørnskov, C. (2008). Social capital and happiness in the United States. *Applied Research in Quality of Life, 3*(1), 43–62.

Bjørnskov, C., Dreher, A., & Fischer, J. A. (2010). Formal institutions and subjective well-being: Revisiting the cross-country evidence. *European Journal of Political Economy, 26*(4), 419–430.

Charron, N., Dijkstra, L., & Lapuente, V. (2014). Regional governance matters: Quality of government within European Union member states. *Regional Studies, 48*(1), 68–90.

Charron, N., Dijkstra, L., & Lapuente, V. (2015). Mapping the regional divide in Europe: A measure for assessing quality of government in 206 European regions. *Social Indicators Research, 122*(2), 315–346.

Diener, E., & Seligman, M. E. (2002). Very happy people. *Psychological Science, 13*(1), 81–84.

Frey, B. S., & Stutzer, A. (2000). Happiness, economy and institutions. *The Economic Journal, 110*(466), 918–938.

Frey, B. S., & Stutzer, A. (2005). Beyond outcomes: Measuring procedural utility. *Oxford Economic Papers, 57*(1), 90–111.

Geys, B., & Qari, S. (2017). Will you still trust me tomorrow? The causal effect of terrorism on social trust. *Public Choice, 173*(3–4), 289–305.

Han, S. (2015). Social capital and subjective happiness: Which contexts matter? *Journal of Happiness Studies, 16*(1), 241–255.

Helliwell, J. F. (2006). Well-being, social capital and public policy: What's new? *The Economic Journal, 116*(510), C34–C45.
Helliwell, J. F., Huang, H., Grover, S., & Wang, S. (2018). Empirical linkages between good governance and national well-being. *Journal of Comparative Economics, 46*(4), 1332–1346.
Koenker, R. (2005). *Quantile Regression*. New York: Cambridge University Press.
Koenker, R., & Bassett, G. (1978). Regression quantiles. *Econometrica, 46*(1), 33–50.
Kuroki, M., et al. (2011). Does social trust increase individual happiness in Japan? *The Japanese Economic Review, 62*(4), 444–459.
Neira, I., Lacalle-Calderon, M., Portela, M., & Perez-Trujillo, M. (2018). Social capital dimensions and subjective well-being: A quantile approach. *Journal of Happiness Studies*, 1–29.
North, D. C. (1986). The new institutional economics. *Journal of Institutional and Theoretical Economics, 142*(1), 230–237.
North, D. C. (1989). Institutions and economic growth: An historical introduction. *World Development, 17*(9), 1319–1332.
North, D. C. (1991). Institutions. *Journal of Economic Perspectives, 5*(1), 97–112.
North, D. C. (1994). Economic performance through time. *American Economic Review, 84*(3), 359–368.
Nunn, N., & Wantchekon, L. (2011). The slave trade and the origins of mistrust in Africa. *American Economic Review, 101*(7), 3221–3252.
Orviska, M., Caplanova, A., & Hudson, J. (2014). The impact of democracy on well-being. *Social Indicators Research, 115*(1), 493–508.
Ott, J. (2010). Greater happiness for a greater number: Some non-controversial options for governments. *Journal of Happiness Studies, 5*(11), 631–647.
Ott, J. C. (2011). Government and happiness in 130 nations: Good governance fosters higher level and more equality of happiness. *Social Indicators Research, 102*(1), 3–22.
Portela, M., Neira, I., & del Mar Salinas-Jiménez, M. (2013). Social capital and subjective wellbeing in Europe: A new approach on social capital. *Social Indicators Research, 114*(2), 493–511.
Robinson, J. A., & Acemoglu, D. (2012). *Why Nations Fail: The Origins of Power, Prosperity, and Poverty*. Crown Business.
Rodríguez-Pose, A., & von Berlepsch, V. (2014). Social capital and individual happiness in Europe. *Journal of Happiness Studies, 15*(2), 357–386.
Sarracino, F. (2010). Social capital and subjective well-being trends: Comparing 11 western European countries. *The Journal of Socio-Economics, 39*(4), 482–517.
Tokuda, Y., Fujii, S., & Inoguchi, T. (2010). Individual and country-level effects of social trust on happiness: The Asia barometer survey. *Journal of Applied Social Psychology, 10*(40), 2574–2593.
Uslaner, E. (2008). Where you stand depends upon where your grandparents sat. *Public Opinion Quarterly, 72*(4), 725–740.
Yamamura, E., Tsutsui, Y., Yamane, C., Yamane, S., & Powdthavee, N. (2015). Trust and happiness: Comparative study before and after the Great East Japan Earthquake. *Social Indicators Research, 123*(3), 919–935.

Jesús Peiró-Palomino is Associate Professor at the Department of Applied Economics II (Estructura Econòmica), University of Valencia. His research interests are institutions and their role in economic development processes, especially at the regional level. He is also interested in the measurement of well-being and social progress, their spatial distribution and their evolution over time. His work has been published in several international scientific journals.

Emili Tortosa-Ausina is Professor of Applied Economics at Universitat Jaume I (Spain). His main fields of research are efficiency and productivity analysis, banking and finance, and regional and urban economics. He has published several books and articles in specialised journals, including European Economic Review, Economic Geography, Environment and Planning A, Journal of Banking and Finance, World Development, Omega, etc.

The Effects of Democracy and Trust on Subjective Well-Being: A Multilevel Study of Latin American Countries

Isabel Neira, Marta Portela, and Maricruz Lacalle-Calderon

1 Introduction

Subjective well-being (SWB) has received increasing attention in the empirical social science literature in recent years. Most of this research has focused on how SWB (usually measured through happiness or life satisfaction) is affected by individuals' traditional factors such as income, marriage, health or level of education (Clark & Oswald, 1994; Easterlin, 1974, 2001; Frey & Stutzer, 2002; Layard, 2005, among others). More recently, however, an attempt to include not only individual characteristics but also the environment in which the individuals live has led to consideration of socio-economic factors at regional-national level. Two factors that currently have great significance are social capital (or trust) (Portela et al., 2013; Puntscher et al., 2015; Rodriguez-Pose & von Berlepsch, 2014) and democracy (Frey & Stutzer, 2000; Graham & Pettinato, 2001; Orviska et al., 2014). All of these studies show that these two factors have positive and significant effects on individual SWB. In the case of social capital, these results are found mainly when social capital is measured through generalized social trust (2006; Helliwell & Putnam, 2004; Sarracino, 2010).

I. Neira (✉)
Quantitative Economics Department, Faculty of Economics and Business Studies, Universidade de Santiago de Compostela, Santiago, Spain
e-mail: isabel.neira@usc.es

M. Portela
Department of Finance, Faculty of Business Administration, Universidade de Santiago de Compostela, Santiago, Spain
e-mail: marta.portela@usc.es

M. Lacalle-Calderon
School of Economics and Business, Depament for Economic Development, Universidad Autónoma de Madrid, Madrid, Spain
e-mail: maicu.lacalle@uam.es

A. Almakaeva et al. (eds.), *Social Capital and Subjective Well-Being*, Societies and Political Orders in Transition,
https://doi.org/10.1007/978-3-030-75813-4_9

Although previous literature has demonstrated a positive effect of trust and democracy on SWB at the micro and macro level, descriptive data on Latin American countries shows a lack of correspondence, or dissociation, between individual well-being and these two institutional factors of the Latin American social context or environment. Most Latin American countries register low levels of satisfaction with democracy and trust (interpersonal trust and trust in government) but high levels of SWB. A similar pattern of SWB in Latin America has been analyzed by Rojas (2016, p. 18), who asserts «an apparent Latin American welfare paradox: the existence of a comparatively high level of happiness coupled with a comparatively low level of economic, health and educational development».

Following the ideas of Rojas (2016) and the Latin Barometer (2016 and 2017), the main objective of this study is to shed light on the complex relationship between SWB and the institutional factors of trust and democracy in the Latin American region. To achieve this objective, we perform both a multilevel analysis and an in-depth descriptive analysis. Instead of using single-level microanalysis[1], we run a multilevel analysis to determine whether the countries' averages for trust (measured by *Interpersonal trust* and *Trust in government*) and democracy (measured by *Satisfaction with democracy* and *Democracy is the best form of government*) affect individual well-being. To do so, we use the Latin Barometer database of 18 Latin American countries for 2016, with 20,204 individual data items. This multilevel analysis also allows us to establish differences within and between countries.

The results from the multilevel analysis are in line with previous research and show a positive correlation of trust and democracy with SWB at the micro and macro level. However, results from the in-depth descriptive analysis shows an important disassociation between the individual data on SWB and the levels of satisfaction with democracy and trust in Latin American countries. This finding indicates the strangeness of the results of previous analyses (that is, the positive correlation among these three variables). Descriptive data show that Latin American citizens register one of the highest levels of SWB in the world, while simultaneously expressing very low levels of satisfaction with democracy and trust.

This study thus contributes to the literature by helping to explain the influence of social capital and democracy on individual SWB through the relational effects between micro and macro levels (people and their environments). The study is also relevant to explaining the complex situation of Latin American countries, which are currently undergoing significant loss of democratic and social values, which seem to be dissociated from the people's level of well-being.

[1] That is, ordered probit estimations, as in previous literature.

2 Theoretical Background

2.1 *Trust and Democracy as Institutional Factors and Their Effects on SWB*

Institutions are generally defined as the rules of the game or humanly devised constraints that shape political, economic and social human interaction (North, 1990). Historically, institutions emerged through a social contract between citizens and the state, the former delegating use of violence to the latter in exchange for protection and social order (Casson et al., 2010). Since each country has its own historical evolution, the institutional framework consists of formal institutions (or official rules), informal institutions and their enforcement characteristics. Formal institutions are «a set of rules, compliance procedures and moral and ethical behavioural norms designed to constrain the behaviour of individuals in the interest of maximising the wealth or utility of the principals» (North, 1990). These institutions are very clearly and formally defined and include laws, constitutions, regulations and all other precisely formulated rules such as legal regulations, rules governing economic activity (e.g., private property rights, labour markets, tax laws) and political freedoms (e.g., democracy or degree of democratization). Informal institutions are much more complex. They refer to informal rules of behaviour and include customs, traditions and codes of conduct such as social trust (for example, interpersonal trust, trust in the government and other official entities such as political parties). Following North (2003), informal institutions are sometimes more important than the formal rules of behaviour. Casson et al. (2010) affirm that informal institutions play an important role in shaping formal institutions in developing countries and may even emerge as preponderant rules when formal institutions fail.

Iinstitutional factors may thus take many forms, two of which are democracy and trust. The complexity and multidimensionality of democracy and trust[2] increases the difficulty of empirically studying their relationship to other variables such as SWB.

Today, institutional factors are considered as very important, not only for economic progress (Acemoglu & Robinson, 2012) but also to increase happiness and well-being. A high degree of democratization and a highly trustworthy environment are two components of a sturdy institutional framework that may result in a considerable level of well-being among citizens of any country. For instance, following Dorn et al. (2007) and Frey and Stutzer (2000), a more democratic system—one in which citizens

[2] Democracy has been defined in so many ways that reaching an agreement on what it is and how to measure it is a very difficult challenge. For further information on these issues, see Coppedge (2012). Trust is one of the three dimensions of social capital. Following Coleman (1988), Bourdieu (1986) and Putnam et al. (1993), most authors agree that the most common empirical indicators of social capital can be grouped into three broad dimensions: trust, networks and social norms (Grootaert & van Bastelaer, 2001; Van Oorschot & Arts, 2005; Portela, et al. 2013; Afandi et al., 2017). The literature on trust distinguishes two types: (a) *horizontal trust*, also known as interpersonal trust, or trust among people; and (b) *vertical trust*, also known as political trust, or the trust people have in their governments or political parties (Rothstein & Eek, 2001; Khodyakov, 2007).

have more say in governmental policies—is likely to produce political outcomes closer to the preferences and wishes of the voters than a system with fewer democratic elements. Further, citizens in a more democratic system have a greater chance to participate in the political decision-making process, a factor that improves their well-being. Ceteris paribus, greater exposure to democracy can help raise individuals' well-being (Dorn et al., 2007; Frey & Stutzer, 2000; Inglehart et al., 2008; Orviska et al., 2014; Owen et al., 2008, among others[3]). The nature of the relationship between democracy and well-being, however, is not without flaws. While some authors find no relationship (Fosu et al., 2006), several others see important problems of endogeneity between these variables (Orviska et al., 2014). At the empirical level, previous studies focus on individual well-being using ordered probit estimations and macro-data on democracy from databases like Freedom House or Polity IV. The results reveal a positive and significant relationship between democracy in a country and individual well-being. Our study contributes to the analysis of this relationship by focusing on individual well-being, using not ordered probit estimations but multilevel analysis (which enables us to capture better both individual behaviour and the average). We also use micro rather macro data on democracy (through «Satisfaction with democracy» and «Democracy is the best form of government»). We are aware that using these types of variables to measure democracy has some conceptual problems. For example, as Linde and Ekman (2003) notes, since such variables may be sensitive to different contexts, even dissatisfaction with the performance of democracy does not necessarily imply dissatisfaction with democracy as such (Linde & Ekman, 2003: 396). Many authors have, however, used satisfaction with democracy as an indicator of democratic performance in a country. The foregoing arguments have motivated some scholars to affirm that the item «satisfaction with democracy» is an indicator of «constitutional reality» (Fuchs et al., 1995: 332).

Several studies also support the positive and robust influence of trust on SWB (Portela et al., 2013; Puntscher et al., 2015; Rodriguez-Pose & von Berlepsch, 2014). Trust affects SWB because trusting others means sharing fundamental values, creating links between people and improving cooperation and efficiency in transactions, whether economic or social. At the micro-level, much empirical work on the effect of social capital on SWB focuses on interpersonal trust and social relationships (Becchetti et al., 2008; Bruni & Stanca, 2008; Klein, 2013). The empirical approaches show a positive correlation of trust (interpersonal and institutional) with individual SWB, based on ordered probit at the individual level. Several cross-sectional studies also analyze the relationship between trust and SWB at aggregate level and find evidence that generalized trust at regional or country level is positively associated with national happiness (Bjørnskov, 2003; Helliwell & Putnam, 2004; Inglehart & Klingemann, 2000).

Research on SWB (in an attempt to include not only individual characteristics but also macro-level determinants) has led to consideration of a multilevel approach to socio-economic factors at regional/national level (Aslam & Corrado, 2012; Han,

[3] See Orviska et al., 2014 for further information on the nature of the relationship, if any, between democracy and well-being.

2015; Neira et al., 2018; Pittau et al., 2010; Rampichini & d'Andrea, 1998). The results indicate a comparative income effect with our closest neighbours; having more income always makes us happier, but, in order to have such an effect, the income level must usually be high relative to the country or region average. Social factors show a double positive effect; well-being is conditioned by both our personal relationships and the environment in which we live. Social capital, specifically trust, has a positive effect on individual well-being. The higher the collective perceptions of institutional trust, the lower the relevance of individual perception of trust in explaining individual happiness and life satisfaction. In the case of Latin-American countries, studies such as Orviska et al. (2014) and Rojas (2016) observe higher-than-expected national levels of happiness when measuring social variables such as trust in democracy, political institutions and the welfare-state in those countries. In the following sections, we analyse this dissociation empirically for the case of Latin American countries.

3 Empirical Approach

3.1 Data

To analyze the role trust and democracy play at both individual and macro levels in SWB in Latin-American countries, we will use data from the *Latin Barometer* 2016. The data were gathered from a sample of 20,204 individuals in May and June 2016 in 18 countries.

Our dependent variable is SWB, measured through «Satisfaction with life» using the following *Latin Barometer* question: «Generally speaking, would you say you are satisfied with your life?»; The choices were: (1) Very satisfied, (2) Quite satisfied, (3) Not very satisfied and (4) Not at all satisfied. These responses have been recoded so that higher values indicate higher levels of satisfaction.

The main independent variables are Trust, measured through «Interpersonal trust» and «Trust in government», and Democracy, measured through «Satisfaction with democracy» and «Democracy is the best form of government». These four proxies are based on the following *Latin Barometer* questions:

- «Generally speaking, would you say that you can trust most people, or that you can never be too careful when dealing with others?» The choices were: (1) One can never be too careful when dealing with others, and (2) One can trust most people.
- «Would you say you have a lot (1), some (2), a little (3) or no trust (4) in the national government?»
- «In general, would you say you are (1) very satisfied, (2) quite satisfied, (3) not very satisfied or (4) not at all satisfied with how democracy works in (country)?»
- «Democracy may have problems, but it is the best system of government». (1) Strongly disagree, (2) Disagree, (3) Agree and (4) Strongly agree.

In all cases, the variables were recoded so that the higher values indicate higher levels of trust and democracy.

At country level[4], the variables represent the cumulative frequency of responses in the country where individual «i» lives. The use of these variables at the macro level allows us to deal with endogeneity problems identified by Frey and Stutzer (2002) and Orviska et al. (2014), who suggest that a satisfied population may foster democracy and democratic institutions (Tables 1 and 2).

3.2 *Methodology*

To incorporate all of these factors, we used a multilevel model. This analysis allowed us to establish differences within and between countries. Random intercept was used to check for unexplained national variability.

We follow Snijders and Bosker (2012) for a general description of the models, with slight changes in notation. An indicator of the SWB of individual i nested in country $j(Y_{ij})$ is supposed to depend on individual (level-one) control variables (C_{ij}) and our quality of institution variables (X_{ij}). The index for individuals ($i = 1, \ldots, n_j$) in these variables starts over for each national group. As the values of a level-two variable do not depend on individual i, level-two variables have the group j index (z_j) only.

The individual-level (micro) model for country j captures the compositional effects through the following equation with three β coefficients[6]:

$$\mathrm{Y_{ij}} = \beta_0 + \beta_{1j}\mathrm{X_{ij}} + \beta_{2j}\mathrm{C_{ij}} + \beta_{3j}\mathrm{Z_j} + \epsilon_{ij}$$

The total error of this model is decomposed into two random effects at individual (ε_{ij}) and national (U_{0j}) levels, with variances of σ_ϵ^2 and σ_u^2, respectively.

4 Results

Table 3 shows the results of the multilevel analysis applied, with the main independent variables (trust and democracy) at micro and macro level. Each column shows a different model specification.

---

[4] Interpersonal trust: country-level mean of value «One can trust most peo-ple» in the variable «Generally speaking, would you say that you can trust most people, or that you can never be too careful when dealing with others?"Trust in government: country-level mean of values «A lot» and «Some» in the variable «How much trust do you have in each of the following institutions? National Government».

[6] Note that a level-two variable does not have an i subscript because, by definition, its values do not vary from individual to individual within a level-two unit.

Table 1 Descriptive statistics of the main variables[5]

Variable	Obs	Mean	Std. Dev	Min	Max
Satisfaction with life	12,348	3.039	0.850	1	4
Age	12,348	2.361	0.975	1	4
Age squared	12,348	6.523	4.826	1	16
Political position					
Left	12,348	0.288	0.453	0	1
Center	12,348	0.372	0.483	0	1
Right	12,348	0.340	0.474	0	1
Educational level					
Basic	12,348	0.363	0.481	0	1
Secondary	12,348	0.411	0.492	0	1
Tertiary	12,348	0.226	0.418	0	1
Subjective income					
It is not sufficient, and we have major problems	12,348	0.123	0.329	0	1
It is not sufficient, and we have problems	12,348	0.333	0.471	0	1
It is just sufficient, and we have no major problems	12,348	0.425	0.494	0	1
It is sufficient, and we can save	12,348	0.119	0.324	0	1
Marital status					
Married/Living with partner	12,348	0.550	0.497	0	1
Single	12,348	0.339	0.473	0	1
Separated/Divorced/Widowed	12,348	0.110	0.313	0	1
Religious					
Not devout at all	12,348	0.124	0.330	0	1
Not very devout	12,348	0.361	0.480	0	1
Devout	12,348	0.374	0.484	0	1
Very devout	12,348	0.141	0.348	0	1
Satisfaction with democracy					
Not at all satisfied	12,348	0.228	0.420	0	1
Not very satisfied	12,348	0.420	0.494	0	1
Quite satisfied	12,348	0.256	0.436	0	1
Very satisfied	12,348	0.095	0.294	0	1
Democracy may have problems, but it is the best system of government					
Strongly disagree	12,348	0.031	0.172	0	1
Disagree	12,348	0.173	0.378	0	1
Agree	12,348	0.558	0.497	0	1
Strongly agree	12,348	0.239	0.426	0	1

(continued)

[5] The mean of the dummy variables indicates the proportion of individuals for which those variables take the value 1.

Table 1 (continued)

Variable	Obs	Mean	Std. Dev	Min	Max
Interpersonal trust					
One can never be too careful	12,348	0.833	0.373	0	1
One can trust most people	12,348	0.167	0.373	0	1
Trust in government					
No trust	12,348	0.363	0.481	0	1
Little trust	12,348	0.349	0.477	0	1
Some trust	12,348	0.211	0.408	0	1
A lot of trust	12,348	0.076	0.265	0	1
Interpersonal trust (% country level)	12,348	0.169	0.060	0.033	0.306
Trust in government (% country level)	12,348	0.271	0.109	0.095	0.547
Satisfaction with democ. (% country level)	12,348	0.343	0.128	0.100	0.580
Democ. is the best form of gov. (% country level)	12,348	0.792	0.065	0.657	0.902

The results in Table 3 show a positive and significant correlation between *Satisfaction with democracy* and *Trust in government* with *Satisfaction with Life* at the micro level. That is, SWB is positively related to the individual's perception of the institutional factors in his/her environment. The variables *Interpersonal trust* and *Democracy is the best forms of government* are non-significant, however, due to the low correlation between those variables and *Satisfaction with Life* at the individual level (0.02 and 0.05, respectively; see Table 4). These results are consistent with the micro-level relationship observed by the well-being literature. Graham and Pettinato (2001), for example, find that satisfaction with democracy correlates with higher levels of happiness, while preferring democracy to other forms of government has no significance.

At the macro level, in contrast, we find no significant correlation between *Satisfaction with democracy* and *Trust in government* with *Satisfaction with Life* (Model 2, Table 3). These results may be due to the high correlation between these two variables (0.87; see Table 5), which may cause multicollinearity problems in Model 2. To solve this problem, we include Models 3–8 in Table 3 to estimate different alternatives. In Models 7 and 8, both variables take positive and significant signs. This result may indicate that individuals are more satisfied with life in countries where the population has higher levels of *Satisfaction with democracy* and *Trust in their government*, despite the very low mean level of the two abovementioned variables in those countries (especially in countries such as Brazil, Venezuela and El Salvador; see Table 2).

One of the most surprising results is the negative correlation between *Democracy is the best form of government* and *Satisfaction with life* (SWB), which yields negative results in all models in Table 3. The low correlation between both variables (see Table 5) and the fact that countries such as Brazil, Venezuela and El Salvador show a

Table 2 Levels (in % of population) in 2016

	% Satisfaction with life (SWB) (%)	% Satisfaction with democracy (%)	% Democracy is the best form of government (%)	% Interpersonal trust (%)	% Trust in government (%)
Argentina	79.80	58.02	90.20	25.44	37.85
Bolivia	66.50	42.71	80.11	15.74	32.02
Brazil	61.86	**10.00**	75.11	3.35	**9.54**
Chile	70.49	30.60	80.58	13.41	27.50
Colombia	82.79	21.61	75.58	15.13	21.79
Costa Rica	87.14	39.30	75.69	10.01	18.66
Dominican Republic	88.20	52.92	77.08	17.37	54.73
Ecuador	70.48	41.99	80.09	21.62	39.48
El Salvador	77.12	**25.22**	65.66	13.84	**16.60**
Guatemala	77.91	33.94	71.44	20.10	27.20
Honduras	73.82	26.77	76.16	13.00	21.14
Mexico	73.62	29.14	71.49	30.60	29.23
Nicaragua	81.19	53.98	87.43	18.37	43.21
Panama	86.82	30.73	75.08	19.25	19.94
Paraguay	68.00	36.08	89.80	19.98	22.31
Peru	66.42	26.04	74.82	15.07	18.90
Uruguay	79.62	52.84	88.82	17.27	46.86
Venezuela	58.25	**23.91**	82.98	14.53	**20.89**
Total	74.53	35.23	79.12	16.95	28.17

Source Latin Barometer (2016)

low degree of satisfaction with their democracies despite a high degree of inclination towards the democratic forms of government explains the singularity of this variable. In sum, although not satisfied with the democracies in their territories and having little trust in the government, most countries consider democratic governments to be the best option.

5 Discussion

Our empirical results are in line with previous analyses performed at international level and show a positive and significant effect of trust and democracy on SWB at the micro and macro levels. However, when we analyse the Latin American data using correlations among the macro-level variables, which represents the behaviour of the average person in each country (Table 6 and Fig. 1), we find a lack of correspondence

Table 3 Multilevel analysis

Dependent variable: Satisfaction with life (SWB)								
Independent variables	Model 1	Model 2	Model 3	Model 4	Model 5	Model 6	Model 7	Model 8
Country-level variables								
Interpersonal trust (% country level)		0.04091	0.34280	0.41869	1.02445			
Trust in government (% country level)		0.10547	0.34355			0.43348	1.01010**	
Satisfaction with democracy (% country level)		1.09208		0.24362		−0.00853		1.19072**
Democracy is the best form of government (% country level)		−2.67163***			−1.49754*		−2.14818**	−2.69185***
Individual-level variables								
Interpersonal trust								
One can never be too careful trusting others			–	–	–	–	–	–
One can trust most people	0.00778	0.00758	0.00756	0.00752	0.00731	0.00771	0.00777	0.00761
Trust in government								
No trust	–	–	–	–	–	–	–	–
A little	−0.01711	−0.01759	−0.01724	−0.01721	−0.01733	−0.01721	−0.01756	−0.01756
Some	0.02534	0.02475	0.02485	0.02498	0.02548	0.02488	0.02462	0.02483
A lot	0.10578***	0.10449***	0.10505***	0.10537***	0.10616***	0.10498***	0.10401***	0.10464***
Satisfaction with democracy								
Not at all satisfied			–	–	–	–	–	–
Not very satisfied	0.00854	0.00812	0.00824	0.00820	0.00865	0.00831	0.00862	0.00811

(continued)

Table 3 (continued)

Dependent variable: Satisfaction with life (SWB)								
Independent variables	Model 1	Model 2	Model 3	Model 4	Model 5	Model 6	Model 7	Model 8
Quite satisfied	0.16175***	0.16112***	0.16118***	0.16112***	0.16234***	0.16126***	0.16206***	0.16108***
Very satisfied	0.31473***	0.31413***	0.31424***	0.31415***	0.31553***	0.31427***	0.31523***	0.31407***
Democracy may have problems, but it is the best system of government								
Strongly disagree	–	–	–	–	–	–	–	–
Disagree	0.02364	0.02270	0.02344	0.02336	0.02379	0.02347	0.02360	0.02264
Agree	0.04640	0.04614	0.04616	0.04607	0.04715	0.04615	0.04699	0.04607
Strongly agree	0.07599	0.07665	0.07578	0.07570	0.07678	0.07580	0.07705	0.07661
Age	−0.01671***	−0.01671***	−0.01671***	−0.01671***	−0.01674***	−0.01671***	−0.01671***	−0.01671***
Age squared	0.00015***	0.00015***	0.00015***	0.00015***	0.00015***	0.00015***	0.00015***	0.00015***
Political position								
Left	–	–	–	–	–	–	–	–
Center	0.02550	0.02569	0.02549	0.02542	0.02555	0.02553	0.02592	0.02566
Right	0.01339	0.01374	0.01349	0.01345	0.01354	0.01347	0.01375	0.01372
Educational level								
Basic			–	–	–	–	–	–
Secondary	0.05029**	0.05124**	0.05007**	0.05013**	0.05076**	0.05009**	0.05081**	0.05129**
Tertiary	0.11255***	0.11265***	0.11218***	0.11229***	0.11255***	0.11224***	0.11221***	0.11274***
Subjective income								
It is not sufficient, and we have major problems	–	–	–	–	–	–	–	–

(continued)

Table 3 (continued)

Dependent variable: Satisfaction with life (SWB)								
Independent variables	Model 1	Model 2	Model 3	Model 4	Model 5	Model 6	Model 7	Model 8
It is not sufficient, and we have problems	0.17777***	0.17681***	0.17761***	0.17758***	0.17745***	0.17767***	0.17733***	0.17681***
It is just sufficient, and we have no major problems	0.36512***	0.36415***	0.36497***	0.36487***	0.36490***	0.36505***	0.36503***	0.36410***
It is sufficient, and we can save	0.46925***	0.46867***	0.46942***	0.46926***	0.46914***	0.46943***	0.46952***	0.46857***
Marital status								
Married /Living with partner	–	–	–	–	–	–	–	–
Single	−0.05993***	−0.05962***	−0.05983***	−0.05984***	−0.05966***	−0.05988***	−0.05968***	−0.05964***
Separated/Divorced/Widowed	−0.09451***	−0.09432***	−0.09460***	−0.09458***	−0.09420***	−0.09462***	−0.09435***	−0.09432***
Religious								
Not devout at all	–	–	–	–	–	–	–	–
Not very devout	0.04585	0.04563	0.04621	0.04613	0.04508	0.04624	0.04567	0.04561
Devout	0.08380***	0.08382***	0.08426***	0.08419***	0.08302***	0.08428***	0.08370***	0.08380***
Very devout	0.18119***	0.18106***	0.18180***	0.18174***	0.18027***	0.18178***	0.18088***	0.18103***
(Intercept)	2.95567***	4.63917***	2.80151***	2.79973***	3.96233***	2.83684***	4.36268***	4.65698***
Regions (σ^2_{U0})	0.04579	0.02365	0.04305	0.04353	0.03467	0.04336	0.02749	0.02369
Individuals (σ^2_{ϵ})	0.61702	0.61702	0.61702	0.61702	0.61702	0.61702	0.61702	0.61702
-2 Log likelihood	29,150.43	29,138.83	29,149.35	29,149.55	29,145.57	29,149.47	29,141.46	29,138.86
ICC	0.0691	0.0369	0.0652	0.0659	0.0532	0.0657	0.0427	0.0370
Observations	12,348	12,348	12,348	12,348	12,348	12,348	12,348	12,348

(continued)

Table 3 (continued)

Dependent variable: Satisfaction with life (SWB)

Independent variables	Model 1	Model 2	Model 3	Model 4	Model 5	Model 6	Model 7	Model 8
Groups	18	18	18	18	18	18	18	18

Sample: 12,348 individuals, observations clustered in 18 countries. Year: 2016

Source Latin Barometer (2016)

$^{***}p < 0.001$, $^{**}p < 0.01$, $^{*}p < 0.05$.

Table 4 Correlation matrix

	Satisfaction with life (SWB)	Satisfaction with democracy	Democracy is the best form of government	Interpersonal trust	Trust in government
Satisfaction with life (SWB)	1.00				
Satisfaction with democracy	0.18	1.00			
Democracy is the best form of government	**0.02**	**0.14**	1.00		
Interpersonal trust	**0.05**	0.13	0.02	1.00	
Trust in government	0.11	0.38	0.13	0.12	1.00

(Individual Level) 2016
Source Latin Barometer (2016)

Table 5 Correlation matrix

	Satisfaction with life (SWB)	Satisfaction with democracy	Democracy is the best form of government	Interpersonal trust	Trust in government
Satisfaction with life (SWB)	1.00				
Satisfaction with democracy	0.47	1.00			
Democracy is the best form of government	**−0.07**	0.60	1.00		
Interpersonal trust	0.24	0.51	0.28	1.00	
Trust in government	0.41	**0.87**	0.45	0.51	1.00

(Country Level) 2016
Source Latin Barometer (2016)

between the level of individual well-being and the levels of the two abovementioned social factors. On average, the mean of SWB in Latin American countries is 3.03 out of 4. In other words, 75% of the population in these countries are satisfied with their lives. In the case of democracy (measured by *Satisfaction with democracy*), however, the value is 2.2 out of 4. This much lower value indicates that only 35.23% of the population is satisfied with democracy. The same happens with trust (1.7 out of 2 for the average person but 17% for the total population). Although *Satisfaction with democracy* and *Trust in government* (1.9 out of 4 for the average person but 28.17%

Table 6 Means or average person's behavior (2016)

Country	Satisfaction with life (SWB) (From 1–4)	Satisfaction with democracy (From 1–4)	Democracy is the best form of government (From 1–4)	Interpersonal trust (Yes = 1; No = 2)	Trust in government (From 1–4)
32 Argentina	3.00	2.66	3.24	1.25	2.14
68 Bolivia	2.84	2.39	2.94	1.16	2.12
76 Brazil	2.59	1.58	3.02	1.03	1.59
152 Chile	2.89	2.14	3.05	1.13	1.95
170 Colombia	3.28	2.00	2.87	1.15	1.85
188 Costa Rica	3.32	2.32	2.88	1.10	1.75
214 Dominican Rep	3.52	2.69	2.83	1.17	2.50
218 Ecuador	2.95	2.39	3.07	1.22	2.29
222 El Salvador	3.08	1.97	2.70	1.14	1.75
320 Guatemala	3.16	2.21	2.77	1.20	2.01
340 Honduras	3.16	1.93	2.84	1.13	1.76
484 Mexico	3.04	2.07	2.91	1.31	2.02
558 Nicaragua	3.15	2.55	2.94	1.18	2.37
591 Panama	3.34	2.21	2.83	1.19	1.80
600 Paraguay	2.85	2.30	3.24	1.20	1.90
604 Peru	2.91	2.13	2.86	1.15	1.75
858 Uruguay	3.03	2.55	3.19	1.17	2.33
862 Venezuela	2.66	1.83	3.30	1.15	1.71
Average	**3.03**	**2.22**	**2.98**	**1.17**	**1.98**

Source Latin Barometer (2016)

for the total population) have a positive and significant effect on *Satisfaction with life*, the values of the former are much lower than those of the latter.

Figure 1a shows that, as *Satisfaction with life* (measured on the x-axis) increases from level 1 to level 4, *Satisfaction with democracy* rises, indicating a positive correlation (0.18, Table 4) on an individual scale. If we look at the finer details, however, we realize that, on average, people who assigned *Satisfaction with life* to level 1 gave

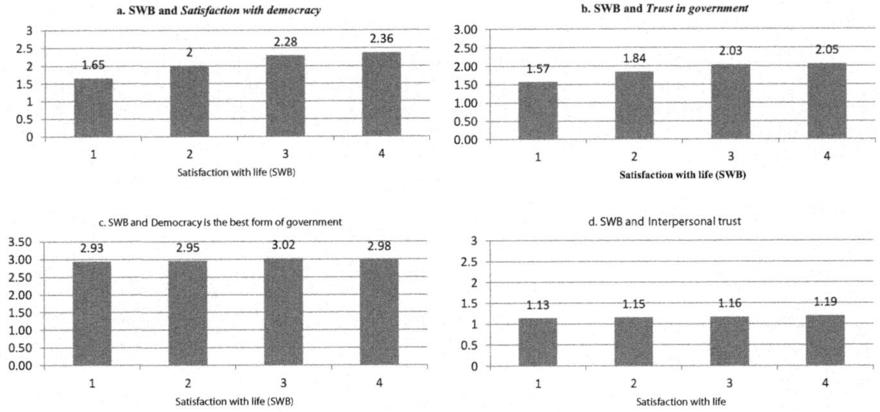

Fig. 1 SWB and institutional factors for the average person

Satisfaction with democracy a 1.65; those who gave *Satisfaction with life* a score of 2 also gave *Satisfaction with democracy* a 2; those who rated *Satisfaction with life* level 3 gave *Satisfaction with democracy* a 2.28; and those who gave *Satisfaction with life* a 4 gave *Satisfaction with democracy* a 2.36. In other words, *Satisfaction with democracy* rises very little—only from 1.65 to 2.36—indicating that the average levels of this variable are very low compared to the population's SWB levels of the population, and practically do not increase. A similar situation can be observed in the other three graphs (b, c, d) in Fig. 1. *Trust in government* varies only slightly, from 1.57 to 2.05, for those who are least and those who are most satisfied with life. *Interpersonal trust* only increases from 1.13 to 1.19, and *Democracy is the best form of government* from 2.93 to 2.98.

As people are more satisfied with their lives, their level of trust and satisfaction with democracy increases, but this increase is very slight. Why do high levels of SWB exist even if individuals are lowly satisfied with their democracies and have very low levels of social capital? Some studies, like Rojas (2016), suggest that the family is the fundamental source of support in these societies, creating strong bonds of trust, while there also exists significant distrust towards everyone else. This «generalized» trust goes hand in hand with costly deals among individuals and high costs for society, whether, for example, in cases of corruption or economic growth. Using Putnam's definition (2000), we argue that high levels of «bonding social capital» are perceived as strong ties within the community (at family level in this case), while «generalized trust» in Latin America refers to bridging social capital indicators that reflect «intergroup» social cohesion and heterogeneous relationships. The continent's history has left a mark on its culture, and the climate of generalized distrust, derived from both relationships, simultaneously determines all relationships among groups as well as perceptions of governments and democracy.

6 Conclusions

The most significant conclusion to be drawn from this study is that, although the models demonstrate a positive correlation between *Satisfaction with Life* and both *Satisfaction with democracy* and *Trust in government*, they do not explain the low variability in the latter two variables. This low variability may be motivated by all citizens' generalized distrust—little trust in the government and low satisfaction with democracy—whereas citizens' positive outlook on the world motivates a slightly higher response on a scale of 1 to 4. To put it another way, the most positive people are more lenient when it comes to evaluating all aspects of society. Following Frey and Stutzer (2002) and Graham and Pettinatio (2001), Orviska et al. (2014), satisfied people are more likely to be kinder in evaluating institutions and governance. We simply find a more positive personal perception of life and democracy. These low values both on an individual scale and for each country collectively do not substantiate a direct and positive relationship between *Satisfaction with democracy* and SWB.

Further research might investigate the following: Firstly, studies could use other databases, such as the World Value Survey, as the low variability of the Latin Barometer scales (from 1 to 4) does not help to explain the differences between the happiest and the least happy people or even an individual's perception of democracy. Secondly, macro-analyses could be performed, taking into account the evolution of the variables during the latest survey waves. We must know whether this situation indicates a decline in the democratic system or is merely a one-off occurrence. Thirdly, more homogenous analyses of the region could consider clusters of countries according to their level of «Institutional quality». All of these challenges would help to create a breakthrough in understanding the complex social phenomenon identified in this region.

References

Acemoglu, D., & Robinson, J. (2012). *Why nations fail: Origins of power*. Crown Publishers (Random House).

Afandi, E., Kermani, M., & Mammadov, F. (2017). Social capital and entrepreneurial process. *International Entrepreneurship and Management Journal, 13*(3), 685–716. https://doi.org/10.1007/s11365-016-0421-8

Aslam, A., & Corrado, L. (2012). The geography of well-being. *Journal of Economic Geography, 12*(3), 627–649. https://doi.org/10.1093/jeg/lbr041

Becchetti, L., Pelloni, A., & Rossetti, F. (2008). Relational goods, sociability, and happiness. *Kyklos, 61*(3), 343–363.

Bjørnskov, C. (2003). The happy few: Cross–country evidence on social capital and life satisfaction. *Kyklos, 56*(1), 3–16.

Bourdieu, P. (1986). The forms of capital. *Handbook of Theory and Research for the Sociology of Education*. https://doi.org/10.1017/CBO9781107415324.004

Bruni, L., & Stanca, L. (2008). Watching alone: Relational goods, television and happiness. *Journal of Economic Behavior and Organization, 65*(3–4), 506–528. https://doi.org/10.1016/j.jebo.2005.12.005

Casson, M. C., Della Giusta, M., & Kambhampati, U. S. (2010). Formal and informal institutions and development. *World Development, 38*(2), 137–141.
Clark, A. E., & Oswald, A. J. (1994). Unhappiness and unemployment. *The Economic Journal, 104*(424), 648–648. https://doi.org/10.2307/2234639
Coleman, J. S. (1988). Social capital in the creation of human-capital. *American Journal of Sociology*. https://doi.org/10.1086/228943
Coppedge, M. (2012). *Democratization and research methods*. Cambridge University Press. https://doi.org/10.1017/CBO9781139016179
Dorn, D., Fisher, J., Gebhard, K., & Souza-Poza, A. (2007). Is it culture or democracy? The impact of democracy and culture on happiness. *Social Indicators Research, 82*, 505–526.
Easterlin, R. (1974). Does economic growth improve the human lot? Some empirical evidence. *Nations and Households in Economic Growth, 89*(2), 89–125. https://doi.org/10.1007/BF00286477
Easterlin, R. A. (2001). Income and happiness: Towards a unified theory. *The Economic Journal, 111*(473), 465–484. https://doi.org/10.1111/1468-0297.00646
Frey, B. S., & Stutzer, A. (2000). Happiness, economy and institutions. *The Economic Journal, 110*, 918–938. https://doi.org/10.1111/1468-0297.00570
Frey, B. S., & Stutzer, A. (2002). What can economists learn from happiness research? *Journal of Economic Literature, 40*(2), 402–435. https://doi.org/10.1257/002205102320161320
Fosu, A., Bates, R., & Hoeffler, A. (2006). Institutions, governance and economic development in Africa: An overview. *Journal of African Economies, 15*(suppl_1), 1–9.
Fuchs, D., Guidorossi, G., & Svensson, P. (1995). Support for the democratic system. *Citizens and the State, 1*, 323–353.
Graham, C., & Pettinato, S. (2001). Happiness, markets, and democracy: Latin America in comparative perspective. *Journal of Happiness Studies, 2*(3), 237–268. https://doi.org/10.1023/A:1011860027447
Grootaert, C., & van Bastelaer, T. (2001). *Understanding and measuring social capital: A synthesis of findings and recommendation from the social capital initiative*. Word Bank Working Paper No. 24.
Han, S. (2015). Social capital and subjective happiness: Which contexts matter? *Journal of Happiness Studies, 16*(1), 241–255. https://doi.org/10.1007/s10902-014-9506-7
Helliwell, J. F. (2006). Well-being, social capital, and public policy: What's new? *Economic Journal, 116*(510), C34–C45.
Helliwell, J. F., & Putnam, R. D. (2004). The social context of well-being. *Philosophical Transactions of the Royal Society B: Biological Sciences, 359*(1449), 1435–1446. https://doi.org/10.1098/rstb.2004.1522
Inglehart, R., Foa, R., Peterson, C., & Welzel, C. (2008). Development, freedom, and rising happiness: A global perspective (1981–2007). *Perspectives on Psychological Science, 3*(4), 264–285. https://doi.org/10.1111/j.1745-6924.2008.00078.x
Inglehart, R., & Klingemann, H. (2000). Genes, culture, democracy, and happiness. In E. Diener & E. M. Suh (Eds.), *Culture and subjective well-being* (pp. 165–183). MIT Press.
Khodyakov, D. (2007). Trust as a process: A three-dimensional approach. *Sociology, 41*(1), 115–132. https://doi.org/10.1177/0038038507072285
Klein, C. (2013). Social capital or social cohesion: What matters for subjective well-being. *Social Indicators Research, 110*(3), 891–911.
Latinobarómetro. (2016). *Latinobarómetro Report 2016*. Latinobarómetro Corporation.
Latinobarómetro. (2017). *Latinobarómetro Report 2017*. Latinobarómetro Corporation.
Layard, R. (2005). *Happiness: Lessons from a new science*. Penguin Books. Allen Lane.
Linde, J., & Ekman, J. (2003) Satisfaction with democracy: A note on a frequently used indicator in comparative politics. *European Journal of Political Research, 42*, 391–408.
Neira, I., Bruna, F., Portela, M., & García-Aracil, A. (2018). Individual well-being, geographical heterogeneity and social capital. *Journal of Happiness Studies, 19*(4), 1067–1090. https://doi.org/10.1007/s10902-016-9840-z

North, D. C. (1990), Institution, institutional change and economic performance. Cambridge: Cambridge University Press.
North, D. (2003). *The role of institutions in economic development*. ECE Discussion Papers Series 2003_2 UNCE.
Orviska, M., Caplanova, A., & Hudson, J. (2014). The impact of democracy on well-being. *Social Indicators Research, 115*(1), 493–508. https://doi.org/10.1007/s11205-012-9997-8
Owen, A. L., Videras, J., & Willemsen, C. (2008). Democracy, participation, and life satisfaction. *Social Science Quarterly, 89*(4), 987–1005. https://doi.org/10.1111/j.1540-6237.2008.00595.x
Pittau, M. G., Zelli, R., & Gelman, A. (2010). Economic disparities and life satisfaction in European regions. *Social Indicators Research, 96*(2), 339–361. https://doi.org/10.1007/s11205-009-9481-2
Portela, M., Neira, I., & Salinas-Jiménez, M. M. (2013). Social capital and subjective wellbeing in Europe: a new approach on social capital. *Social Indicators Research, 114*(2), 493–511.
Puntscher, S., Hauser, C., Walde, J., & Tappeiner, G. (2015). The impact of social capital on subjective well-being: A regional perspective. *Journal of Happiness Studies, 16*(5), 1231–1246. https://doi.org/10.1007/s10902-014-9555-y
Putnam, R. D., Leonardi, R., & Nanetti, R. (1993). *Making democracy work: Civic traditions in modern Italy*. Princeton University Press.
Rampichini, C., & d'Andrea, S. S. (1998). A hierarchical ordinal probit model for the analysis of life satisfaction in Italy. *Social Indicators Research, 44*(1), 41–69. https://doi.org/10.1023/A:1006888613727
Rodríguez-Pose, A., & von Berlepsch, V. (2014). Social capital and individual happiness in Europe. *Journal of Happiness Studies, 15*(2), 357–386. https://doi.org/10.1007/s10902-013-9426-y
Rojas, M. (2016). *Handbook of happiness research in Latin America*. Springer.
Rothstein, B., & Eek, D. (2001). *The causal mechanism between trust in authorities and trust in others: An experimental approach.*
Sarracino, F. (2010). Social capital and subjective well-being trends: Comparing 11 Western European countries. *Journal of Socio-Economics, 39*(4), 482–517. https://doi.org/10.1016/j.socec.2009.10.010
Snijders, T. A. B., & Bosker, R. J. (2012). *Multilevel analysis: An introduction to basic and advanced multilevel modeling*. Sage Publishers.
van Oorschot, W., & Arts, W. (2005). The social capital of European welfare states: The crowding out hypothesis revisited. *Journal of European Social Policy, 15*(1), 5–26. https://doi.org/10.1177/0958928705049159

Isabel Neira is associate Professor of Applied Economics (Econo-metrics) at Universidad de Santiago de Compostela (Spain). Specialist in well-being, social capital, welfare and entrepreneurship. She has published several articules in journals such as Social Indicators Resarch and Journal of Happiness Studies. The total number of citations in google scholar is 1353 since 2013, an index h of 19, index i10 of 43 and an index of 21.17 in Research Gate (https://www.researchgate.net/profile/Isabel_Neira); https://orcid.org/0000-0003-0619-5964.

Marta Portela got Ph.D. in Economics from the Universidad de Santiago de Compostela (USC) (Spain). Assistant full-time profes-sor of Accounting and Finance at USC. Research in social capital, well-being, happiness economics and entrepreneurship. Senior Re-searcher in project The Global Entrepreneurship Research Associa-tion for the realization of GEM-GALICIA. She has 544 citations in google scholar. Her h index is 10 and her i10 index is 12. Profile in Research Gate https://www.researchgate.net/profile/Marta_Portela_Maseda; https://orcid.org/0000-0002-0399-0818.

Maricruz Lacalle-Calderon is associate professor at the Depart-ment of Development Economics, Universidad Autónoma de Ma-drid (Spain), as well as founder and academic director of the "Inter-national Master in Microfinance and Financial Inclusion" at this University. Her main research topics include microfinance, poverty, and economic development. She has published several articles in journals such as Review of Development Economics, The Developing Economies; Canadian Journal of Development Studies, among others. She has also edited and published books as the Handbook of Microcredit in Europe (Edward Elgar, 2010). She has 653 citations in google scholar since 2014. Her h index is 12 and her i10 index is 14. Profile in Research Gate https://www.researchgate.net/profile/Maricruz_Lacalle-Calderon; https://orcid.org/0000-0001-6662-4527.

Degree of Benefit? The Interconnection Among Social Capital, Well-Being and Education

Janine Jongbloed and Ashley Pullman

1 Introduction

Overall levels of educational attainment, and in particular tertiary credentials, are a common measure of national development, one of "the best readily available indicators" (Inglehart, 2008, p. 132) of modernization. Education is also central to individual and societal well-being beyond its impact on national and individual economic outcomes. In particular, higher levels of education are associated with greater levels of social trust and improved social relatedness, two forms of individual social capital (Huang et al., 2009), and well-being (Woessmann & Schuetz, 2006). Given the employment and life-course outcomes associated with tertiary education–from improved earnings to greater employment stability (Pallas, 2000)–the correlation between rising levels of social capital and well-being among this highly educated group may be due to a range of confounding effects. In turn, the association between social capital and well-being may differ between individuals with and without tertiary education.

Rising levels of overall education at the state level are also linked to higher levels of social capital (Helliwell & Putnam, 2007) and well-being (Vila, 2000, 2005) within societies. Yet how increased levels of tertiary education at the state level change the interrelations between social capital and subjective well-being is unclear. Just as rising overall income at the country-level is not necessarily associated with

J. Jongbloed (✉)
Institut de Recherche Sur l'Éducation: Sociologie et Économie de l'Éducation (IREDU), Université Bourgogne Franche-Comté, Dijon, France
e-mail: janine.jongbloed@u-bourgogne.fr

A. Pullman
Education Policy Research Initiative, Graduate School of Public and International Affairs, University of Ottawa, Ottawa, Canada
e-mail: apullman@irpe-epri.ca

A. Almakaeva et al. (eds.), *Social Capital and Subjective Well-Being*, Societies and Political Orders in Transition,
https://doi.org/10.1007/978-3-030-75813-4_10

greater well-being on average (Easterlin, 1995), an increased proportion of individuals with tertiary education may not actually improve individual-level social capital and well-being. When framed as a positional good (Salinas-Jiménez et al., 2011), tertiary education may have a relative rather than an absolute relationship with both social capital and well-being. In contrast, some researchers have found that there is a significant positive association between national performances on PISA tests and overall happiness scores (Kirkcaldy et al., 2004). Thus, along with providing insight on the moderating effect of individual-level tertiary education on the relationship between social capital and well-being, the following study also seeks to understand how overall levels of tertiary education at the country-level change the nature of the relationship between social capital and well-being.

Social capital is not a single attribute; rather, the term social capital captures a variety of entities that have two important characteristics in common: "they all consist of some aspect of a social structure, and they facilitate certain actions of individuals who are within the structure" (Coleman, 1990, p. 302). Building upon prior research, we assess two elements of social capital: generalized social trust (Beilmann et al., 2017) and social relatedness (Carmo & Nunes, 2013; Conzo et al., 2016). It is important not to assume that tertiary education has the same relationship with different forms of social capital, both at the individual and state level. Notably, Inglehart (2008) and Marks (1997) argue that higher levels of tertiary attainment support the development of post-materialist values. With an emphasis on individual autonomy and self-expression (Inglehart & Welzel, 2007; Zagórski, 2011), this value shift may influence the association between certain forms of social capital and well-being.

More specifically, tertiary education may improve civic engagement (e.g., Brand, 2010; Burden, 2009) but has "little effect on *schmoozing*–informal social connectedness" (Putnam, 2000, p. 186). Huang et al. (2009) theorize that this discrepancy is due to a "trade off" between education and different forms of social capital in which "the emphasis on the role of schooling as a source of human capital could be detrimental to the contribution of schooling on cultivating social capital for collective welfare" (p. 461). In contrast, patterns of modernization are associated with shifts towards "rational, tolerant, trusting, and participatory" values (Inglehart & Baker, 2000, p. 19), which align with forms of social capital related to generalized trust. In this sense, improved social trust signals the ability of tertiary education to impact values, which may or may not actually improve social relatedness.

This chapter uses the European Social Survey (ESS) to examine the relationships among tertiary education, social capital, and subjective well-being in 27 countries. Prior studies suggest that tertiary education is significantly associated with social trust and that social trust is similarly associated with self-reported well-being. For its part, social relatedness is intricately tied to well-being and is even conceptualized as one part of the well-being construct in 'self-determination' and 'flourishing' understandings of well-being (Ryan & Deci, 2000). However, given its theorized influence on individual autonomy and self-expression (Inglehart & Welzel, 2007), the relationship between social relatedness and well-being is not as clearly linked to tertiary education.

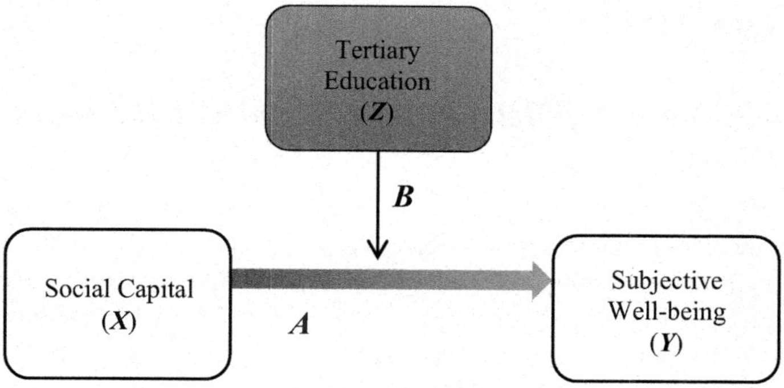

Fig. 1 Schema illustrating the proposed relationship between social capital and subjective well-being as moderated by tertiary education in individual- and cross-level interactions

As shown in Fig. 1, we hypothesize that the relationship between social capital–in this case, social trust and social relatedness–and subjective well-being is moderated in different ways by tertiary attainment. Specifically, we predict a 'trade-off' between individual human capital and interpersonal social capital, where either one or the other plays a dominant role. Furthermore, we expand on a modernization perspective by studying how overall levels of tertiary education within a country affect the relationships between different forms of social capital and well-being. Based on these aims, our research questions are as follows:

(1) How do individual levels of social capital, as defined by both social trust and social relatedness, and subjective well-being descriptively differ by individual tertiary educational attainment within 27 European countries?
(2) Does tertiary education influence the relationship between social capital and subjective well-being? In other words, does education at the individual level moderate the relationships between social trust and well-being and social relatedness and well-being?
(3) Does the inclusion of an indicator measuring overall societal levels of tertiary educational attainment have an influence on the relationship between social capital and well-being? In other words, does education at the country level moderate the relationships between social trust and well-being and social relatedness and well-being?

In order to answer these research questions, the next section provides an overview of prior research on the relationships among well-being, social capital, and education. Following, the data and methods section details how key concepts within this study are operationalized and our quantitative approach. After providing an overview of the main findings, the discussion and conclusion section details answers to the original research questions, as well as future areas of research and overall limitations.

2 Literature Review

2.1 The Relationship Between Social Capital and Subjective Well-Being

A multi-dimensional construct of 'subjective well-being' captures both individual-level feeling and functioning and is defined as an individual's cognitive and affective evaluation of his or her life (Diener et al., 1999; Klein, 2013). High subjective well-being involves feeling "many pleasant and few unpleasant emotions," and being satisfied with one's life (Diener, 2000, p. 34). Although this concept is used extensively across many studies, it does not cover the entire spectrum of the definition of a 'good life' or of good mental health; however, it does allow for important insights into whether or not individuals give mainly positive or negative evaluations of their lives.

Prior research has examined how different forms of social capital relate to subjective well-being (Haller & Hadler, 2006; Helliwell et al., 2014; Portela et al., 2013; Puntscher et al., 2015). Both 'bonding' (e.g., strong ties) and 'bridging' (e.g., weak ties) forms of social capital are compared, the first concerning "relationships with family and close friends, who tend to be quite homogeneous," and the second surrounding social trust and "relationships with distant others, including friends, colleagues and associates, who tend to have varied backgrounds, values and experiences" (Pereira et al., 2017, p. 385). In this sense, social capital entails both structural and cognitive components, one "associated with group membership," and the other "linked with the expectations, obligations, and trust embedded in relationships" (Pereira et al., 2017, p. 384).

Both social trust (Rodríguez-Pose & Berlepsch, 2014) and social relatedness, as measured by feeling appreciated (Adler & Fagley, 2005) and level of social support (Siedlecki et al., 2014), are significantly related to subjective well-being; yet, social context plays an important role (Diener, 2012; Yamaoka, 2008). As measured by both social trust and social support, there may be stronger associations between social capital and well-being in high-income countries (Calvo et al., 2012), especially those in Western Europe (Sarracino, 2012). Lesser known is if education level within a country moderates the relationship between social capital and well-being. Nevertheless, the Human Development Index (HDI)–which includes a measure of education level–is significantly associated with greater well-being cross-nationally, a model that also finds no association in terms of overall levels social capital, as measured by overall level of press freedom, when modelled simultaneously with the HDI (Vemuri & Costanza, 2006).

2.2 The Relationship Between Education and Subjective Well-Being

Tertiary credentials are associated with a range of individual life outcomes, including enhanced physical and mental health (Delhey, 2010; Field, 2009; Groot & Brink, 2007; Lynch & Hippel, 2016; Tuijnman, 1990), and benefits inside and outside of the labour market (Grossman, 2005; Haveman & Wolfe, 1984; McMahon & Oketch, 2013; Oreopoulos & Salvanes, 2011; Vila, 2000). Although the link between education and life satisfaction and/or personal happiness is well established (Woessmann & Schuetz, 2006), the exact nature of this relationship is unclear. Education is often included as a control variable within well-being research and is not discussed in depth (Barrington-Leigh,2013; Bonikowska et al., 2013; Hou, 2014). Depending on the analysis and other factors considered within these studies, tertiary credentials may appear to directly or indirectly influence subjective well-being.

Although differing by the conception of well-being employed (Jongbloed, 2018a; Nikolaev, 2018), research examining the direct relationship between tertiary education and certain forms of well-being is somewhat dubious and suggests that "educational attainment is not strongly or consistently related to life satisfaction" (Fahey & Smyth, 2004, p. 17). There is often little to no direct association, or even a significant *negative* association, between education and life satisfaction (Nikolaev, 2018). Contrastingly, research examining the indirect relationship between education and well-being highlights biases within these results. By accounting for indirect effects–for example, through income–the magnitude and even the sign of the education coefficient may change (Powdthavee et al., 2015).

Research investigating the association between education and broader conceptions of well-being suggest that individuals with high attainment report greater eudaimonic well-being, more meaning in their lives, and fewer negative emotions (Jongbloed, 2018a; Nikolaev, 2018). Other attributes, such as self-efficacy, autonomy, mental health, and confidence, are also positively associated with education (Chevalier & Feinstein, 2006; Field, 2009; Galton & Page, 2015). In terms of psychological health, individuals with more education report lower psychological distress, increased emotional health, and lower rates of depression, anxiety, anger, and malaise (Pallas, 2000). These studies lend support to the contention that education not only shapes "preferences, expectations, feelings, and emotional states" but also "perceptions of self and society" (Tuijnman, 1990, p. 286).

2.3 The Relationship Between Education and Social Capital

Tertiary-level credentials also link to social capital, both at the individual and societal levels (Helliwell & Putnam, 2007). Besides income, education level is one of the most influential socio-demographic factors associated with social capital in Europe (Kaasa, & Parts, 2008). Individuals with tertiary education report higher levels of social capital in terms of: social trust and tolerance; membership in voluntary organizations; community involvement and political participation; and access to social support from relatives and friends (Borgonovi & Burns, 2015; Kingston et al., 2003; Nieminen et al., 2008). Prior studies suggest that tertiary education improves social capital by changing individual perceptions of cultural and social structures (Huang et al., 2011). Particularly relevant to our study, individuals with tertiary credentials report greater levels of social trust (Easterbrook et al., 2016; Helliwell & Putnam, 2007; Huang et al., 2012).

Although meta-analyses have confirmed the robustness of the relationship between education and social capital across studies (Huang et al., 2009), the causal nature of this association is contested in three ways: (1) the direction of the relationship; (2) the extent to which it exists for all forms of social capital; and (3) the influence of often omitted variables. As is also argued concerning the education-health gradient (Lynch & Hippel, 2016), there is evidence that individuals with high levels of social capital at a young age are more likely to have greater levels of educational attainment (Roth, 2013). Additionally, while education is a "strong and robust correlate" of individual social capital, social relatedness shows a weaker association compared to social trust (Huang et al., 2009, p. 454). As discussed in the introduction, there is weak evidence that education improves "informal social connectedness" (Putnam, 2000, p. 186). Rather the nature of social capital may change for highly educated individuals, such as increased social connectedness via technology (Fischer, 2005). Finally, the relationship between education and social trust may appear stronger when other correlates are omitted, such as increased optimism among tertiary graduates (Uslaner, 2002) and environmental factors early in the life course (Oskarsson et al., 2017).

Past research is mixed in regards to the relationship between how overall levels of tertiary education within a country are associated with social capital. Borgonovi and Burns (2015) argue that, although there is little to no association between country-level social trust and tertiary education, overall levels of assessed cognitive skills are positively associated with trust. Additionally, the relationship between social capital and education becomes more complicated when considering well-being. Although education has a positive association with individual-level social capital (e.g., Helliwell & Putnam, 2007) and subjective well-being (e.g., Rodríguez-Pose & Berlepsch, 2014), once a model also includes social capital variables, education may have a significant *negative* impact on subjective well-being (e.g., Portela et al., 2013). Furthermore, the multiple associations covered in this literature review highlight that tertiary education is likely associated with subjective well-being directly, while also moderating the relationship between social capital and well-being. That is, the association between social trust and social relatedness and well-being may differ for those with higher levels of education.

3 Analytical Approach

3.1 Data and Sample Selection

Initiated by the European Science Foundation in 2002, the aim of the ESS is to capture cross-national attitudes, values, and beliefs within the European Union every two years. This study uses the sixth wave (2012/2013) of the ESS, a face-to-face survey that focuses specifically on personal and social well-being and includes several measures of social trust and social relatedness, along with socio-demographic information, including level of education. The sampling strategy uses a strict random probability design in 29 separate countries,[1] a universe that aims to represent non-institutionalized individuals age 15 and over regardless of their legal status, nationality, and language.

To study a comparable group of respondents cross-nationally, we limit our analysis to respondents age 25 to 65 who were active in the labour market during the survey period. We exclude Albania and Kosovo due to the small number of respondents with tertiary education within the ESS data. Following ESS guidelines, we apply post-stratification and population size weights in all analyses (ESS, 2014b). The post-stratification weight corrects for within-country non-response bias due to age, gender, education, and region, while the population size weight corrects for differing population sizes in a cross-national analysis. For further information on the ESS wave six survey design, see the ESS documentation freely available online (ESS, 2012, 2014a, 2014b).

3.2 Dependent Variable

Beyond only a consideration of an individual's evaluation of his or her life satisfaction, the dependent variable representing well-being includes three ESS items measuring both positive and negative emotions–that is, self-reported life satisfaction and levels of happiness and depression–and aligns with the concept of 'subjective well-being' outlined above (Diener et al., 2010). We first standardize responses to each question (i.e., to have a mean of zero and a standard deviation of one) and then use polychoric factor analysis to construct the measure of well-being and Bartlett's factor scores to scale responses. As shown in Table 1, the coefficient of reliability is 0.70.

---

[1] Participating countries include: Albania, Belgium, Bulgaria, Cyprus, Czech Republic, Denmark, Estonia, Finland, France, Germany, Hungary, Iceland, Ireland, Israel, Italy, Kosovo, Lithuania, Netherlands, Norway, Poland, Portugal, Russian Federation, Slovakia, Slovenia, Spain, Sweden, Switzerland, Ukraine, and the United Kingdom.

3.3 Independent Variables

The main independent variables of interest are tertiary attainment and two measures of social capital: social trust and social relatedness. Building on the conception that university is a "critical stage" (Huang et al., 2009, p. 462) influencing social capital, an ESS item measuring self-reported highest education level captures tertiary attainment. We transform this ordinal scale into a dichotomous variable categorizing ESS respondents with and without university-level credentials (i.e., a degree at the undergraduate or graduate level). Aligning with 'bridging' forms of social capital, three ESS questions measure 'social trust' and capture beliefs that other people can be trusted, are fair, and are helpful, a composite measure used within prior research (e.g., Poortinga, 2006). Following Conzo et al. (2017), four ESS items operationalize a 'bonding' form of capital termed 'social relatedness.' These questions ask respondents to report the extent to which they feel appreciated and respected by others and provide and receive help. We use polychoric factor analysis and Bartlett's factor scores to construct both social capital scales, which are grand-mean centered in the analyses.[2] As shown in Table 1, the coefficients of reliability range from 0.79 to 0.70.

Analyses also include several control variables known to be influential on well-being, social capital, and time use–the latter of which may influence social relatedness. Dummy variables measure: gender, if the respondent reported being married or in a common-law relationship, the presence of children in the home, and if the respondent was in school during the survey period. Continuous variables measure age/age^2 and the number of hours typically worked in a respondent's main job, including overtime. Categorical variables measure income group and professional status. See the Appendix for an overview of the variables, scale construction, and levels of missing values.

Table 1 Reliability and correlation table of main individual-level variables

	Well-being	Tertiary education	Social trust	Social relatedness
Well-being	(0.70)			
Tertiary education	0.11	(NA)		
Social trust	0.31	0.15	(0.79)	
Social relatedness	0.40	0.07	0.19	(0.70)

Note Correlations with tertiary education calculated using the point-biserial correlation coefficient. Coefficients of reliability shown in parentheses

[2] Grand mean centering subtracts the overall mean (i.e., across all countries) from each score, a procedure that changes the mean of all scores to zero. In contrast, group mean centering subtracts the mean of each cluster (i.e., individual countries) from each score within it. Both aim to produce "meaningful zero points" and improve interpretability (Enders & Tofighi, 2007). Because the derived social capital variables are constructed using responses across all countries, sensitivity analysis (available upon request) showed that grand and group mean centering produce almost identical estimates. Our choice to use grand mean centering is based on the recommendation that it is best suited in analysis involving a level-two variable (Peugh, 2010).

3.4 Modelling Approach

As part one of the findings section will illustrate, overall levels of social capital and well-being differ by country. Thus, we use linear multi-level modelling with random country intercepts and an unstructured covariance matrix to examine the relationship between the dependent variable–self-reported well-being–and our main independent variables of interest. Multi-level modelling allows us to correct for country-level clustering, a violation of the assumptions of ordinary least squares regression, through a two-level modelling structure with the addition of a composite residual term in the mixed model (Raudenbush & Bryk, 2002). While level one assesses country-variant terms, level two examines how country-invariant covariates explain variance within the level-one model.

After describing country differences in how overall levels of social capital and well-being differ for ESS participants with and without tertiary education, part two of our analysis graphically represents how tertiary education at the individual level moderates both forms of social capital. Separate multi-level models without level-two covariates operationalize these moderated relationships through two-way fixed interaction terms; that is, we separately model one interaction term between individual-level tertiary education and social trust and another interaction term between education and social relatedness. Given the influence of additional socio-demographic and employment factors, section two also assesses how tertiary education functions as a moderator with and without the inclusion of additional fixed control variables. Following best practice, the interaction model includes all constitutive terms (Brambor et al., 2006).

Part three further refines the multi-level models by introducing a level-two country-invariant variable measuring the overall level of tertiary education. We derive the country-level indicator from the ESS data as the percentage of respondents within each country with tertiary education, a measure that correlates at 0.62 with 2012 attainment data from the United Nations Statistics Division. To assess how average levels of tertiary education at the country level change the individual-level relationship between both measures of social capital and well-being, fixed cross-level interaction terms are introduced into the model. These indicators measure two-way interactions between social trust indicators at level one and overall country-level tertiary education at level two.

Importantly, the multiplicative interaction models in parts two and three of our findings are symmetric. Therefore, these models cannot differentiate between a hypothesis asserting that education at the individual or country level modifies the effect of social capital on well-being from its opposite where social capital modifies the effect of education on well-being (Brambor et al., 2006). Although the direction of causality cannot be determined empirically, theoretical argumentation in combination with the empirical results provide strong evidence for a particular interpretation, a point that will be further developed in the discussion and conclusion.

Model development included running an unconditional means model with no predictors at level one or two to understand within- and between-country variation that covariates in later models may explain. This initial model generated an inter-class correlation of 0.16. Thus, only an estimated 16% of the total score variation in subjective well-being is attributable to differences among countries. We further evaluate each multi-level model through pseudo R^2 and goodness-of-fit measures, assessing the deviance and how the proportional reduction in the level-1 variance component (R^2_r) and the variance reduction on the intercept (R^2_{u0}) changes in reference to a means-only model.

4 Results

4.1 Descriptive Overview

Figures 2, 3, and 4 illustrate that social trust, social relatedness, and subjective well-being differ between ESS respondents with and without tertiary degrees on average and across most national contexts. As illustrated in Fig. 2, among all countries modelled, respondents without tertiary education report levels of subjective well-being that are 5.9% lower on average. Nevertheless, the difference in well-being by education level ranges considerably amongst countries, from little to no difference by education level in Finland and Denmark, to approximately 21% lower self-reported subjective well-being among non-tertiary graduates in Hungary. Notably, there is a less pronounced difference among respondents with and without tertiary education at high ends of the well-being index.

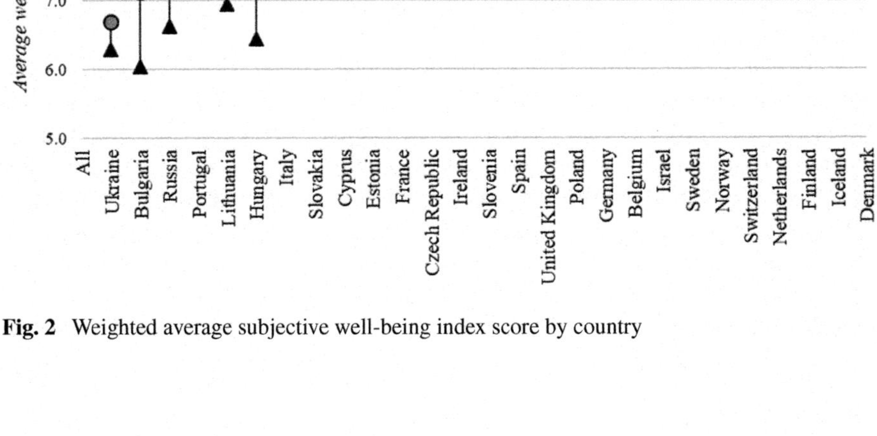

Fig. 2 Weighted average subjective well-being index score by country

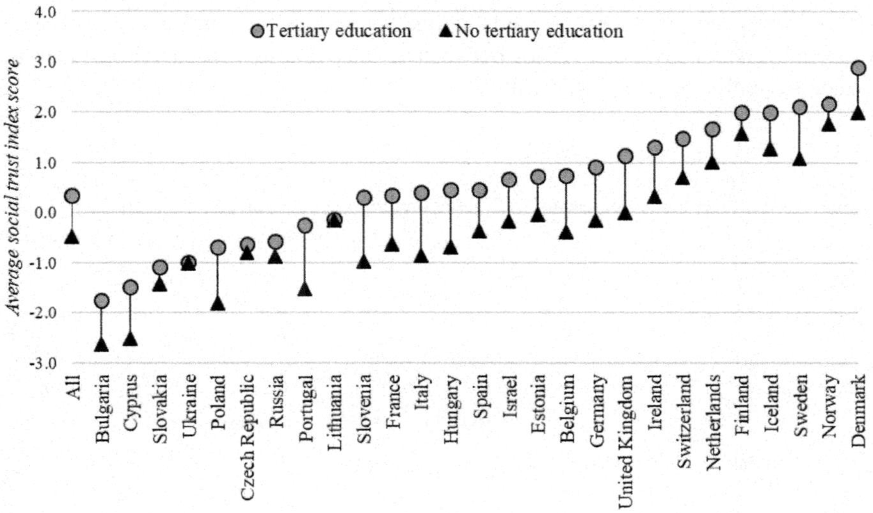

Fig. 3 Weighted average social trust index score by country

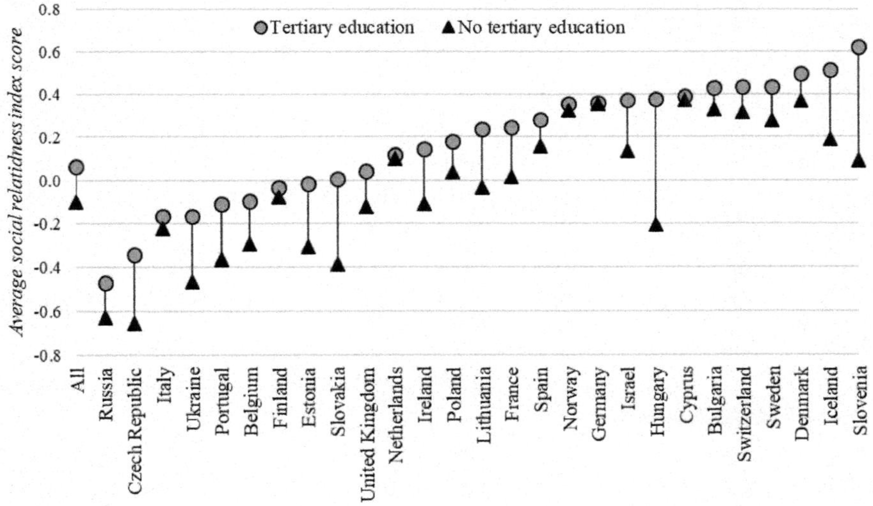

Fig. 4 Weighted average social relatedness index score by country

Shown in Figs. 3 and 4, on average, ESS respondents with tertiary education report higher index levels across both social capital measures. Nonetheless, respondents with and without tertiary education report similar levels of social trust in some Eastern (e.g., Slovakia, Ukraine, Czech Republic, Russia, and Lithuania) and Northern (e.g., Norway and Finland) European countries. There is also little to no difference in social relatedness by education level in several countries, including Italy, Finland,

Netherlands, Norway, Germany, and Cyprus. In contrast, there is a sizable difference in social relatedness index scores between tertiary and non-tertiary holders in the Czech Republic, Slovenia, and Hungary.

Table 2 Multilevel model regressing well-being on tertiary education and social trust

	Model 1	Model 2	Model 3	Model 4	Model 5
Level 1					
Tertiary education	0.301***	0.310***	0.273***	0.101	0.092
	(0.093)	(0.087)	(0.070)	(0.089)	(0.094)
Social trust	0.212***	0.226***	0.224***	0.216***	0.198***
	(0.011)	(0.009)	(0.009)	(0.010)	(0.017)
Tertiary*social trust interaction		−0.060**	−0.056**	−0.054*	
		(0.021)	(0.022)	(0.023)	
Demographic controls			*Included*	*Included*	*Included*
Employment controls				*Included*	*Included*
Level 2					
% of pop. with tertiary education					−0.007
					(0.017)
Cross-level interaction with social trust					0.000
					(0.000)
Constant	8.091***	8.099***	7.540***	7.106***	7.316***
	(0.160)	(0.158)	(0.154)	(0.171)	(0.553)
Variance components					
Constant variance	0.525	0.530	0.549	0.572	0.559
	(0.123)	(0.125)	(0.131)	(0.134)	(0.124)
Residual variance	3.998	3.994	3.881	3.804	3.807
	(0.200)	(0.198)	(0.202)	(0.212)	(0.214)
Pseudo R^2 & Goodness-of-fit					
R^2_r	0.068	0.069	0.095	0.113	0.113
R^2_{u0}	0.354	0.347	0.324	0.296	0.313
Deviance	98,982	98,958	98,288	97,816	97,837
N	23,133				

Note Robust standard errors in parentheses
$^{+}p < 0.10$, $^{*}p < 0.05$, $^{**}p < 0.01$, $^{***}p < 0.001$

4.2 The Moderating Role of Education

Adding control variables and interaction terms consecutively, Tables 2 and 3 show the results of multilevel models examining the associations among education, social capital (i.e., social trust and social relatedness), and well-being. Both social capital coefficients are significant and positive across all models, a trend that suggests that they both enhance well-being. The larger coefficient for social relatedness highlights a more prominent association with well-being compared to social trust. In Models 2, 3, and 4, the interaction terms between individual-level tertiary education and

Table 3 Multi-level model regressing well-being on tertiary education and social relatedness

	Model 1	Model 2	Model 3	Model 4	Model 5
Level 1					
Tertiary education	0.366***	0.368***	0.344***	0.153*	0.150*
	(0.066)	(0.062)	(0.050)	(0.069)	(0.075)
Social relatedness	0.582***	0.597***	0.581***	0.562***	0.560***
	(0.027)	(0.030)	(0.029)	(0.029)	(0.056)
Tertiary*s. relatedness interaction		−0.071**	−0.074***	−0.072**	
		(0.024)	(0.023)	(0.024)	
Demographic controls			*Included*	*Included*	*Included*
Employment controls				*Included*	*Included*
Level 2					
% of pop. with tertiary education					−0.000
					(0.018)
Cross-level interaction with s. relatedness					−0.000
					(0.001)
Constant	8.055***	8.058***	7.577***	7.200***	7.204***
	(0.171)	(0.170)	(0.169)	(0.192)	(0.602)
Variance components					
Constant variance	0.675	0.674	0.703	0.700	0.700
	(0.181)	(0.181)	(0.185)	(0.188)	(0.188)
Residual variance	3.717	3.715	3.632	3.571	3.573
	(0.182)	(0.181)	(0.189)	(0.201)	(0.201)
Pseudo R2 & Goodness-of-fit					
R^2_r	0.134	0.134	0.153	0.167	0.167
R^2_{u0}	0.169	0.170	0.134	0.138	0.138
Deviance	95,345	95,336	94,816	94,435	94,444
N	22,688				

Note Robust standard errors in parentheses
$^{+}p < 0.10$, $^{*}p < 0.05$, $^{**}p < 0.01$, $^{***}p < 0.001$

both forms of social capital are statistically significant and *negative*.[3] This suggests that the relationship between social capital and well-being is weaker for those with tertiary education. Although there is less of a social capital gradient in well-being for those with advanced credentials, the individual-level interaction terms only modestly contribute to the overall explanatory power of the models.

Looking at the results for social trust more specifically, Fig. 5 illustrates the conditional marginal effects of an individual-level interaction term between tertiary education and social trust both with and without additional control variables. The top graph demonstrates how overall levels of well-being differ on average between respondents with and without tertiary education across different levels of social trust, as estimated by an individual-level interaction term in Model 2 in Table 2 without additional demographic or employment control variables. It demonstrates that the relationship between tertiary education and well-being is stronger among individuals with lower social trust index scores; however, at high ends of the scale (i.e., scores greater than 4), there is no significant difference in well-being among individuals with and without tertiary education. However, as shown in the bottom of the graph, the conditional marginal effect comparing respondents with and without tertiary education is less pronounced when Model 4 in Table 2 accounts for employment and demographic controls. Although a small difference may exist at the lowest end of the social trust index, the 95 percent confidence interval passes zero at most levels of social trust once controls are included in the model.

Taking these results together, Fig. 5 demonstrates that average levels of well-being are more strongly impacted by social trust for those *without* tertiary education. Although other influential factors attenuate this finding in Model 4, differences in well-being between respondents with and without tertiary education are only significant at mid-to-lower levels of social trust in Model 2. That is, respondents who self-report high levels of social trust have similar levels of well-being regardless of their education level.[4] Thus, the negative individual-level interaction term indicates that the impact of social trust on well-being is smaller overall for those with tertiary education, while on the other hand, the conditional marginal effects suggest that highly educated respondents have greater well-being regardless of their level of social trust. This moderation effect suggests a 'trade-off' between individual human capital and interpersonal social capital, where one has a greater effect where the other is weaker, and vice versa.

Next, we turn to equivalent models examining social capital in the form of social relatedness. The top portion of Fig. 6 graphically represents the results of Model 2 in

[3] In robustness checks, the significance of the main variables and interaction terms does not change in models incorporating both forms of social capital in the same model. The results of these models are available upon request.

[4] As emphasized earlier in the chapter, these models cannot differentiate between a hypothesis asserting that education at the individual or country level modifies the effect of social capital on well-being from its opposite where social capital modifies the effect of education on well-being (Brambor et al., 2006). However, our theoretically based argument is that education is the moderating variable.

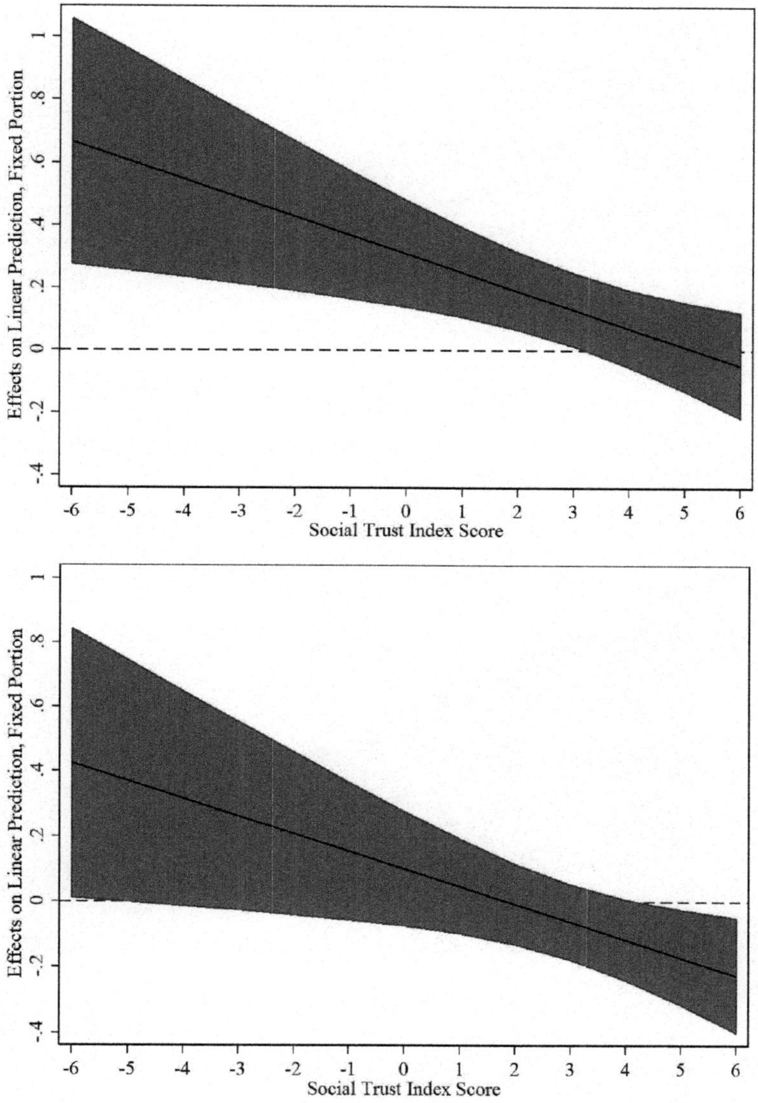

Fig. 5 Conditional marginal effects illustrating the moderation effect of tertiary education attainment on the association between social trust and well-being at the individual level, without (top) and with (bottom) control variables. *Note* 95% confidence interval in grey

Table 3 through the conditional marginal effect of the difference in the level of well-being between respondents with and without tertiary education by level of social relatedness. As the slope never passes zero (i.e., the dotted line), respondents with tertiary education have higher levels of well-being regardless of their self-reported level of social relatedness. However, like the results for social trust, the negative

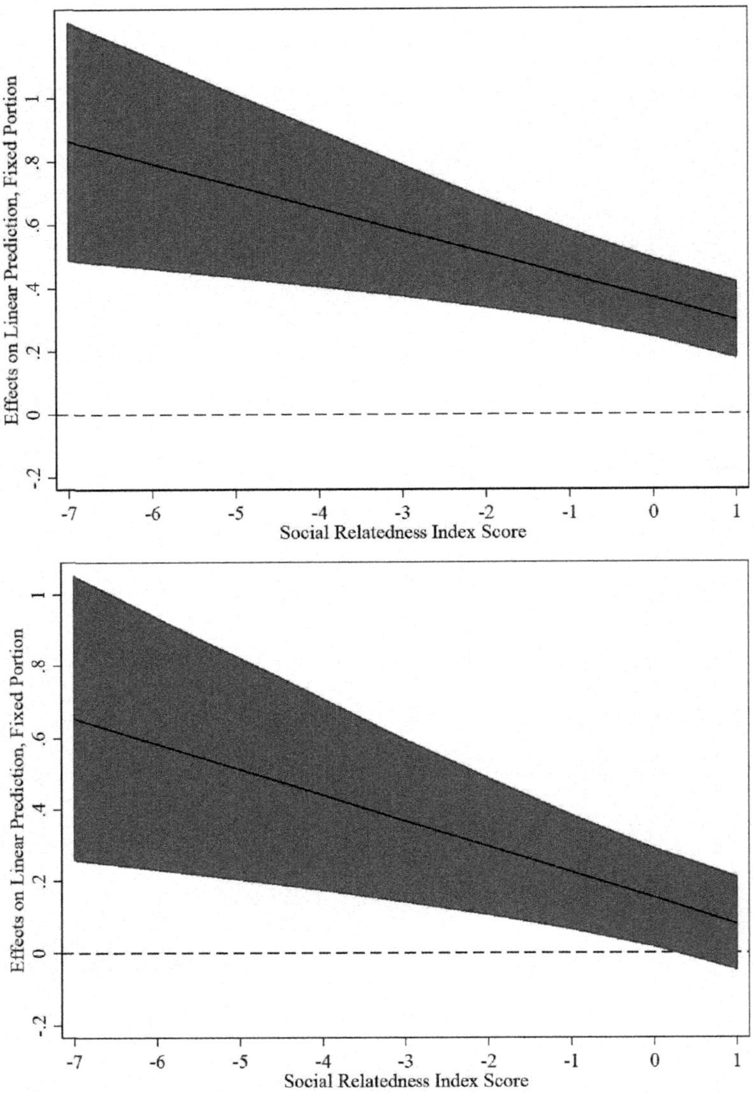

Fig. 6 Conditional marginal effects illustrating the moderation effect of tertiary education attainment on the association between social relatedness and well-being at the individual level, without (top) and with (bottom) control variables. *Note* 95% confidence interval in grey

slope suggests that high levels of social relatedness have a weaker relationship with well-being for individuals with tertiary education compared to individuals without tertiary education. In other words, the results show that the difference in well-being by education level is smaller for respondents with high self-reported social relatedness. Although those with tertiary education have higher levels of well-being overall, respondents without tertiary education 'catch up' in overall levels of well-being when they report high levels of social relatedness. The bottom portion of Fig. 6 demonstrates how this relationship changes once all control variables are included in Model 4. Unlike social trust, the results of Model 4 are similar to Model 2, as the 95 percent confidence interval passes zero only at very high social relatedness index scores.

4.3 The Role of National Context

Model 5 in Tables 2 and 3 further explores the association between overall levels of tertiary education and individual levels of well-being in each country using multilevel modeling with cross-level interaction terms. As neither the constitutive nor the interaction term are significant, we find that overall national levels of tertiary education *do not* moderate the relationship between individual-level social relatedness or trust and well-being. This suggests that as overall levels of tertiary education increase at the country-level in Europe, respondents do not report greater well-being and the relationship between social capital and well-being is unchanged. In part, these results likely connect to the low level of variance in subjective well-being amongst countries. As the baseline inter-class correlation reported above (i.e., 0.16) demonstrates, differences in well-being are more variable within than between countries. However, as we discuss next, it is important to consider why education at an individual level changes the relationship between social capital and well-being but has no effect at a national level.

5 Discussion

This chapter focused on two forms of social capital and their associations with individual well-being, testing if individual tertiary educational attainment moderates these relationships. Social capital, as defined by both social trust and social relatedness, and subjective well-being descriptively differ between respondents with and without tertiary education across contexts and within the majority of the 27 European countries under study. Notably, there is a less pronounced difference by education level at high ends of the well-being index, a finding that is consistent with previous research demonstrating that overall inequality in well-being is lowest in countries with high levels overall (Ovaska & Takashima, 2010). Further, educational inequalities in well-being are also minimized in these contexts (Jongbloed, 2018b). The results also indicate other important country differences in terms of social capital; although an education gradient exists for both social capital measures, the distribution is more or less pronounced in certain country contexts. Countries with the lowest and highest levels of social trust in Europe–generally Eastern versus Northern countries–show a weaker education gradient in social trust, while this is only true among countries with the highest social relatedness average index scores.

Concerning the moderating effect of education, tertiary education significantly influences the relationship between both forms of social capital and subjective well-being. Our findings illustrate that social capital in the form of generalized social trust correlates more strongly with subjective well-being for respondents without tertiary education–well-being is therefore more variable by level of trust among this group. Likewise, social capital in the form of social relatedness has a stronger association with subjective well-being for those without tertiary education. Contrastingly, the association between both forms of social capital and well-being is weaker for respondents with tertiary education, a relationship that is more pronounced in the case of social relatedness than social trust. Notably, these findings relate to prior research which highlights that low-income families and individuals may report higher access to social capital due to greater reliance on informal networks (Boisjoly et al., 1995; Zhang et al., 2011). The negative moderation effect in our research supports the suggestion of a 'trade-off' between individual human capital and interpersonal social capital, where either one or the other comes to play a more important role in determining individual well-being, depending on comparative levels of these two factors.

Finally, the models presented here briefly take into consideration how educational context shapes the association between social capital and well-being. The inclusion of an indicator measuring overall societal levels of tertiary educational attainment did not have an influence on either personal well-being or the relationship between both forms of social capital and well-being. Insofar as these relationships remain unchanged, the influence of tertiary education on the relationship between social capital and well-being appears to be 'absolute' rather than 'relative.' This contrasts prior research by Salinas-Jiménez et al. (2013), who find that education has a larger association with well-being when fewer people attain higher levels. Preliminary analyses into how a country's educational context impacts the influence of tertiary education on well-being suggests that tertiary degree holders self-report higher levels of well-being in contexts where a greater percentage of the population holds a tertiary credential. Of note, an individual- and society-level tertiary education attainment interaction term (results not shown here) is significant and positive when controlling for social trust, but not significant when controlling for social relatedness. This provides some suggestion that tertiary education has a stronger association with well-being in societies where overall levels of tertiary education are higher, further supporting an interpretation of an absolute rather than a relative effect of education (Helliwell & Putnam, 2004), although further investigation into how social relatedness influences this relationship is necessary.

As these empirical models cannot disentangle if education or social capital functions as the moderator (Brambor et al., 2006), theoretical guidance is necessary for interpretation. Treating education as a background factor, prior research largely focuses on how tertiary education is associated with higher levels of social capital–that is, impacting the chance for higher levels on average–and provides support for a causal story in which education plays the moderating role (e.g., Huang et al., 2009). However, this argument, like that concerning education and health (Lynch & Von Hippel, 2016), could also function in the opposite direction. Social capital might also moderate the association between tertiary education and well-being. That is, the line of causality may function from tertiary education to well-being, with social capital modifying this relationship. In this case, reduced social capital in the form of generalized social trust or social relatedness may cause subjective well-being to be more strongly associated with tertiary education levels.

A second limitation concerns variable selection. One might argue that the analyses should also include personal values. This variable, as well as a three-way interaction with social capital and tertiary education, would examine to what extent differences in the effects of social capital on well-being by educational category are indeed due to varying value sets, and not another third variable. Our aim was to first clearly delineate the relationships among education, well-being, and social capital before adding complexity into the models with further variables tapping into personal values. As a new field of research, further theorization and empirical investigation are necessary to understand how shifts in value orientations may also be associated with the relationships we study.

A final limitation is our choice to focus on only two forms of social capital and only two educational groups. Evidently, further nuance can be added to our findings in future research, extending these models to more detailed categories of educational attainment, in particular comparing vocational education and training and academic streams of post-secondary education across countries. What is more, a third type of social capital—'linking' capital, which measures social participation in a civic sense–might show quite different patterns. Because this type of social capital captures "membership in groups wherein members with varying amounts of power join together to undertake civic action or promote social change" (Ioakimidis & Heijke, 2016, p. 217), tertiary education may enhance, rather than trade off with, this form of social capital. This is an important avenue for future research.

6 Conclusion

We began this chapter by summarizing previous research that illustrates both how social capital is associated with personal well-being and how this relationship may differ by educational level. These relationships are important and highly relevant because both education and social capital are integral to personal well-being and societal functioning. Indeed, in terms of non-market outcomes, social capital advantages for individual well-being may be equivalent to extremely large increases in economic rewards in the workplace (Helliwell & Huang, 2010). To further investigate the relationship among tertiary education, social capital, and subjective well-being, we test the hypothesis that tertiary education moderates the relationship between two broad forms of social capital, social trust and social relatedness, and well-being. Our results indicate a 'trade-off' between individual human capital and interpersonal social capital, with social capital being more instrumental in predicting subjective well-being for those without tertiary education. Beyond this, the analysis also highlights that overall levels of tertiary education at the national level does not change the strength of the relationship between individual-level social capital and well-being.

In sum, only tertiary education at the individual level operates as a non-pecuniary moderator, shaping the social capital-well-being association. Individual-level tertiary education plays a significant role both in predicting well-being and the slope of the relationship between social capital and subjective well-being. Although respondents with tertiary education exhibit higher levels of well-being across self-reported levels of social capital, the extent to which increased social trust and social relatedness are associated with greater well-being is weaker for these highly educated respondents. In contrast, those with less education report greater well-being benefits through social capital, thus 'catching up' to the more educated when they have higher social capital levels. Through these findings, this study provides new evidence that social capital in the form of generalized social trust, and–even more so–social relatedness, impacts well-being in different ways across educational groups within societies.

Appendix: Description of Key Variables

Dependent variable: Subjective well-being

Variable	ESS variables	Level of missing	Scale
Subjective well-being	Stflife, happy, fltsd	Less than 1%	A single measure of well-being was constructed using polychoric factor analysis and scaled using Bartlett's factor scores. The coefficient of reliability is 0.70

Main independent variables

Variable	ESS variables	Level of missing (%)	Scale
Tertiary education	Eisced	0.64	1 = undergraduate or graduate degree 0 = no degree
Social trust	(1) ppltrst: generalized social trust "Would you say that most people can be trusted, or that you can't be too careful in dealing with people?' (range 0–10)	(1) 0.31	A single measure of social trust was constructed using polychoric factor analysis, scaled using Bartlett's factor scores, and is grand-mean centered within analyses. The coefficient of reliability is 0.79

(continued)

(continued)

Variable	ESS variables	Level of missing (%)	Scale
	(2) pplfair: “do you think that most people would try to take advantage3 of you if they got the chance, or would they try to be fair?” (range 0–10)	(2) 0.83	
	(3) pplhlp: “Would you say that most of the time people try to be helpful or that they are mostly looking out for themselves?” (range 0–10)	(3) 0.44	
Social networks	(1) flapppl: Feel appreciated by people you are close to (range 0–10)	(1) 0.74	A single measure of informal social networks was constructed using polychoric factor analysis, scaled using Bartlett’s factor scores, and is grand-mean centered within analyses. The coefficient of reliability is 0.71
	(2) rehlppl: Receive help and support from people you are close to (range 0–10)	(2) 0.79	
	(3) prhlppl: Provide help and support to people you are close to (range 0–10)	(3) 0.73	
	(4) trtrsp: Feel people treat you with respect (range 0–6)	(4) 0.09	

Level-two variable

Variable	Variable description	Source
Percent with tertiary ed	% of individuals aged 25–65 working at least one hour a week who have a tertiary education credential (ISCED5) in 2012	ESS

Level-one control variables

Variable	ESS Variable Name	Coding
Gender	Gndr	1 = Male 0 = Female
Marital status	Maritalb	1 = partnered 0 = non-partnered
Work hours	Wkhtot	Continuous Grand-mean centered
Currently in education	Edctn	1 «In School» 0 «Not in school»
Professional status	Isco08	1 «Professional» 0 «Not professional»

(continued)

(continued)

Variable	ESS Variable Name	Coding
Missing professional status	Isco08	1 «Occupation mission» 0 «Not missing»
Middle income	Hinctnta (4th to 7th decile) *Comparison group = income low (1st to 3rd decile)*	1 = yes 0 = no
High income	Hinctnta (8th to 10th decile) *Comparison group = income low (1st to 3rd decile)*	1 = yes 0 = no
Income missing	Hinctnta (missing = 17.67%) *Comparison group = income low (1st to 3rd decile)*	1 = yes 0 = no
Children	Chldhm	1 "has children" 0 "no children"
Age	Agea	Continuous Grand-mean centered
Age-squared	Agea	Continuous Grand-mean centered

References

Adler, M. G., & Fagley, N. S. (2005). Appreciation: Individual differences in finding value and meaning as a unique predictor of subjective well-being. *Journal of Personality, 73*(1), 79–114.

Barrington-Leigh, C. P. (2013). The quebec convergence and canadian life satisfaction, 1985–2008. *Canadian Public Policy, 39*(2), 193–219. https://doi.org/10.3138/CPP.39.2.193.

Beilmann, M., Kööts-Ausmees, L., & Realo, A. (2017). The relationship between social capital and individualism-collectivism in Europe. *Social Indicators Research, 137*(2), 641–664.

ESS. (2012). *ESS round 6: European social survey round 6 data (Data file edition 2.3)*. Bergen, Norway: Norwegian Social Science Data Services.

ESS. (2014a). *ESS round 6: European social survey: ESS-6 2012 documentation report (Edition 2.3)*. Bergen, Norway: Norwegian Social Science Data Services.

ESS. (2014b). *Weighting European social survey data*. Bergen, Norway: Norwegian Social Science Data Services.

Boisjoly, J., Duncan, G. J., & Hofferth, S. (1995). Access to social capital. *Journal of Family Issues, 16*(5), 609–631.

Borgonovi, F., & Burns, T. (2015). *The educational roots of trust*. Paris: OECD Education Working Papers. Retrieved from https://doi.org/10.1787/5js1kv85dfvd-en

Brambor, T., Clark, W. R., & Golder, M. (2006). Understanding interaction models: Improving empirical analyses. *Political Analysis, 14*(1), 63–82.

Brand, J. E. (2010). Civic returns to higher education: A note on heterogeneous effects. *Social Forces, 89*(2), 417–433.

Burden, B. C. (2009). The dynamic effects of education on voter turnout. *Electoral Studies, 28*(4), 540–549.

Calvo, R., Zheng, Y., Kumar, S., Olgiati, A., & Berkman, L. (2012). Well-being and social capital on planet earth: Cross-national evidence from 142 countries. *PLoS ONE, 7*(8), e42793. https://doi.org/10.1371/journal.pone.0042793

Carmo, R. M., & Nunes, N. (2013). Class and social capital in Europe: A transnational analysis of the European social survey. *European Societies, 15*(3), 373–387.

Chevalier, A., & Feinstein, L. (2006). Sheepskin or prozac? The causal effect of education on mental health (No. 71; CEE Working Papers, Issue August). http://search.proquest.com/docview/1011397521?accountid=13042

Coleman, J. S. (1990). *Foundations of social theory*. Belknap Press of Harvard University Press.

Conzo, P., Aassve, A., Fuochi, G., & Mencarini, L. (2017). The cultural foundations of happiness. *Journal of Economic Psychology, 62*(C), 268–283.

Conzo, P., Aassve, A., Fuochi, G., & Mencarini, L. (2017). The cultural foundations of happiness. *Journal of Economic Psychology, 62*(October), 268–283. https://doi.org/10.1016/j.joep.2017.08.001

Delhey, J. (2010). From materialist to post-materialist happiness? National affluence and determinants of life satisfaction in cross-national perspective. *Social Indicators Research, 97*(1), 65–84.

del Mar Salinas-Jiménez, M., Artés, J., & Salinas-Jiménez, J. (2011). Education as a positional good: A life satisfaction approach. *Social Indicators Research, 103*(3), 409–426.

Diener, E. (2000). Subjective well-being: The science of happiness and a proposal for a national index. *The American Psychologist, 55*(1), 34–43.

Diener, E. (2012). New findings and future directions for subjective well-being research. *American Psychologist, 67*(8), 590–597.

Diener, E., Suh, E. M., Lucas, R. E., & Smith, H. L. (1999). Subjective well-being: Three decades of progress. *Psychological Bulletin, 125*(2), 276–302.

Diener, E., Wirtz, D., Tov, W., Kim-Prieto, C., Choi, D., Oishi, S., & Biswas-Diener, R. (2010). New well-being measures: Short scales to assess flourishing and positive and negative feelings. *Social Indicators Research, 97*(2), 143–156.

Easterbrook, M. J., Kuppens, T., & Manstead, A. S. (2016). The education effect: Higher educational qualifications are robustly associated with beneficial personal and socio-political outcomes. *Social Indicators Research, 126*(3), 1261–1298.

Easterlin, R. A. (1995). Will raising the incomes of all increase the happiness of all? *Journal of Economic Behavior and Organization, 27*(1), 35–47.

Enders, C. K., & Tofighi, D. (2007). Centering predictor variables in cross-sectional multilevel models: A new look at an old issue. *Psychological Methods, 12*(2), 121–138.

Fahey, T., & Smyth, E. (2004). Do subjective indicators measure welfare? Evidence from 33 European societies. *European Societies, 6*(1), 5–27. https://doi.org/10.1080/1461669032000176297

Field, J. (2009). Good for your soul? Adult learning and mental well-being. *International Journal of Lifelong Education, 28*(2), 175–191.

Fischer, C. S. (2005). Bowling alone: What's the score? *Social Networks, 27*(2), 155–167.

Galton, M., & Page, C. (2015). The impact of various creative initiatives on wellbeing: a study of children in English primary schools. *Cambridge Journal of Education, 45*(3), 349–369. https://doi.org/10.1080/0305764X.2014.934201

Groot, W., & van den Brink, H. M. (2007). The health effects of education. *Economics of Education Review, 26*(2), 186–200.

Grossman, M. (2005). *Education and nonmarket outcomes* (NBER Working Paper Series No. 11582). Cambridge, MA: National Bureau of Economic Research.

Haller, M., & Hadler, M. (2006). How social relations and structures can produce happiness and unhappiness: An international comparative analysis. *Social Indicators Research, 75*(2), 169–216.

Haveman, R. H., & Wolfe, B. L. (1984). Schooling and economic well-being: The role of nonmarket effects. *The Journal of Human Resources, 19*(3), 377–407.

Helliwell, J. F., & Putnam, R. D. (2004). The social context of well-being. *Philosophical Transactions of the Royal Society of London, 359*(1449), 1435–1446.
Helliwell, J. F., & Putnam, R. D. (2007). Education and social capital. *Eastern Economic Journal, 33*(1), 1–19.
Helliwell, J. F., Huang, H., & Wang, S. (2014). Social capital and well-being in times of crisis. *Journal of Happiness Studies, 15*(1), 145–162.
Hou, F. (2014). Keep Up with the joneses or keep on as their neighbours: Life satisfaction and income in Canadian Urban neighbourhoods. *Journal of Happiness Studies, 15*, 1085–1107. https://doi.org/10.1007/s10902-013-9465-4
Huang, J., Van den Brink, H. M., & Groot, W. (2009). A meta-analysis of the effect of education on social capital. *Economics of Education Review, 28*(4), 454–464.
Huang, J., van den Brink, H. M., & Groot, W. (2011). College education and social trust: An evidence-based study on the causal mechanisms. *Social Indicators Research, 104*(2), 287–310.
Huang, J., van den Brink, H. M., & Groot, W. (2012). Does education promote social capital? Evidence from IV analysis and nonparametric-bound analysis. *Empirical Economics, 42*(3), 1011–1034.
Inglehart, R. F. (2008). Changing values among western publics from 1970 to 2006. *West European Politics, 31*(1–2), 130–146.
Inglehart, R. F., & Baker, W. E. (2000). Modernization, cultural change, and the persistence of traditional values. *American Sociological Review, 65*(1), 19–51.
Inglehart, R. F., & Welzel, C. (2007). *Modernization, cultural change and democracy: The human development sequence*. Cambridge University Press.
Ioakimidis, M., & Heijke, H. (2016). Income inequality and social capital, are they negatively related?: European cross-country analyses 2006–2012. *The Journal of Developing Areas, 50*(1), 215–235.
Jongbloed, J. (2018a). Higher education for happiness? Investigating the impact of education on the hedonic and eudaimonic well-being of Europeans. *European Educational Research Journal, 17*(5), 733–754. https://doi.org/10.1177/1474904118770818
Jongbloed, J. (2018b). *Les systèmes éducatifs engendrent-ils des inégalités de bien-être ? Une recherche comparative internationale/Do educational systems generate well-being inequalities? An international comparative analysis*. Doctoral dissertation. Université Bourgogne Franche-Comté, France.
Kaasa, A., & Parts, E. (2008). Individual-level determinants of social capital in Europe: Differences between country groups. *Acta Sociologica, 51*(2), 145–168.
Kingston, P. W., Hubbard, R., Lapp, B., Schroeder, P., & Wilson, J. (2003). Why education matters? *Sociology of Education, 76*(1), 53–70.
Kirkcaldy, B., Furnham, A., & Siefen, G. (2004). The relationship between health efficacy, educational attainment, and well-being among 30 nations. *European Psychologist, 9*(2), 107–119. https://doi.org/10.1027/1016-9040.9.2.107
Klein, C. (2013). Social capital or social cohesion: What matters for subjective well-being? *Social Indicators Research, 110*(3), 891–911.
Lynch, J. L., & Von Hippel, P. T. (2016). An education gradient in health, a health gradient in education, or a confounded gradient in both? *Social Science and Medicine, 154*, 18–27.
Marks, G. N. (1997). The formation of materialist and postmaterialist values. *Social Science Research, 68*(26), 52–68.
McMahon, W. W., & Oketch, M. (2013). Education's effects on individual life chances and on development: An overview. *British Journal of Educational Studies, 61*(1), 79–107.
Nieminen, T., Martelin, T., Koskinen, S., Simpura, J., Alanen, E., Härkänen, T., & Aromaa, A. (2008). Measurement and socio-demographic variation of social capital in a large population-based survey. *Social Indicators Research, 85*(3), 405–423.
Nikolaev, B. (2018). Does higher education increase hedonic and eudaimonic happiness? *Journal of Happiness Studies, 19*(2), 483–504.

Oreopoulos, P., & Salvanes, K. G. (2011). Priceless: The nonpecuniary benefits of schooling. *The Journal of Economic Perspectives, 25*(1), 159–184.

Oskarsson, S., Thisted Dinesen, P., Dawes, C. T., Johannesson, M., & Magnusson, P. K. E. (2017). Education and social trust: Testing a causal hypothesis using the discordant twin design. *Political Psychology, 38*(3), 515–531.

Ovaska, T., & Takashima, R. (2010). Does a rising tide lift all the boats? Explaining the national inequality of happiness. *Journal of Economic Issues, 44*(1), 205–224.

Pallas, A. M. (2000). The effects of schooling on individual lives. In M. T. Hallinan (Ed.), *Handbook of the Sociology of Education* (pp. 499–525). Kluwer Academic/Plenum Publishers.

Pereira, M. C., Coelho, F., & Lourenço, Ó. (2017). Who feels credit constrained in Europe? The role of social capital. *Journal of Consumer Affairs, 51*(2), 380–405. https://doi.org/10.1111/joca.12123.

Peugh, J. L. (2010). A practical guide to multilevel modeling. *Journal of School Psychology, 48*(1), 85–112.

Poortinga, W. (2006). Social capital: An individual or collective resource for health? *Social Science and Medicine, 62*(2), 292–302.

Portela, M., Neira, I., & del Mar Salinas-Jiménez, M. (2013). Social capital and subjective wellbeing in Europe: A new approach on social capital. *Social Indicators Research, 114*(2), 493–511.

Powdthavee, N., Lekfuangfu, W. N., & Wooden, M. (2015). What's the good of education on our overall quality of life? A simultaneous equation model of education and life satisfaction for Australia. *Journal of Behavioral and Experimental Economics, 54*, 10–21. https://doi.org/10.1016/j.socec.2014.11.002

Puntscher, S., Hauser, C., Walde, J., & Tappeiner, G. (2015). The impact of social capital on subjective well-being: A regional perspective. *Journal of Happiness Studies, 16*(5), 1231–1246.

Putnam, R. D. (2000). *Bowling alone: America's declining social capital.* Palgrave Macmillan.

Raudenbush, S. W., & Bryk, A. S. (2002). *Hierarchical linear models: Applications and data analysis methods.* Sage.

Rodríguez-Pose, A., & Von Berlepsch, V. (2014). Social capital and individual happiness in Europe. *Journal of Happiness Studies, 15*(2), 357–386.

Roth, T. (2013). The role of social capital in the explanation of educational success and educational inequalities. *Irish Educational Studies, 32*(3), 335–354.

Ryan, R. M., & Deci, E. L. (2000). Self-determination theory and the facilitation of intrinsic motivation, social development, and well-being. *The American Psychologist, 55*(1), 68–78. http://www.ncbi.nlm.nih.gov/pubmed/11392867

Salinas-Jiménez, M., Artés, J., & Salinas-Jiménez, J. (2013). How do educational attainment and occupational and wage-earner statuses affect life satisfaction? *Journal of Happiness Studies, 14*, 367–388. https://doi.org/10.1007/s10902-012-9334-6

Sarracino, F. (2012). Money, sociability and happiness: Are developed countries doomed to social erosion and unhappiness? *Social Indicators Research, 109*(2), 135–188.

Siedlecki, K. L., Salthouse, T. A., Oishi, S., & Jeswani, S. (2014). The relationship between social support and subjective well-being across age. *Social Indicators Research, 117*(2), 561–576.

Tuijnman, A. (1990). Adult education and the quality of life. *International Review of Education, 36*(3), 283–298.

Uslaner, E. M. (2002). *The moral foundations of trust.* Cambridge University Press.

Vemuri, A. W., & Costanza, R. (2006). The role of human, social, built, and natural capital in explaining life satisfaction at the country level: Toward a national Well-Being Index (NWI). *Ecological Economics, 58*(1), 119–133.

Vila, L. E. (2000). The non-monetary benefits of education. *European Journal of Education, 35*(1), 21–32.

Vila, L. E. (2005). The outcomes of investment in education and people's well-being. *European Journal of Education, 40*(1), 3–11. https://doi.org/10.1111/j.1465-3435.2005.00206.xa

Woessmann, L., & Schuetz, G. (2006). *Efficiency and equity in European education and training systems.* Brussels, Belgium: European Parliament.

Yamaoka, K. (2008). Social capital and health and well-being in East Asia: A population-based study. *Social Science and Medicine, 66*(4), 885–899.
Zagórski, K. (2011). Income and happiness in time of post-communist modernization. *Social Indicators Research, 104*(2), 331–349.
Zhang, S., Anderson, S. G., & Zhan, M. (2011). The differentiated impact of bridging and bonding social capital on economic well-being: An individual level perspective. *Journal of Sociology and Social Welfare, 38*, 119.

Janine Jongbloed is a Postdoctoral Research Fellow in the Department of Educational Studies at the University of British Columbia (UBC) in Canada and an Associate Researcher with the Institute for Research in the Sociology and Economics of Education (IREDU) in France. Her research interests include the nonmarket effects of tertiary education; educational participation and patterns over the life-course; and comparative studies of educational and welfare production regimes.

Ashley Pullman is a Senior Research Associate at The Graduate School of Public and International Affairs at the University of Ottawa in Canada. She specializes in policy-relevant quantitative research and evaluation using survey and population-level administrative data to conduct quasi-experimental, longitudinal, and latent modelling in topics related to education, training, and skill.

Occupation and Subjective Well-Being: A Knowledge Economy Perspective

Irina Vartanova and Vladimir Gritskov

1 Introduction

In recent decades, the amount of cheap unqualified labor has been in decline, even during the global economic crisis, while the knowledge economy has become a source of new well-paid jobs (Hurley et al., 2013). According to some forecasts, such as by Frey and Osborne (Frey & Osborne, 2017), 47% of the US jobs are susceptible to full automation in the next one or two decades. The jobs at risk include most of transportation and logistics occupations, office and administrative support workers, and production occupations. The probability of job computerization is highly correlated with the required education and salary.

Despite the country-by-country differences in the employment changes (Fernandez-Macias, 2012), the overall number of jobs for highly qualified knowledge workers is increasing. It is only a matter of time when machines will substitute manual routine tasks completely in developed countries. The knowledge work will be the main source of employment then. Besides unemployment and other problems arising from this prediction, an open question also remains if it will be beneficial for subjective well-being (SWB) of workers. The main research question is whether knowledge workers have higher SWB in comparison with other occupations and if so, why?

The chapter aims to fill the gap in research studying the link between the nature of work and SWB with a special focus on jobs that will be in high demand in the future.

I. Vartanova (✉)
Institute for Futures Studies, Stockholm, Sweden
e-mail: irina.vartanova@iffs.se

HSE University, Moscow, Russia

V. Gritskov
St Petersburg University, St Petersburg, Russia
e-mail: v.gritskov@spbu.ru

A. Almakaeva et al. (eds.), *Social Capital and Subjective Well-Being*, Societies and Political Orders in Transition,
https://doi.org/10.1007/978-3-030-75813-4_11

We analyze the association between knowledge work and SWB, consider the main possible reasons for it, and explore relative importance of these reasons in several European countries with different level of economic development.

2 The Nature of Work in the Knowledge Economy

The idea of converting knowledge into capital has been developed in the concepts of information society and the knowledge economy (Machlup, 1962; Webster, 2002). In the new type of knowledge economy, value added production is shifted from tangible assets to information technology and knowledge. The key role here is assigned to workers whose main functions are to create, reproduce, and apply accumulated knowledge–they are called knowledge workers.

Occupational identity of knowledge workers is different from the identity of manual workers and includes jobs that are referred as professionals (accountancy, legal professions or scientific work) and also more contemporary type of work such as consultancy, software development, or public relations (Newell et al., 2002). By the nature of their work, knowledge workers are not only distinguished from manual workers, but also from information officers whose job roll requires them to process, save and pass information on to others not necessarily trying to understand it.

Several publications are devoted to conceptualization of the knowledge work (Pyöriä, 2005; Timonen & Paloheimo, 2008), its characteristics (Huang, 2014; Ramirez & Steudel, 2008), and organizational behavior of individuals who engage in such occupations (Kelloway & Barling, 2000). The specified characteristics of knowledge work include high requirements for education, job complexity and processing of large amounts of information, problem-solving capabilities, the non-routine nature of this work and especially, and the increased autonomy over work (Davenport, 2005; Florida, 2002; Morgeson & Humphrey, 2006; Ramirez & Steudel, 2008; Robertson & Swan, 2003; Sajeva, 2007; Tsoukas & Vladimirou, 2001).

3 Subjective Well-Being and Work

Life satisfaction as one of indicators of subjective well-being is shaped during the life span in the space that can be divided in two large domains: work and life outside of work (Guest, 2002). There is a body of literature exploring how various aspects of work are related to SWB. Empirical findings suggest that job satisfaction (Van Praag et al., 2003), work-life balance (Guest, 2002), and income (Clark et al., 2008; Diener et al., 2013), among others, are strong predictor of overall subjective well-being.

Autonomy is a key factor of job quality due to its link to SWB. According to self-determination theory, autonomy is one of the basic human needs (Deci & Ryan, 1995). Empirical evidence for the link between autonomy and SWB has been shown in different cultural contexts which support the universal nature of the need (Chirkov et al., 2003). Work autonomy does not merely impact job satisfaction. It promotes feeling of agency that is known to have an impact on life satisfaction (Inglehart et al., 2008; Welzel & Inglehart, 2010).

Autonomy connection with another key factor of life satisfaction–work-life conflict–is not straightforward. On the one hand, work autonomy promotes work-life balance due to the flexibility in managing workloads (Ahuja et al., 2007; Maruyama et al., 2009). On other hand, it often leads to longer working time and higher involvement in working problems even in spare time (Fontinha et al., 2019; Shevchuk et al., 2019).

Based on the discussed theoretical arguments the following hypotheses are put forward:

H1. Knowledge workers have a higher level of life satisfaction in comparison with services and manual workers.
H2.1. Job satisfaction mediates the relationship between occupation and life satisfaction.
H2.2. Income, autonomy, and work-life conflict mediate the relationship between occupation and life satisfaction.

4 Country Level

The cultural revolution that signify the transition to a post-industrial society combines the development of the information society based on the knowledge economy and the spread of self-expression values (Inglehart & Welzel, 2005). The economic prosperity allows people to shift the main concern from economic security to the quality of life and freedom. Agency in conjunction with creating and reproducing new knowledge become the basis of productive activity and bring SWB (Welzel & Inglehart, 2010). Delhey has shown that happiness recipes vary in different countries depending on the level of economic prosperity. In postindustrial societies, personal autonomy and creativity are stronger predictors of happiness than in poor countries where income plays more important role (Delhey, 2010). We aim to extend these findings and check if economic factors could explain the differences in several reasons explaining why knowledge workers may have higher SWB when compared with other occupations.

The contextual factors regarding the effect of work-life conflict on SWB are less clear. Even though a country variation in the average level of work-life conflict has been noted, it is rather explained by welfare regime and working life regulations (Crompton & Lyonette, 2006; Lunau et al., 2014) than economic development (Schöneck, 2018). Reported moderators of the link between work-life conflict and SWB are scarce and mostly of cultural nature, such as individualism and support for gender equality (Haar er al., 2014; Hagqvist et al., 2017).

On the contextual level, the following hypothesis are to be checked:

H3.1. The mediating effect of autonomy is stronger in higher developed countries compared to lower developed ones.

H3.2. The mediating effect of income and overall job satisfaction is stronger in less developed countries compared to higher developed ones.

We do not have prior expectations about country differences in the mediating effect of work-life conflict. While researchers have shown that work-life conflict might be stronger predictor for SWB in more gender egalitarian societies (Hagqvist et al., 2017), the reported variation is small and suggests that the link has universal nature.

5 Data and Method

To examine the hypotheses presented above, we use the 5th round (2010) of the European Social Survey (ESS). The sample we use for analysis includes working population in 26 countries: Belgium (830), Bulgaria (904), the United Kingdom (1182), Hungary (742), Germany (1505), Greece (1054), Denmark (824), Israel (1011), Ireland (945), Spain (905), Cyprus (538), Lithuania (616), the Netherlands (932), Norway (918), Poland (851), Russia (1335), Slovakia (808), Slovenia (615), Ukraine (712), Finland (885), France (863), Croatia (542), Czech Republic (1192), Switzerland (854), Sweden (832), and Estonia (855). The data source fits well for testing the suggested hypotheses. The sample is representative to the countries labor markets, and the questionnaire includes information about respondents' occupation, which could be used to understand the nature of their work.

We use life satisfaction as the main outcome variable in our models. It is a key indicator of SWB and represents a cognitive assessment of one's life circumstances (Linley et al., 2009). The cognitive component of SWB is relatively stable and has a higher correlation with objective characteristics of life domains when compared to the affective component which is shown to be closer related to personality traits (Schimmack, 2008). Life satisfaction is measured with a single item: "All things considered, how satisfied are you with your life as a whole nowadays?". Response options range from 0—"extremely dissatisfied" to 10—"extremely satisfied", in an 11-point scale.

To operationalize the concept of knowledge worker, we use respondent's occupation coded according to the International Standard Classification of Occupations (ISCO-88). The variable is based on respondents' description of their job title, main content of work and education requirements. We include series of dummy variables for the major occupational groups in the models. The armed forces category is omitted from analysis since it includes only a small number of respondents. We analyze the results with the focus on the groups of interest and compare SWB of knowledge workers represented by professionals (group 2 in ISCO-88) with service and sales workers (group 5), and manual work occupations including craft workers and machine operators (groups 7 and 8).

Mediating variables include job satisfaction, work autonomy, income, and work-life conflict. The job satisfaction measure includes responses to the question: "All things considered, how satisfied are you with your present job?". The response scale contains 11 points ranging from 0—"extremely dissatisfied" to 10—"extremely satisfied". The income measure relies on respondents estimates of overall household income chosen on the scale of country-specific income deciles. The variable is weighted by the proportion of household income that respondents provide themselves with the weights equal 0 for none, 0.17—very small, 0.33—under a half, 0.5—about half, 0.67—over a half, 0.83—very large, and 1 for sole income earners. The ESS round 5 includes several questions that allow us to measure work autonomy and work-life conflict (Table 1), and we include them in the model as latent factors.

The analyzed models also include established predictors of SWB and demographic variables such as sex, age, age squared, marital status, living in the rural area, and subjective religiosity.

We use a structural equation modeling (SEM) approach to test the hypotheses about mediation effects. Mediation holds when a third variable–mediator–intervening in the effect of a predictor on an outcome variable (Preacher & Hayes, 2008). SEM allows to distinguish between the direct and indirect effects of a predictor on an outcome variable and takes into account the measurement error of the latent variables if any included in the model. We use maximum likelihood with robust standard errors and the Satorra-Bentler correction for models estimation to account for possible non-normality in the variables distributions (Satorra & Bentler, 1994).

In this study, two of the considered mediators are latent constructs and measured with multiple indicators. Measurement equivalence across different countries should be established before the mediation effects could be compared.

Table 1 Wording for the items measuring autonomy and work-life conflict

Factor	Label	Item	Scale
Autonomy	A1	How much the management at your work allows/allowed you: … to decide how your own daily work is/was organized?	0—I have/ had no influence to 10—I have/had complete control
	A2	… to influence policy decisions about the activities of the organization?	
	A3	… to choose or change your pace of work?	
Work-life conflict	C1	How often do you: … keep worrying about work problems when you are not working?	1—Never to 5—Always
	C2	… find that your job prevents you from giving the time you want to your partner or family?	
	C3	… feel too tired after work to enjoy the things you would like to do at home?	

6 Measurement Invariance of Autonomy and Work-Life Conflict

We conducted a multigroup confirmatory factor analysis to assess the fit of the measurement model for autonomy and work-life conflict latent constructs. We first analyzed the basic structural equivalence model which only requires that latent variables have a similar structure of items in compared groups without any equality constrains for their intercepts and factor. The base two factors model with three items loaded on each factor reveals poor fit (Chi sq. = 2461.5, df = 208, CFI = 0.949, RMSEA = 0.116). The analysis of misspecifications based on modification indices and estimated parameters changes (Saris et al., 2009) indicated that item C1– "worrying about work problems"–from the work-life conflict measure is also highly loaded on the autonomy factor. This finding is consistent with the theory about the nature of knowledge work, according to which the problem solving is its large part. Thinking about a problem is not bound to a specific time or place. High work autonomy entails the feeling of responsibility and might inspire working outside normal business hours (Hackman & Oldham, 1976). Searching for a solution to a problem may continue in spare time, not necessarily leading to work interference with personal life. For this reason, item C1 is additionally loaded on the autonomy factor. The modified measurement model shows good fit (Table 2).

We then tested for measurement invariance of the two latent factors to ensure their comparability in different countries (Davidov et al., 2014). Metric equivalence suggests equality of factor loadings meaning that a latent variable measures the same concept and has the same unit size in the compared groups. It is required for meaningful comparison of regression coefficients between groups. Scalar equivalence is determined by equality of items intercepts and provides correspondence of the same scores on the latent variable between groups (Steenkamp & Baumgartner, 1998).

Table 2 shows fit indices for structural, metrics, and scalar equivalence of the measurement model with the work autonomy and work-life conflict latent factors. Scalar equivalence serves the baseline to determine how introducing stricter constraints affect the model fit. Most indices for metric equivalence change within the recommended cutoff values with only CFI being on the border line (0.01) (Chen, 2007). The measurement model reveals no scalar invariance, however metric equivalence is sufficient for the aims of the current paper as it ensures comparability of regression coefficients for work autonomy and work-life balance between the countries.

7 Results

To test the specified hypotheses, we estimated a set of models with gradual increase of complexity. Model 1 represents path analysis of occupation as a predictor of life satisfaction with the focus on the main (unmediated) effect (hypothesis 1). Model

Table 2 Measurement equivalence of the work autonomy and work-life conflict factors model

Model	Chi sq	df	CFI	RMSEA	SRMR	Satorra-Bentler diff. test	CFI delta	RMSEA delta	SRMS delta
Structural equivalence	521.2	182	0.989	0.048	0.025				
Metric equivalence	948.7	307	0.978	0.051	0.042	429.9** (125)	−0.011	0.003	0.017
Scalar equivalence	2848.5	407	0.918	0.087	0.062	2345.8** (100)	−0.06	0.036	0.020

** $p < 0.01$

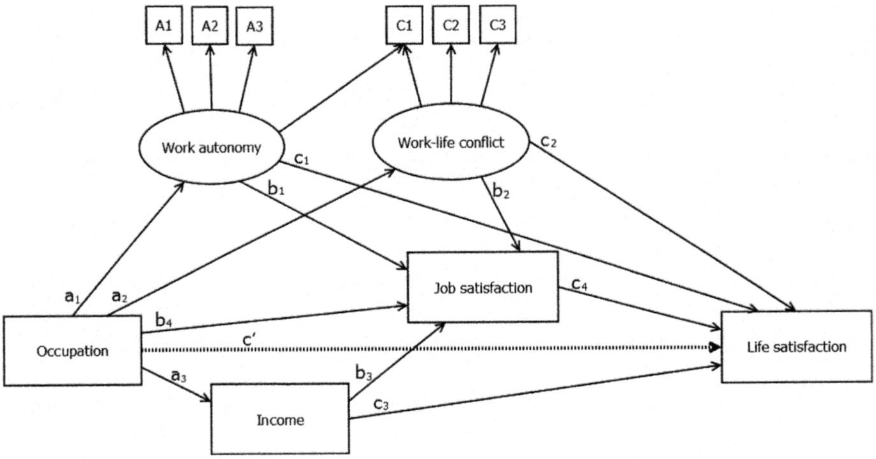

Fig. 1 Representation of the full model. Occupation effect on life satisfaction is mediated by autonomy, work-life conflict, income, and overall life satisfaction. *Note* Control variables are not shown but included in the estimated model as predictors for the outcome and mediator variables

2 additionally includes job satisfaction as a mediator between occupation and life satisfaction (hypothesis 2.1). Indirect effect of occupation on life satisfaction mediated by job satisfaction is of the main of interest. Model 3 represents full structural model with all mediator variables (hypothesis 2.2, see Fig. 1). The model 3 includes multiple double mediation effects which were estimated as

$$f = a_i * b_i * c_4 + a_i * c_i$$

All models also include control variables as predictors for the outcome and mediator variables to eliminate their confounding effect on the path coefficients of interest.

Figure 2 plots unstandardized coefficients and their 95% confidence intervals for the professional effect on life satisfaction relative to the reference category represented by manual workers. Model 1 estimates the main effect without mediation. Model 2 shows indirect effect of professionals on life satisfaction mediated by job satisfaction and the remaining direct effect. Model 3 decomposes further the indirect path through the autonomy, work-life conflict (WLC), income, and job satisfaction (JS) mediator variables. The countries are ordered by the knowledge index provided by the World Bank.[1] Coefficients with $p > 0.05$ are faded.

Only in 14 out of the 26 countries life satisfaction of professionals is significantly higher than that of blue collars (model 1). The effect of occupation is insignificant in the Nordic countries as well as in most of the developed countries.

In most of the countries in which the effect of occupation is significant, it is partially explained by job satisfaction (model 2). In several East European countries,

[1] http://data.worldbank.org/data-catalog/KEI.

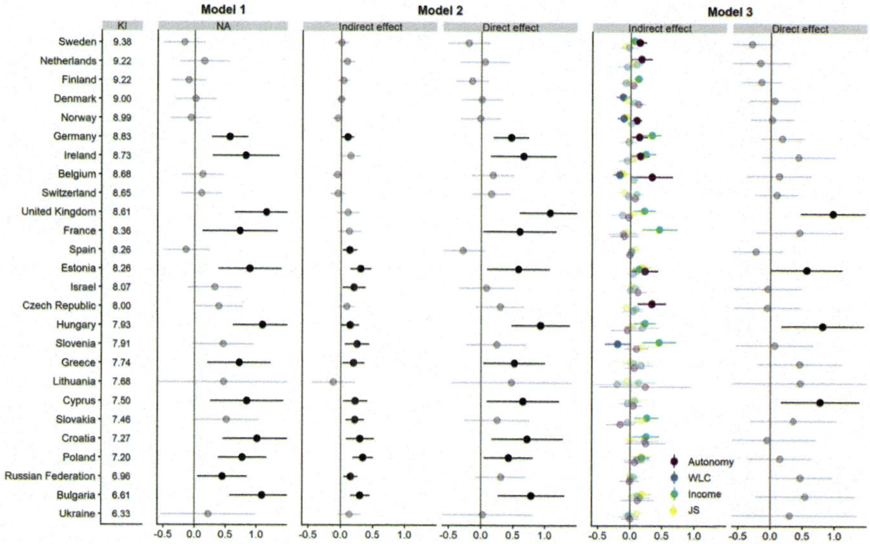

Fig. 2 Unstandardized coefficients and 95% CI of the occupation effect (professionals relative to manual workers) on life satisfaction

there is a mediating effect of job satisfaction while the total effect of occupation on SWB is insignificant. We explore the effect of occupation in more details in the model 3 which includes all mediating variables. Most consistent positive indirect effect has been found for income. Work autonomy is significant in its intervening effect only in 8 countries, predominantly in Northern and Western Europe. The hypothesis about the mediating role of work-life conflict is generally not supported with the effect being significant only in a few countries (Denmark, Norway, Belgium, and Slovenia).

Figure 3 displays the relative effect of professionals on life satisfaction compared to service workers. Model 1 estimates the main effect without mediation. Model 2 shows indirect effect of professionals on life satisfaction mediated by job satisfaction and the remaining direct effect. Model 3 decomposes further the indirect path through the autonomy, work-life conflict (WLC), income, and job satisfaction (JS) mediator variables. The countries are ordered by the knowledge index provided by the World Bank.[2] Coefficients with $p > 0.05$ are faded.

The main results are largely similar except for the work autonomy mediation effect, which is weaker in most of the countries.

To explore country differences in the mediation effect of autonomy, work-life conflict, and income in more detail, we analyzed the two pathways of each mediation process separately. The "leading to" paths represented by a_i on the diagram (Fig. 1) show the difference professional and manual work in the level of considered mediators. The "going out" paths are marked by bi and represent relevance of the mediators for job satisfaction. Figure 4 shows countries estimates and their 95%

[2] http://data.worldbank.org/data-catalog/KEI.

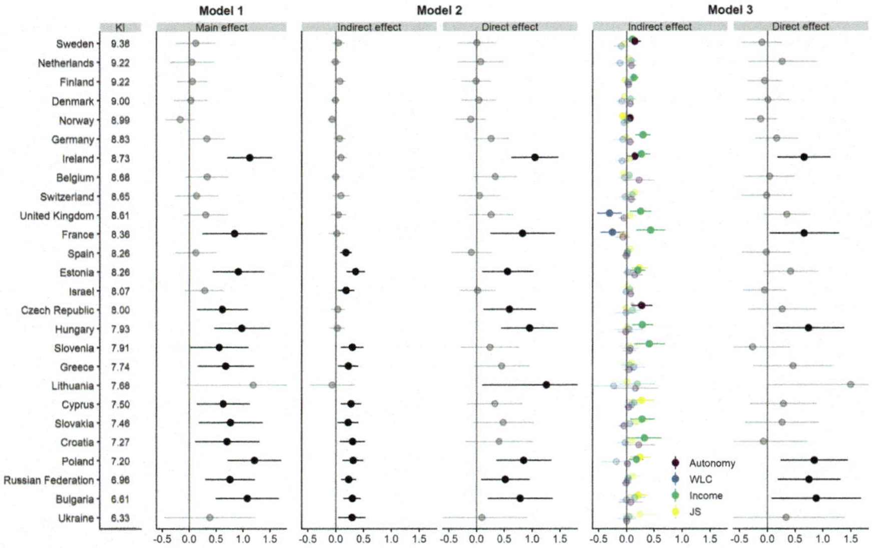

Fig. 3 Unstandardized coefficients of the occupation effect (professionals relative to service workers) on life satisfaction

confidence intervals of these paths for each mediation process. Each country is also positioned on the X-axis according to its knowledge index score.

The work autonomy level is higher among professionals compared to manual workers in all the countries although the effect is insignificant in Ukraine. However, the size of these differences is correlated with the level of economic development. In the South and East European countries, these differences are more salient than in the Western and Nordic countries. Although there is no significant effect of occupation on work-life conflict in most of the studied countries, the distribution of the effect in different countries does not look random and is noticeably related to the knowledge index score. In the less prosperous countries, professionals have even higher work-life balance than manual workers while in the knowledge economies professionals experience more interference of work with their personal life than blue collar workers. Income differences between the worker groups are also larger in more prosperous societies.

Analysis of the "going out" paths reveals that the positive association of work autonomy with job satisfaction is stronger in the countries with a more developed knowledge economy while the income effect on job satisfaction is weaker in these countries than in the less developed economies. The association between the income effect on job satisfaction and the economic development is less obvious. However, the positive effect is insignificant in most of the reach countries while is solid in most of the Eastern and Southern European countries. Work-life conflict is negatively associated with job satisfaction in all the countries irrespective of their economic development.

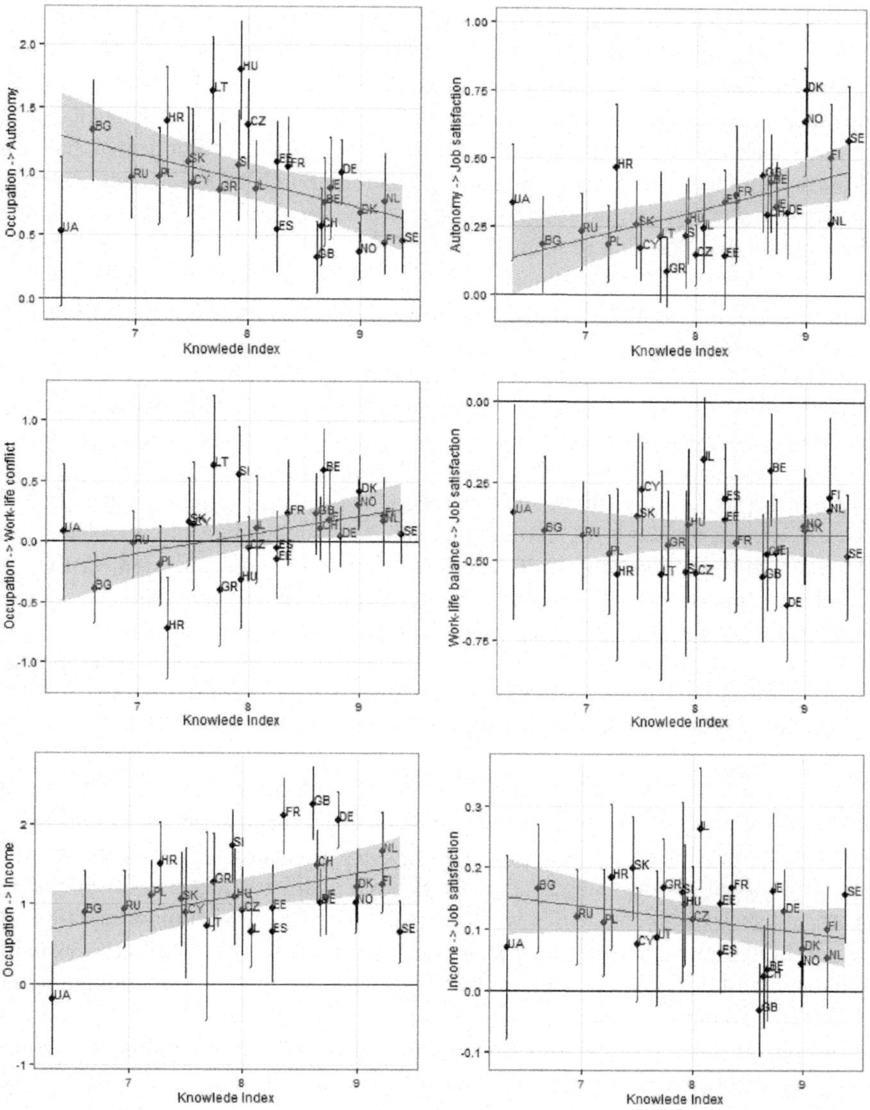

Fig. 4 Mediation effects decomposition. Estimates and their 95% confidence intervals of the autonomy, work-life conflict and income mediation pathways plotted versus knowledge index for each country

8 Discussion

Knowledge workers have higher life satisfaction than manual and service workers only in less economically developed countries. Job satisfaction partially explains these differences. The hypothesis about the mediating role of income is confirmed and its strength is only weakly correlated with economic prosperity. This somehow conflicts with the earlier finding that income has stronger effect on SWB in poorer countries (Delhey, 2010) although a more recent study has shown that financial satisfaction might be a universal predictor of life satisfaction (Ng & Diener, 2014).

The analysis of the other two mediators reveals more complicated patterns. Working autonomy seems to be a poor explanation of higher life satisfaction among knowledge workers. In the countries where the autonomy level of professionals is distinctly higher than that of manual workers, it is less critical for job and life satisfaction. However, in the developed countries where autonomy is of high value, as it has been noted before (Delhey, 2010), the differences between occupations are small. Particularly in the Nordic countries, autonomy is not a distinctive feature of the knowledge work. It seems likely that in the prosperous societies with a high general level of SWB and strong employment protection, additional time, efforts, and money invested in education do not bring additional increase in life satisfaction.

We have also not found a clear statistical evidence that work-life conflict could explain the small effect of occupation on life satisfaction in the developed countries. However, the work-life conflict mediating effect is noticeably correlated with the economic development level. The coefficient even shifts the sign; in the less developed countries the effect is positive while in the knowledge economies professionals have lower work-life balance than blue collars and that is detrimental for their SWB. This systematic pattern is difficult to ignore, and it could have several policy implications. Like special programs of autonomy increase are used for low qualified jobs, regulations for work-life balance will be increasingly required for knowledge workers.

To conclude, we would like to discuss some limitations of the study. Despite the fact that we analyze occupation as a predictor of life satisfaction, it is impossible to establish the direction of the link and to justify the causal nature of the relationship. Empirical findings suggest that SWB has a positive effect on performance at work and success (Oishi, 2012), which may in turn make impact on occupation and career. Longitudinal data are needed to examine if the diminishing differences in life satisfaction of different occupations and higher appreciation of work autonomy are driven by economic changes.

Moreover, the list of explored mediators of the association between occupation and life satisfaction is clearly non-exhaustive. The direct effect of occupation on life satisfaction that is unexplained by the effects of mediators remains strong in many countries. One of possible explanations could be higher prestige of the knowledge work when compared to the service worker. Other mediators that may have a negative impact on SWB among professionals are important to examine. Specifically, relatively higher demands and expectations among knowledge workers when compared to blue collar ones could be such negative mediators.

Acknowledgements The chapter was prepared within the framework of the HSE University Basic Research Program.

References

Ahuja, M. K., McKnight, D. H., Chudoba, K. M., George, J. F., & Kacmar, C. J. (2007). IT road warriors: Balancing work-family conflict, job autonomy, and work overload to mitigate turnover intentions. *MIS Quarterly, 31*, 1–17.

Chen, F. F. (2007). Sensitivity of goodness of fit indices to lack of measurement invariance. *Structural Equations Modeling, 14*, 464–504.

Chirkov, V. I., Ryan, R. M., Kim, Y., & Kaplan, U. (2003). Differentiating autonomy from individualism and independence: A self-determination theory perspective on internalization of cultural orientations and wellbeing. *Journal of Personality and Social Psychology, 84*, 97–110.

Clark, A. E., Frijters, P., & Shields, M. (2008). Relative income, happiness, and utility: An explanation for the Easterlin paradox and other puzzles. *Journal of Economic Literature, 46*(1), 95–144.

Crompton, R., & Lyonette, C. (2006). Work-life 'balance' in Europe. *Acta Sociologica, 49*(4), 379–393.

Davenport, T. (2005). *Thinking for a living: How to get better performance and results from*. Harvard Business School Press.

Davidov, E., Meuleman, B., Cieciuch, J., Schmidt, P., & Billiet, J. (2014). Measurement equivalence in cross-national research. *Annual Review of Sociology, 40.*

Deci, E. L., & Ryan, R. M. (1995). Human autonomy: The basis for true self-esteem. In M. Kernis (Ed.), *Efficacy, agency, and self-esteem* (pp. 31–49). Plenum.

Delhey, J. (2010). From materialist to post-materialist happiness? National affluence and determinants of life satisfaction in cross-national perspective. *Social Indicators Research, 97*(1), 65–84.

Diener, E., Tay, L., & Oishi, S. (2013). Rising income and the subjective well-being of nations. *Journal of Personality and Social Psychology, 104*(2), 267–276.

Fernandez-Macias, E. (2012). Job polarization in Europe? Changes in the employment structure and job quality, 1995–2007. *Work and Occupations,* (39), 157–182.

Florida, R. (2002). *The rise of the creative class*. Basic Books.

Fontinha, R., Easton, S., & Van Laar, D. (2019). Overtime and quality of working life in academics and nonacademics: The role of perceived work-life balance. *International Journal of Stress Management, 26*(2), 173–183.

Frey, C. B., & Osborne, M. A. (2017, September). The future of employment: how susceptible are jobs to computerisation? *Technological Forecasting & Social Change*, 254–280. Retrieved June 16, 2014, from http://www.oxfordmartin.ox.ac.uk/downloads/academic/The_Future_of_Employment.pdf.

Guest, D. (2002). Perspectives on the study of work-life balance. *Social Science Information,* (41), 255–279.

Haar, J. M., Russo, M., Suñe, A., & Ollier-Malaterre, A. (2014). Outcomes of work–life balance on job satisfaction, life satisfaction and mental health: A study across seven cultures. *Journal of Vocational Behavior, 85*(3), 361–373.

Hackman, J., & Oldham, G. (1976). Motivation through the design of work: Test of a theory. *Organizational Behavior and Human Performance, 16*, 250–279.

Hagqvist, E., Gådin, K. G., & Nordenmark, M. (2017). Work–family conflict and well-being across Europe: The role of gender context. *Social Indicators Research, 132*(2), 785–797.

Huang, T.-P. (2014). Comparing motivating work characteristics, job satisfaction, and turnover intention of knowledge workers and blue-collar workers, and testing a structural model of the variables' relationships in China and Japan. *The International Journal of Human Resource Management, 22*(4), 924–944.

Hurley, J., Fernández-Macías, E., & Storrie, D. (2013). *Employment polarisation and job quality in the crisis: European jobs monitor 2013*. Eurofound.

Inglehart, R., & Welzel, C. (2005). *Modernization, cultural change and democracy: The human development sequence*. Cambridge University Press.

Inglehart, R., Foa, R., Peterson, C., & Welzel, C. (2008). Development, freedom and rising happiness. *Perspectives on Psychological Science, 3*, 264–285.
Kelloway, E. K., & Barling, J. (2000). Knowledge work as organizational behavior. *International Journal of Management Reviews, 2*, 287–304.
Linley, P. A., Maltby, J., Wood, A. M., Osborne, G., & Hurling, R. (2009). Measuring happiness: The higher order factor structure of subjective and psychological well-being measures. *Personality and Individual Differences, 47*, 878–884.
Lunau, T., Bambra, C., Eikemo, T. A., van Der Wel, K. A., & Dragano, N. (2014). A balancing act? Work–life balance, health and well-being in European welfare states. *European Journal of Public Health, 24*(3), 422–427.
Machlup, F. (1962). *The production and distribution of knowledge in the United States*. Princeton University Press.
Maruyama, T., Hopkinson, P. G., & James, P. W. (2009). A multivariate analysis of work-life balance outcomes from a large scale telework programme. *New Technology, Work, and Employment, 24*, 76–88.
Morgeson, F., & Humphrey, S. (2006). The work design questionnaire (WDQ): Developing and validating a comprehensive measure for assessing job design and the nature of work. *Journal of Applied Psychology, 26*(3), 573–596.
Newell, S., Robertson, M., Scarbrough, H., & Swan, J. (2002). *Managing knowledge work*. Palgrave.
Ng, W., & Diener, E. (2014). What matters to the rich and the Poor? subjective well-being, financial satisfaction, and postmaterialist needs across the world. *Journal of Personality and Social Psychol, 2*(107), 326–338.
Oishi, S. (2012). *The psychological wealth of nations: Do happy people make a happy society?* Wiley-Blackwell.
Preacher, K. J., & Hayes, A. F. (2008). Asymptotic and resampling strategies for assessing and comparing indirect effects in multiple mediator models. *Behavior Research Methods, 40*(3), 879–891.
Pyöriä, P. (2005). The concept of knowledge work revisited. *Journal of Knowledge Management, 9*(3), 116–127.
Ramirez, Y. W., & Steudel, H. J. (2008). Measuring knowledge work: The knowledge work quantification framework. *Journal of Intellectual Capital, 9*(4), 564–584.
Robertson, M., & Swan, J. (2003). Control—what control?' Culture and ambiguity within a knowledge intensive firm. *Journal of Management Studies, 40*(4), 831–858.
Sajeva, S. (2007). Identifying factors affecting motivation and loyalty of knowledge workers. *Economics and Management, 12*, 643–652.
Saris, W. E., Satorra, A., & van der Veld, W. M. (2009). Testing structural equation models or detection of misspecifications? *Structural Equations Modeling, 16*, 561–582.
Satorra, A., & Bentler, P. M. (1994). Corrections to test statistics and standard errors in covariance structure analysis. In A. von Eye & C. C. Clogg (Eds.), *Latent variables analysis: Applications for developmental research* (pp. 399–419). SAGE Publications.
Schöneck, N. M. (2018). Europeans' work and life—out of balance? An empirical test of assumptions from the "'acceleration debate."' *Time & Society, 27*(1), 3–39.
Schimmack, U. (2008). The structure of subjective well-being. In M. Eid & R. J. Larsen (Eds.), *The science of subjective well-being* (pp. 97–120). The Guilford Press.
Shevchuk, A., Strebkov, D., & Davis, S. N. (2019). The autonomy paradox: How night work undermines subjective well-being of internet-based freelancers. *ILR Review, 72*(1), 75–100.
Steenkamp, J. B., & Baumgartner, H. (1998). Assessing measurement invariance in crossnational. *Journal of Consumer Research, 25*(1), 78–107.
Timonen, H., & Paloheimo, K. (2008). The emergence and diffusion of the concept of knowledge work. *The Electronic Journal of Knowledge Management, 6*(2), 177–190.
Tsoukas, H., & Vladimirou, E. (2001). What is organizational knowledge? *Journal of Management Studies, 38*(7), 973–993.

Van Praag, B. M., Frijters, P., & Ferrer-i-Carbonell, A. (2003). The anatomy of subjective well-being. *Journal of Economic Behavior and Organization,* (51), 29–49.
Webster, F. (2002). *Theories of the information society*. Routledge.
Welzel, C., & Inglehart, R. (2010). Agency, values, and well-being: A human development. *Social Indicators Research, 97*, 43–63.

Irina Vartanova is a researcher at the Institute for Futures Studies. She has a Ph.D. in psychology and is an expert in the statistical analysis of large survey data. Her research focuses on social norms and value change.

Vladimir Gritskov is a lecturer at St Petersburg University (Russia). He designs courses for universities on decision making, soft skills, and the entrepreneurial mindset. His research interests lie in work analysis, decision making, and rationality in knowledge work and management.

Social Capital and Loneliness in Welfare State Regimes Before and After the Global Financial Crisis: Results Based on the European Social Survey

Fredrica Nyqvist, Mikael Nygård, and Thomas Scharf

1 Introduction

Considering worldwide demographic changes marked by rising proportions of older people, research and policy are increasingly interested in understanding how best to meet the needs of aging populations. This entails identifying resources that can contribute to extending the number of years lived in good health. Healthy aging is highly influenced by the social environment in which the older person lives, with social capital offering scholars a means to understand the relevance of the social environment for well-being. In this chapter we therefore focus on social capital and its meaning for improving overall well-being, such as absence of loneliness, in older people while acknowledging its individual- and macro-level predictors. While access to social capital is realized and distributed through welfare institutions, such as state, family and the market, we include a broad classification of welfare systems, i.e. welfare regimes, as a macro-level predictor of loneliness as well as a moderator between social capital and loneliness.

Since 2000, European governments have faced increasing financial pressures, implementing austerity policies that have increased pressure on state budgets and undermining economic and social security amongst older people. Such strategies might also have influenced the role of social capital in relation to loneliness, pointing to the need to assess change over time. The aim of this chapter is therefore to study the

F. Nyqvist (✉) · M. Nygård
Faculty of Education and Welfare Studies, Social Policy, Åbo Akademi University, Vaasa, Finland
e-mail: Fredrica.Nyqvist@abo.fi

M. Nygård
e-mail: Mikael.nygard@abo.fi

T. Scharf
Newcastle University, Population Health Sciences Institute, Newcastle upon Tyne, UK
e-mail: thomas.scharf@ncl.ac.uk

A. Almakaeva et al. (eds.), *Social Capital and Subjective Well-Being*,
Societies and Political Orders in Transition,
https://doi.org/10.1007/978-3-030-75813-4_12

relationship between social capital and loneliness across different welfare regimes over time. We focus on two time points, one before and one after the Global Financial Crisis of 2008–2009.

The first section of this chapter lays out the theoretical framework, drawing upon theories on loneliness, social capital and welfare regimes. The second section outlines the source of evidence, with data drawn from the European Social Survey of 2006 and 2014. The final section discusses and summarizes the key findings.

2 Loneliness and Social Capital

Loneliness has been extensively studied in recent decades, with evidence pointing to a range of negative effects associated with being lonely, including poor physical and psychological health and increased mortality (Holt-Lunstad et al., 2015). Previous research has also identified multiple risk factors for loneliness, including female gender, advanced old age, low socio-economic status, and limited social resources, such as poor quality and quantity of social contacts (de Jong Gierveld, 1998; Pinquart & Sorensen, 2001). Loneliness amongst older people in particular has become an issue of public concern, since societal and structural changes encompassing increasing proportions of older people, growing urbanization, the increasing spatial separation of family members, and growth of solitary living provide the potential for an increased prevalence of loneliness. However, contrary to assumptions, there is no clear picture of decreasing or increasing prevalence of loneliness over time at a population level (Dykstra, 2009). For example, while loneliness rates have been stable amongst older people in The Netherlands (Honigh-de Vlaming et al., 2014), Sweden (Dahlberg et al., 2018; Nyqvist et al., 2017) and the UK (Victor et al., 2002), a small increase has been noticed in Belgium (Vanderleyden & Heylen, 2007).

A growing body of evidence points to cross-national variation in loneliness rates in later life (e.g. de Jong Gierveld & Tesch-Römer, 2012; Fokkema et al., 2012; Hansen & Slagsvold, 2015; Lykes & Kemmelmeier, 2014; Sundström et al., 2009; Yang & Victor, 2011). In Europe, the focus of our study, a north–south gradient in loneliness has been found, with southern European countries tending to report higher levels of loneliness than northern countries. Further, higher levels of loneliness have also been found in Eastern than in West European countries (de Jong Gierveld & Tesch-Römer, 2012; de Jong Gierveld et al., 2012; Hansen & Slagsvold, 2015). It has been suggested that countries differ in cultural values and norms so that more family-oriented welfare societies, for example Spain, where interpersonal interaction with family is highly valued, as compared to more individualistic countries, such as Finland, were autonomy is valued, affect loneliness levels (Lykes & Kemmelmeier, 2014). In countries with strong norms of familial responsibility, expectations of support may be higher than in countries with a more individualistic orientation. If these support expectations are not met, then the prevalence of loneliness might be higher.

Empirically, while loneliness seems to vary across space and groups of people, there is less evidence for variation in loneliness over time. It is nonetheless evident that the understanding of loneliness is complex and, as suggested by de Jong Gierveld and Tesch-Römer (2012), an integrative model including both micro- and macro-level factors should be considered when studying loneliness. The starting point in this study is, therefore, that individual-level characteristics, such as socio-economic status, health and social resources, are relevant in determining whether people feel lonely or not. While these issues have been extensively studied in past decades (de Jong Gierveld, 1998; Pinquart & Sörensen, 2001), the theoretical concept of social capital has been under-researched (Litwin & Schiovitz-Erza, 2011; Nyqvist et al., 2016) in comparison with related and distinct concepts of social networks and social support. Social capital is generally described as a social resource that can be used in explaining health and well-being inequalities (Islam et al., 2006). According to Putnam (2000), social capital is a public good and can be defined as "features of social organization, such as trust, norms, and networks, that can improve the efficiency of society by facilitating coordinated actions" (Putnam 1993, p 167). Social capital includes both cognitive and structural components (Islam et al., 2006; Putnam, 2000). While structural social capital describes the networks, relationships, and institutions that link people and groups together, the cognitive dimension reflects the values, trust, confidence and norms that characterize these relationships. In this chapter, we follow Putnam in viewing social capital as a resource that is acquired through involvement in social activities, i.e. structural social capital, which may foster cognitive social capital, including interpersonal trust.

However, individuals' social resources might also be conditioned by welfare-institutional arrangements (de Jong Gierveld & Tesch-Römer, 2012). Extensive social welfare provision for older populations through, for example, comprehensive pension systems or income maintenance programs, decreases the risk of an older person living in poverty and hence may increase the ability to be socially integrated. Further, the welfare state might also influence loneliness by supporting services that enable older people to interact socially and to engage in leisure activities. Welfare states could also address the cognitive component of loneliness by addressing equality and fairness in services provided to older people, which could in turn influence trust levels (Kumlin & Rothstein, 2005). Trust is an important characteristic necessary in order to be able to interact with other people and to develop supportive relations. Individual social capital, including structural and cognitive resources, are thus formed in the exchange with a person's welfare state context. The theoretical assumption is that in more redistributive welfare regimes, people are less dependent on individual social resources for health and well-being as compared to welfare regimes where health and well-being are to a greater extent dependent on family ties, the voluntary sector and the market. Our theoretical model is depicted in Fig. 1.

Putnam (2000) showed that the USA experienced a decline in social capital during the twentieth century due to its changing demographic composition, increasing numbers of women in the workforce and increased mobility of families. While these findings have been supported by some research, other studies provide less support for the erosion of social capital in the US (e.g. Paxton, 1999). In Europe, the

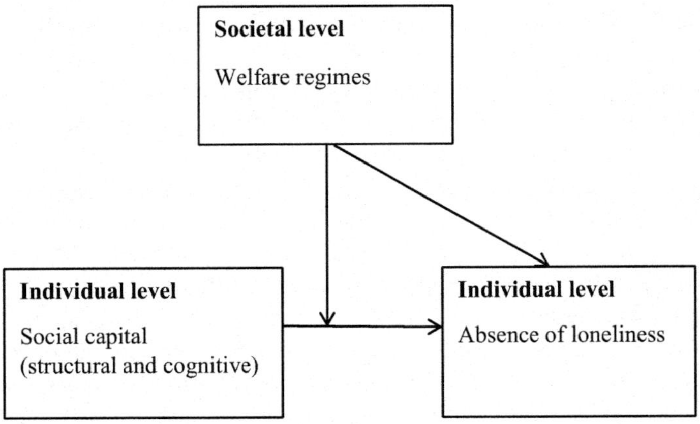

Fig. 1 Theoretical model used in this study [inspired by the model developed by de Jong Gierveld and Tesch-Römer (2012)]

evidence is also mixed and seems to depend on the measures of social capital that are used. The evidence is equivocal when it comes, for example, to interpersonal trust. Some studies report a decline in interpersonal trust after the economic crisis of 2008 in such countries as Sweden, Spain, the UK, Germany and Russia (Green et al., 2011; Kumlin et al., 2018). While The Netherlands reported a decline in trust from 2008 to 2010, trust levels returned to previous levels in 2013 (Kumlin et al., 2018). Sarracino and Mikucka (2017) reported an increasing trend in interpersonal trust between 1990 and 2012, especially in Denmark, Belarus and Switzerland, and a strong negative trend in Bulgaria, Slovakia and Ireland. Although the evidence suggests that social contacts differ across countries so that the Mediterranean countries, characterized by high familialism, usually report the highest levels of social contacts (Sheepers et al., 2002) in comparison with the Nordic countries (Kääriäinen & Lehtonen, 2006), there is limited and ambiguous evidence regarding the impact of the Global Financial Crisis on social contacts in different welfare contexts (Reeskens & van Oorschot, 2014). Divergent hypotheses, such as *crowding in* and *crowding out*, have been used as explanations concerning whether informal contacts can replace the role of welfare states in times of retrenchment. The crowding-out hypothesis suggests that generous and universal welfare states have negative impacts on informal social relations, since the welfare state is responsible for those in need and thus crowds out informal support networks. The crowding-in argument proposes that well-developed welfare states redistribute the resources necessary for social contacts to be developed and flourish. Although evidence generally suggests that comprehensive welfare states do not crowd out interpersonal trust (Rothstein & Stolle, 2008), the crowding-out hypothesis has found some support when it comes to social contacts (Reeskens & van Oorschot, 2014).

3 Welfare State Change and its Implications for Loneliness in Older People

The welfare state regime literature is closely linked to the work of Esping-Andersen (1990, 1999). Put simply, it argues that countries can be clustered on the basis of certain commonalities in terms of their welfare-institutional configurations and outcomes (Arts & Gelissen, 2002; Kumlin & Rothstein, 2005). While Esping-Andersen (1990) initially operated with three regimes, the Social-Democratic, the Conservative and the Liberal regime, later endeavours added Eastern-European and Southern-European regimes (Hemerijck, 2013). Consequently, this chapter operates with five European welfare state regimes: Nordic, Continental, Anglo-Saxon, Eastern-European and Southern-European.

Since the 1990s, European welfare states have been transformed by changing social needs, demographic aging and mounting economic challenges (Hemerijck, 2013). For instance, some countries not formerly committed to public welfare services, such as Germany, have invested more intensely in public services to families and older adults as part of a social investment paradigm (Kuitto, 2016; Morel et al., 2012; Nygård et al., 2015). However, they have also faced increasing financial strains due to higher unemployment, maturated welfare commitments and faltering growth, especially during the period of economic crisis after 2008. Consequently, in the wake of the crisis, most governments have pursued austerity measures to restore fiscal balance through spending limits or expenditure and welfare cuts (Farnsworth & Irving, 2015; Ólafsson et al., 2019; Taylor-Gooby et al., 2017). This raises the question regarding the extent to which welfare commitments to older persons and notably services preventing loneliness may have been undermined during the recessionary period.

Traditionally, the *Nordic regime* has been characterized by high levels of state involvement in social welfare, although a trend towards greater marketization can be observed since the 1990s (Kuisma & Nygård, 2015). It has combined individual social rights and substantial state involvement in social welfare, for example relatively generous pensions and universal provision of defamilizing public services (Bambra, 2007), and is marked by relatively low levels of inequality and poverty amongst older people (Fritzell et al., 2012). This can also be expected to influence loneliness of aging adults, since universal welfare states—perhaps somewhat contrary to intuition—not only tend to foster high social capital, but also to facilitate social participation through an enabling welfare system (Kumlin & Rothstein, 2005). However, with the exception of Iceland and to some extent Norway, these countries have responded to the crisis by cutting public expenditure (Farnsworth & Irving, 2015), thus weakening the universal character of welfare states and increasing older people's exposure to loneliness.

Also the *Continental regime* combines extensive state involvement in social welfare with involvement of corporate actors, notably the churches and different NGOs. However, the focus on status-maintaining social rights (Esping-Andersen, 1990), with relatively generous pensions for 'insiders' and lower means-tested benefits for 'outsiders', and limited provision of public social services, has been linked to higher inequality and poverty levels in old age (Schludi 2005). Furthermore, the higher degree of familization in these countries (Bambra, 2007), in combination with a less socially-enabling welfare state, would suggest that the prevalence of loneliness amongst older people is higher and conditioned by family ties. Many of the countries in this regime have maintained statutory obligations to provide for one's older parents, something which intuitively would make loneliness also dependent on family networks. Also in this regime, effects of austerity measures and structural reforms to curb pension expenditures have been significant (Farnsworth & Irving, 2015). This may have contributed to reducing the welfare state's capacity to counteract loneliness amongst older adults.

The *Anglo-Saxon regime* has traditionally had a less-pronounced state involvement and relied more squarely on the market, for instance in terms of private pensions and services. Increasing reliance on privately-funded pensions, together with modest and means-tested public social benefits (Clasen, 2005), has led to relatively high levels of inequality and poverty amongst older adults (Fritzell et al., 2012). We can also expect a higher prevalence of loneliness in older persons here, due to a less socially-enabling welfare state. However, the higher degree of familization in Ireland would suggest family ties have a greater conditioning effect on loneliness than is the case in the UK. We can also expect austerity measures to have been significant, especially in the UK, although successive governments have been reluctant to advocate cuts in state pensions for electoral reasons (Taylor-Gooby et al., 2017).

In the *Southern-European regime*, the family, local communities and the Catholic Church, with its principles of subsidiarity and humanitarianism, have generally played a more important role for social welfare than the state. Limited provision of public social services and modest pension benefits for older people has been linked to high inequality and widespread poverty (Ferrera, 1996). The high degree of familization (Bambra, 2007) in combination with a socially disenabling welfare state would suggest the prevalence of loneliness to be highly, and perhaps exclusively, conditioned by family or other social ties. Although older people with a work history have generally received generous pensions in countries such as Greece, Italy and Spain, and some improvements were also made in public services prior to the crisis, cuts in healthcare and welfare services made during the crisis have undermined older people's quality of life (Guillén & Pavolini, 2017). These factors may also have weakened these welfare states' capacity to prevent loneliness.

The *Eastern-European regime* consists of countries with highly divergent historical and institutional legacies, but with a half century of communist rule in common (Siegert, 2009). They are characterized by a rapid transformation from universal social protection systems during communism to more differentiated regimes in the post-communist era (Aidukaite, 2009). While the communist era largely implied modest benefits, albeit with broad coverage and public services for the whole population, the development after 1991 has been towards some corporatist elements, for example earnings-related pensions for some groups, mixed with liberal elements, such as means-tested benefits for older people. This points to considerable variation between countries in this welfare state regime in terms of welfare generosity and outcomes. While some countries, such as the Czech Republic or Poland, leaned towards a corporatist model, others, such as Hungary and the Baltic countries, have been more influenced by market-based elements (Aidukaite, 2009; Saxonberg & Szelewa, 2007). This also makes it harder to postulate commonalities regarding outcomes relating to loneliness. What may be of special interest here is not only the rapid transformation of society and the welfare state after the fall of communism (Siegert, 2009), but also the shift to austerity that can be observed for many of these countries (Farnsworth & Irving, 2015). This may have had a curtailing effect on social participation and a triggering effect on loneliness in older people, especially in countries with a marked transformation towards liberalism, such as Hungary or Lithuania, whereas predominantly Catholic countries with a more 'continental' form of social protection, such as Poland, would suggest loneliness in older people to be a lesser problem.

Acknowledging the critique of welfare regime theory, arguing that it is simplistic, gender-biased or overly static (Arts & Gelissen, 2002; Baldwin, 1996; Bambra, 2007), it still can serve as a tool for dealing with the complexity linked to welfare-institutional configurations (Hemerijck, 2013) and enabling assumptions on the role that such configurations play in the lives of older persons. This would be the case when more suitable alternatives for assessing country-level factors are absent, due, for example, to limited data availability (cf. Bryan & Jenkins, 2015).

To sum up, a relatively complex social capital and loneliness picture has been discussed. Several studies suggest that the level of universalism has positive implications on interpersonal trust, while high levels of social contacts have been found in less-developed welfare states. Although previous studies have shown a strong relation between social capital and health (Kawachi et al., 2008), few studies have acknowledged the significance of the broader institutional context, i.e. welfare regimes, for the maintenance of social capital and its potential for health and well-being in later life, including the absence of loneliness. In this study, we follow a different course than most previous analyses and evaluate welfare states' impact in improving overall well-being amongst older people, here measured as the absence of loneliness. We argue that welfare states have an important role in promoting national populations' happiness, health and wealth (Rothstein & Stolle, 2008). Consequently, "absence of loneliness" rather than loneliness can be used as the appropriate indicator. Our focus on older people is motivated by previous research, which demonstrated greater benefits of social capital for older rather than younger people (Muckenhuber et al., 2013). Moreover, the prevalence of loneliness is higher amongst older people (Dykstra, 2009), suggesting that loneliness may be particularly relevant for studies in this age group. It has been argued that social capital is under threat due to the pressure of modernization (Putnam, 2000), including higher levels of individualism, and this may be aggravated further by European nations' austerity programs (e.g. Blyth, 2013). Indeed, aspects of social capital have declined in many western countries, although divergent trends have been noticed for both interpersonal trust and social contacts across European countries.

This study aims, therefore, to assess social capital and the absence of loneliness amongst older people across European welfare regimes between 2006 and 2014 and to investigate the influence of social capital on loneliness. Based on previous theoretical discussion and research, while we expect relatively stable levels of absence of loneliness across the two time periods, we hypothesize divergent trends in social capital across time and welfare regimes. Although we expect absence of loneliness to vary across welfare regimes, so that older people in more universal welfare regimes report higher levels of absence of loneliness, we expect to find weaker welfare regime effects in 2014 as compared to 2006 due to changing welfare state contexts in times of economic crisis. Finally, we anticipate that the effect of social capital on the absence of loneliness varies across welfare regimes and also across the two time periods. Our theoretical expectation is that in welfare regimes traditionally marked by generous welfare supports older people are less dependent on individual resources for the absence of loneliness as compared to other regimes where absence of loneliness may to a greater extent be conditioned by family and other social ties.

4 Methods

The data source is the European Social Survey, ESS round 3, 2006, and round 7, 2014. These waves were selected since they help to monitor the levels of loneliness and social capital, respectively, in different welfare states before and after the Global Financial Crisis. The samples are representative of each country's adult population resident within private households, and the response rates vary between 30% and 70% in each country and wave. The countries participating in the third and seventh round of the ESS (with sample size for individuals aged 60 and over in parentheses for 2006 and 2014) were: Austria (512/538), Belgium (457/506), Denmark (480/452), Estonia (460/710), Finland (595/796), France (542/641), Germany (813/997), United Kingdom (780/853), Hungary (554/681), Ireland (439/790), The Netherlands (554/588), Norway (410/402), Poland (369/481), Portugal (840/525), Slovenia (391/418), Spain (485/553), Sweden (526/622), and Switzerland (585/443), thus making a total of 20,789 individuals aged 60 and over. Complete information on the survey is available from http://www.europeansocialsurvey.org.

Loneliness was used as an outcome variable and is measured with the single-item question: "how much of the time during the past week did you feel lonely?" The response alternatives were "none or almost none of the time", "some of the time", "most of the time", and "almost all of the time". The response alternatives "some of the time", "most of the time", and "almost all of the time" were collapsed into one category.

We selected social contacts, i.e. structural social capital, through the question: "how often do you meet socially with friends, relatives or work colleagues?" The response alternatives were "low" (never, less than once a month), "moderate" (once a month, several times a month) and "high" (once a week, several times a week, every day). Interpersonal trust or the cognitive aspect of social capital was measured with the question: "would you say that most people can be trusted, or that you cannot be too careful when dealing with people?" The original response categories, which ranged from 0 (you cannot be too careful) to 10 (most people can be trusted), were divided into three: low (0–3), moderate (4–7) and high (8–10) trust.

The 18 countries were divided into five welfare regime types: "Anglo-Saxon" (Ireland, UK), "Continental" (Austria, Belgium, France, Germany, Netherlands, Switzerland), "Eastern-Europe" (Estonia, Hungary, Poland, Slovenia), "Nordic" (Denmark, Finland, Norway, Sweden), and "Southern" (Portugal, Spain).

The analyses were also adjusted for relevant control variables, such as gender, age, education, self-rated health and living situation. Living situation included the categories: "lives with wife/husband/partner" or "does not". In the ESS, participants were asked to state their highest level of education achieved and included three categories: "primary" (less than lower secondary; lower secondary), "secondary" (upper secondary, post-secondary), and "tertiary" (lower and higher). Self-rated health was assessed with the question: "How is your (physical and mental) health in general?" The five-graded response scale was dichotomised into "good" ("very good", "good") and "poor" health ("fair", "bad" and "very bad").

5 Data Analyses

The association between social capital and the absence of loneliness was analyzed using multivariate logistic regression, treating the welfare regime variable as a fixed effect. The results were presented as odds ratios (OR) and their 95% confidence intervals (CI) for 2006 and 2015, respectively. To test whether possible associations between social capital variables and absence of loneliness varied in different welfare regimes, joint effects with welfare regime and each social capital variable were calculated, which correspond to models that include both the main effect and the interaction effect. The effects were estimated in separate models for each joint effect, adjusting for age, gender, educational level, living situation and self-rated health. Design weights and population size weights were applied, as recommended by the Weighting European Social Survey Data manual. The statistical program IBM SPSS statistics, version 24, was used for the analyses.

6 Results

Descriptive characteristics for social capital variables and loneliness are reported in Table 1. We report significant changes in social capital and loneliness across the welfare regime types between 2006 and 2014.

While countries clustered in the Southern regime have high levels of social contacts amongst older people, older people in the Nordic regime report high levels of interpersonal trust as compared with other regime types (Table 1). Countries in the Eastern regime have the lowest levels of social contacts. In 2006, older people in the Eastern regime reported the lowest levels of interpersonal trust. However, due to

Table 1 Average levels of social contact (1 = never, 7 = every day), social trust (0 = you can't be too careful, 10 = most people can be trusted) and share (%) of older people (≥60) reporting absence of loneliness in 18 European countries, European Social Survey, 2006 and 2014

	Social contacts		Diff	Social trust		Diff	Absence of loneliness		Diff
	2006	2014		2006	2014		2006	2014	
Nordic (n = 4283)									
Finland	4.84	4.73	−0.11	6.53	6.81	0.27	74.00	81.60	7.60
Denmark	5.20	5.11	−0.09	6.87	6.93	0.06	82.30	86.20	3.90
Norway	5.10	5.03	−0.07	6.87	6.71	−0.16	78.00	81.30	3.30
Sweden	4.98	5.11	0.14	6.25	6.12	−0.12	74.80	74.70	−0.10
	5.01	*4.96*	*−0.05*	*6.61*	*6.63*	*0.02*	*77.20*	*80.60*	*3.40***
Anglo-Saxon (n = 2862)									
United Kingdom	5.10	4.89	−0.21	5.51	5.55	0.04	74.20	74.40	0.20
Ireland	4.78	4.46	−0.33	5.47	5.00	−0.47	71.50	67.30	−4.20
	4.99	*4.69*	*−0.30****	*5.50*	*5.30*	*−0.20**	*73.30*	*71.10*	*−2.20*
Continental (n = 7269)									
Austria	4.81	4.69	−0.12	4.51	4.83	0.33	67.60	69.70	2.10
Belgium	4.89	4.93	0.03	4.81	4.96	0.15	72.40	71.90	−0.50
France	4.99	4.98	−0.01	4.39	4.61	0.23	68.80	66.70	−2.10
Germany	4.31	4.46	0.15	4.49	5.09	0.60	67.60	81.30	13.70
The Netherlands	5.13	5.13	0.00	5.67	6.03	0.37	71.70	82.40	10.70
Switzerland	5.03	4.87	−0.16	5.48	5.89	0.41	78.30	82.20	3.90
	4.80	*4.80*	*−0.01*	*4.87*	*5.23*	*0.36****	*70.90*	*76.50*	*5.60****

(continued)

Table 1 (continued)

	Social contacts		Diff	Social trust		Diff	Absence of loneliness		Diff
	2006	2014		2006	2014		2006	2014	
Southern ($n = 2404$)									
Portugal	5.91	5.70	−0.21	4.02	3.32	−0.71	41.10	57.90	16.80
Spain	5.34	5.18	−0.16	4.86	4.50	−0.36	64.30	71.20	6.90
	5.67	*5.42*	*−0.25****	*4.37*	*3.94*	*−0.43****	*50.60*	*64.90*	*14.30****
Eastern ($n = 3971$)									
Hungary	3.23	2.93	−0.31	3.96	3.86	−0.10	55.60	52.10	−3.50
Estonia	4.33	3.82	−0.51	5.36	5.68	0.32	57.30	59.20	1.90
Poland	3.76	3.71	−0.05	3.77	3.77	0.00	56.80	62.40	5.60
Slovenia	4.05	4.13	0.08	3.84	3.89	0.05	56.90	70.00	13.10
	3.85	*3.62*	*−0.23****	*4.27*	*4.43*	*0.16*	*56.60*	*60.10*	*3.50**

ESS 2006 n = 9792, ESS 2014 n = 10,997; T-test was used to compare changes in means of social contacts and social trust in five welfare regimes, whereas Chi-square was used for assessing changes in absence of loneliness in five welfare regimes. Significance levels: *$p < 0.5$, **$p < 0.01$, ***$p < 0.001$

a pronounced decrease in Portugal and Spain, older people in the Southern regime reported the lowest levels of interpersonal trust in 2014. The Anglo-Saxon and Continental regimes were somewhere in between. Further, absence of loneliness was more frequent in the Nordic, Continental and Anglo-Saxon regimes than in the Southern and Eastern regimes.

With the exception of the Continental regime, trends regarding *social contacts* were negative in the various welfare regimes, however, at a non-significant level in the Nordic regime. The most visible decline occurred in the Anglo-Saxon regime. When assessing the countries individually, while the trend was most negative in Estonia followed by Ireland and Hungary, a positive trend was noticed in Sweden, Belgium, Germany and Slovenia.

A mixed pattern was identified for *interpersonal trust*. The trend was especially positive in the Continental regime. While countries clustered in the Southern regime reported a decline, countries in the Anglo-Saxon regime reported mixed results. An increase in interpersonal trust in the UK contrasted with a decrease in Ireland.

The *absence of loneliness* indicator showed a positive trend between 2006 and 2014, an exception being the Anglo-Saxon regime. The most visible change occurred in the countries clustered in the Southern regime. While a negative trend was reported in Ireland, Hungary and France, rather flat trends were exhibited in Belgium and Sweden.

Tables 2 and 3 show results from the multivariate logistic regression models of absence of loneliness amongst older people in Europe in 2006 and 2014.

In all models, social contacts and high interpersonal trust were significantly associated with the absence of loneliness. Moderate interpersonal trust was associated with absence of loneliness in 2006. Although moderate trust was associated with absence of loneliness in model 2 in 2014, the association lost its significance in model 3 when welfare regimes were added to the model. The estimates for social contacts were somewhat lower in 2014 than in 2006.

We estimated the effects of welfare regimes in model 3 in Tables 2 and 3. The odds for absence of loneliness were significantly higher especially in the Nordic, but also in the Anglo-Saxon and Continental regimes, than in the Southern regime in both 2006 and 2014. However, while the odds for the absence of loneliness were significantly higher for the Eastern regime compared with the Southern regime in 2006, in 2014 the odds were lower, although not on a statistically significant level. Further, the estimates of the welfare regimes decreased in 2014, implying a weaker influence of welfare contexts on the absence of loneliness in 2014 than in 2006. Including the welfare regimes significantly ($p < 0.05$ based on likelihood ratio test) improved model fit in both 2006 and 2014, but the improvement was smaller in 2014.

Finally, estimates for the joint effects of welfare regime and each social capital variable in 2006 and 2014 are presented in Table 4.

More frequent social contacts were positively associated with absence of loneliness in all five welfare regimes in 2006. However, in 2014, social contacts were statistically significant only in the Anglo-Saxon, Eastern and Southern regimes. Expressing high interpersonal trust was associated with absence of loneliness in the Continental, Eastern and Southern regimes in 2006. In 2014, the association was no

Table 2 Odds ratios and 95% confidence intervals for the absence of loneliness in 2006, n = 9792

	Model 1		Model 2		Model 3	
	OR	95% CI	OR	95% CI	OR	95% CI
Frequency of being social						
Low	1.00		1.00		1.00	
Moderate	1.87***	(1.53–2.15)	1.77***	(1.49–2.09)	1.76***	(1.48–2.09)
High	2.02***	(1.74–2.36)	1.95***	(1.67–2.28)	1.97***	(1.67–2.31)
Interpersonal trust						
Low			1.00		1.00	
Moderate			1.18**	(1.05–1.33)	1.14*	(1.01–1.28)
High			1.67***	(1.41–1.98)	1.54***	(1.29–1.83)
Welfare regimes						
Nordic					2.14***	(1.66–2.77)
Anglo-Saxon					1.94***	(1.61–2.34)
Continental					1.43***	(1.24–1.71)
Eastern					1.34**	(1.09–1.65)
Log likelihood	8638.47		8557.30		8495.96	
Cox & Snell R2	0.172		0.175		0.181	
Nagelkerke R2	0.241		0.244		0.253	

Note Age, gender, educational level, living situation and self-rated health are controlled for in all models. Welfare regimes are dummy variables. Significance levels: *$p < 0.05$, **$p < 0.01$, ***$p < 0.001$

Table 3 Odds ratios and 95% confidence intervals for the absence of loneliness in 2014, n = 10,997

	Model 1		Model 2		Model 3	
	OR	95% CI	OR	95% CI	OR	95% CI
Frequency of being social						
Low	1.00		1.00		1.00	
Moderate	1.42***	(1.21–1.67)	1.38***	(1.18–1.62)	1.30**	(1.10–1.53)
High	1.65***	(1.42–1.91)	1.57***	(1.35–1.82)	1.47***	(1.26–1.72)
Interpersonal trust						
Low			1.00		1.00	
Moderate			1.16**	(1.04–1.31)	1.11	(0.99–1.25)
High			1.62***	(1.38–1.91)	1.51***	(1.28–1.79)
Welfare regimes						
Nordic					1.47**	(1.15–1.88)
Anglo-Saxon					1.24*	(1.04–1.49)
Continental					1.21*	(1.03–1.42)
Eastern					0.94	(0.79–1.13)
Log likelihood	9724.028		9662.67		9641.711	
Cox & Snell R2	0.162		0.165		0.166	
Nagelkerke R2	0.234		0.239		0.241	

Note Age, gender, educational level, living situation and self-rated health are controlled for in all models. Welfare regimes are dummy variables. Significance levels: $*p < 0.05$, $**p < 0.01$, $***p < 0.001$

Table 4 Odds ratios (OR) and 95% confidence intervals (95% CI) for the joint effects of welfare regime and social contacts and interpersonal trust on the absence of loneliness in 2006 and 2014

	Social contacts				Interpersonal trust			
	2006		2014		2006		2014	
	OR	95% CI	OR	95% CI	OR	95% CI	OR	95% CI
Nordic								
Low	1.00		1.00		1.00		1.00	
Medium	**2.54**	(1.01–6.40)	1.55	(0.64–3.75)	1.23	(0.60–2.51)	1.02	(0.53–1.99)
High	**3.39**	(1.40–8.19)	1.89	(0.81–4.41)	1.19	(0.57–2.48)	1.14	(0.57–2.28)
Anglo-Saxon								
Low	1.00		1.00		1.00		1.00	
Medium	**1.72**	(1.06–2.80)	1.30	(0.86–1.96)	0.89	(0.63–1.24)	0.76	(0.56–1.05)
High	**1.87**	(1.25–2.78)	**1.84**	(1.26–2.69)	1.26	(0.83–1.93)	1.08	(0.74–1.60)
Continental								
Low	1.00		1.00		1.00		1.00	
Medium	**2.06**	(1.60–2.66)	1.09	(0.91–1.46)	1.14	(0.97–1.35)	**1.20**	(1.01–1.42)
High	1.32	(0.99–1.76)	1.15	(0.86–1.53)	**1.45**	(1.11–1.89)	**1.77**	(1.35–2.31)
Eastern								
Low	1.00		1.00		1.00		1.00	
Medium	**1.62**	(1.15–2.29)	**1.52**	(1.13–2.03)	1.22	(0.90–1.64)	1.23	(0.96–1.58)
High	1.20	(0.85–1.70)	1.32	(0.99–1.76)	**2.15**	(1.30–3.55)	1.18	(0.78–1.79)

(continued)

Table 4 (continued)

	Social contacts				Interpersonal trust			
	2006		2014		2006		2014	
	OR	95% CI	OR	95% CI	OR	95% CI	OR	95% CI
Southern								
Low	1.00		1.00		1.00		1.00	
Medium	1.44	(0.85–2.44)	1.24	(0.78–1.96)	1.20	(0.91–1.58)	1.12	(0.87–1.45)
High	**1.76**	(1.12–2.74)	**1.81**	(1.23–2.67)	**1.96**	(1.27–3.02)	**2.13**	(1.30–3.48)

Note Estimates for the joint effect of welfare regime and each social capital variable were calculated, while adjusting for the main effects of all the other explanatory variables. Statistically significant results are emboldened ($p < 0.05$)

longer significant in the Eastern regime. The association between social capital and absence of loneliness was weaker in the Nordic, Anglo-Saxon and Eastern regimes in 2014 than in 2006. However, in the Continental and Southern regimes, the association between interpersonal trust and absence of loneliness was strengthened, and also for social contacts in the Southern regime.

7 Discussion and Conclusions

We conclude this chapter by bringing together the main findings, discussing the results and suggesting ideas for future research. Our starting point was that both individual-level social capital resources and welfare state contexts are important in understanding loneliness amongst older people, an assumption confirmed in our results. Social contacts and interpersonal trust were associated with absence of loneliness. Older adults, especially in the Nordic, Anglo-Saxon and Continental regimes, felt less lonely than those in the Eastern and Southern regimes. Our hypothesis suggested relatively stable levels of loneliness across time and our results showed somewhat higher levels of absence of loneliness in 2014 than in 2006. We also assumed that the role of welfare contexts in explaining the absence of loneliness might have changed due to the Global Financial Crisis of 2008 and the resulting recession, putting welfare states under pressure to adjust their institutional arrangements. The results suggested a somewhat weaker influence of welfare regimes in 2014 than in 2006. We also assumed that the influence of social capital on the absence of loneliness might vary across welfare regimes and across the two time periods.

The results revealed that the influence of social capital on absence of loneliness did indeed differ across welfare regimes and across time periods. However, a rather mixed picture emerged, with both increasing and decreasing trends. These main findings will be discussed next.

Although the main focus of this study was on the relationship between social capital and absence of loneliness across two time periods, the erosion of social capital in modern societies has been extensively discussed in the literature (Putnam, 2000). Consequently, we assessed changes in two measures of social capital in our initial analysis. Overall, while a negative trend for social contacts was observed, trends for interpersonal trust were more mixed. The *crowding-out* hypothesis has previously found some support when it comes to social contacts with family and friends (Scheepers et al., 2002), suggesting that welfare states with comprehensive social and health policies release individuals from obligations towards family, friends and neighbors. However, when Eastern European countries are included in the research (Kumlin et al., 2018), they usually report lower levels of contacts, which again supports the idea that social contacts are promoted in developed welfare states equipped with generous and universal social policies, an exception being the Southern regime. It is likely that the negative trends in social contacts between our study periods might arise from individualization and modernization processes, such as the rise of information and computer technology (e.g. Beck & Beck-Gernsheim, 2002; Putnam,

2000). While meaningful contacts with family, friends and neighbors are important for well-being, these types of networks have also been in transition in late modern society where traditional sources for social integration are less self-evident for realizing one's ambitions. Also, the ways in which older people interact socially have changed (Hunsaker & Hargittai, 2018) and this might not be reflected in our analyses of social contacts.

Theoretically, social contacts and interpersonal trust are connected and, even if Putnam (2000) argued that social participation fosters trust, alternative explanations have been emphasized suggesting that trust is a prerequisite for being socially engaged (Hooghe & Stolle, 2003). One could, therefore, argue that negative trends in social contacts imply negative trends in interpersonal trust. This was observed for the Anglo-Saxon regime and for the two countries clustered in the Southern regime, whereas the Eastern regime in particular reported divergent trends, so that a negative trend was observed for social contacts and a positive trend for interpersonal trust. There seems thus to be no uniform trend across European regimes. Nonetheless, the countries clustered in the Nordic regime have been described as highly trusting (Kumlin & Rothstein, 2005) and this was also shown in our analyses for both study years. Previous research suggests that universal welfare institutions enhance trust in both state institutions as well as social trust towards other people in general, whereas means-testing and selective programs undermine trust (Rothstein & Stolle, 2008). Social trust is, therefore, empirically related to good governance. In our study, the Eastern and Southern countries were usually placed in the category of low-trusting countries. An exception in our data was Estonia, which reported high trust levels in both study years in line with Switzerland and Austria. A clear decline in trust was noticed for Spain and Portugal in the Southern regime as well as Ireland in the Anglo-Saxon regime, countries that were severely hit by the 2008 Global Financial Crisis. Although some previous research suggests a positive correlation between economic performance and trust (Knack & Keefer, 1997; Neira et al., 2009), other studies report mixed trends when assessing social trust before and after the crisis. (Kumlin et al., 2018; Sarracino & Mikucka, 2017).

Notwithstanding such points, the main focus of this study was on the relationship between social capital and absence of loneliness. Although we analyzed resources for the absence of loneliness, we confirmed the established findings of previous studies focusing on other well-being measures such as happiness, quality of life and life satisfaction (Helliwell et al., 2014). We confirmed that individual social capital resources, such as social contacts and interpersonal trust, are closely related to absence of loneliness. We also explored an integrative model of loneliness by including welfare regime types, explaining the influence of contextual factors on becoming lonely or not in 2006 and 2014.

According to our findings, the association between social capital and absence of loneliness is not independent of welfare regimes, with the moderating effect of welfare regimes varying across time periods. In general, the impact of welfare regimes on the absence of loneliness decreased slightly between 2006 and 2014. This might suggest a weakening capacity of welfare states to prevent loneliness of older people through different social programs. The evidence also points to some signs of convergence, especially for the Anglo-Saxon and Continental regimes. Our results also indicate that social contacts and interpersonal trust are important resources for the absence of loneliness in the Southern regime in both study periods, and it seems that the association has somewhat strengthened in 2014. It seems logical to assume that the countries clustered in the Southern regime that were severely hit by the economic crisis after 2008 continue to be highly dependent on individual social resources for the absence of loneliness. A similar strengthening effect was observed in the Continental regime for interpersonal trust. Traditionally, these regimes have shown higher degrees of familialism (Esping-Andersen, 1999), suggesting that well-being is conditioned to a higher degree by various social resources rather than welfare supports provided by the state. According to our results, social capital resources have become even more important for the absence of loneliness in recent years in these two regimes. Whether this has to do with increasing inequality arising from cuts in state welfare provision, higher need of family support or other factors should be assessed in future studies.

In addition, the Nordic regime is still a forerunner when it comes to social investment as well as compensatory policies targeted towards older people (Kuitto, 2016), indicating that older people in the Nordic countries are less dependent on individual resources for their well-being. Contrary to what might be expected, an impact of social contacts on absence of loneliness was observed in the Nordic regime in 2006 but not in 2014. According to some sources, social contacts should have become more important for the absence of loneliness in 2014 as state support has been cut in welfare services, public transport and other measures supporting older adults' welfare. We can only speculate whether the change is related to changes in individual social expectations towards family and friends, quality of living conditions or level of social integration in society in general (de Jong Gierveld & Tesch-Römer, 2012). This issue needs further theoretical and empirical clarification. The results for the other regime types revealed a rather complex picture. While higher frequency of social contacts was associated with loneliness in the Anglo-Saxon regime, in the Eastern regime loneliness was associated with moderate frequency of social contacts. Moreover, interpersonal trust was associated with absence of loneliness in 2006 in the Eastern regime, but not in 2014. Although the inclusion of two time points is an advantage over existing cross-sectional studies, future work would nonetheless benefit from the inclusion of more time points over a longer overall period to reveal a more detailed picture of any fluctuating trends across welfare regimes.

To conclude, the evidence in our study suggests that social capital continues to be an important resource for absence of loneliness amongst older people in Europe. We have also shown that the welfare state has a tangible impact on this aspect of well-being and that, according to the measures reported here, the economic crisis did have a slightly weakening although not devastating well-being impact. The relative high state involvement in social welfare in the Nordic welfare regime seems especially successful in enhancing well-being amongst older people.

References

Aidukaite, J. (2009). Old welfare state theories and new welfare regimes in Eastern Europe: Challenges and implications. *Communist and Post-Communist Studies, 42*(1), 23–39.

Arts, W., & Gelissen, J. (2002). Three worlds of welfare capitalism or more? A state-of-the-art report. *Journal of European Social Policy, 12*(2), 137–158.

Baldwin, P. (1996). Can we define a European welfare state model? In B. Greve (Ed.), *Comparative welfare systems* (pp. 29–44). Macmillan.

Bambra, C. (2007). Defamilisation and welfare state regimes: A cluster analysis. *International Journal of Social Welfare, 16*(4), 326–338.

Beck, U., & Beck-Gernsheim, E. (2002). *Institutionalized individualism and its social and political consequences*. University of Michigan Press.

Blyth, M. (2013). *Austerity: The history of a dangerous idea*. Oxford University Press.

Bryan, M. L., & Jenkins, S. P. (2015). Multilevel modelling of country effects: A cautionary tale. *European Sociological Review, 32*(1), 3–22.

Clasen, J. (2005). *Reforming European welfare states*. Oxford University Press.

Dahlberg, L., Andersson, L., & Lennartsson, C. (2018). Long-term predictors of loneliness in old age: Results of a 20-year national study. *Aging & Mental Health, 22*(2), 190–196.

de Jong Gierveld, J. (1998). A review of loneliness: Concept and definitions, determinants and consequences. *Reviews in Clinical Gerontology, 8*(1), 73–80.

de Jong Gierveld, J., Dykstra, P. A., & Schenk, N. (2012). Living arrangements, intergenerational support types and older adult loneliness in Eastern and Western Europe. *Demographic Research, 27*, 167–200.

de Jong Gierveld, J., & Tesch-Römer, C. (2012). Loneliness in old age in Eastern and Western European societies: Theoretical perspectives. *European Journal of Ageing, 9*(4), 285–295.

Dykstra, P. A. (2009). Older adult loneliness: Myths and realities. *European Journal of Ageing, 6*(2), 91. https://doi.org/10.1007/s10433-009-0110-3

Esping-Andersen, G. (1990). *The three worlds of welfare capitalism*. Polity Press.

Esping-Andersen, G. (1999). *Social foundations of postindustrial economies*. Oxford University Press.

Farnsworth, K., & Irving, Z. (2015). Austerity: More than the sum of its parts. In K. Farnsworth & Z. Irving (Eds.), *Social policy in times of austerity* (pp. 9–21). Policy Press.

Ferrera, M. (1996). The 'Southern model' of welfare in social Europe. *Journal of European Social Policy, 6*(1), 17–37.

Fokkema, T., De Jong Gierveld, J., & Dykstra, P. A. (2012). Cross-national differences in older adult loneliness. *The Journal of Psychology, 146*(1–2), 201–228.

Fritzell, J., Bäckman, O., & Ritakallio, V.-M. (2012). Income inequality and poverty: Do the Nordic countries still constitute a family of their own? In J. Kvist, J. Fritzell, B. Hvinden, & O. Kangas (Eds.), *Changing social equality* (pp. 165–185). Policy Press.

Green, A., Janmaat, G., & Cheng, H. (2011). Social cohesion: Converging and diverging trends. *National Institute Economic Review, 215*(1), R6–R22.

Guillén, A., & Pavolini, E. (2017). Spain and Italy. In P. Taylor-Gooby, B. Leruth, & L. Chung, (Eds.), *After Austerity. Welfare state transformation in Europe after the Great Recession* (pp. 136–154). Oxford University Press.

Hansen, T., & Slagsvold, B. (2015). Late-life loneliness in 11 European countries: Results from the generations and gender survey. *Social Indicators Research, 124*(1), 1–20.

Helliwell, J. F., Huang, H., & Wang, S. (2014). Social capital and well-being in times of crisis. *Journal of Happiness Studies, 15*(1), 145–162.

Hemerijck, A. (2013). *Changing Welfare States*. Oxford University Press.

Holt-Lunstad, J., Smith, T. B., Baker, M., Harris, T., & Stephenson, D. (2015). Loneliness and social isolation as risk factors for mortality: A meta-analytic review. *Perspectives on Psychological Science, 10*(2), 227–237.

Honigh-de Vlaming, R., Haveman-Nies, A., Bos-Oude Groeniger, I., de Groot, L., & van't Veer, P. (2014). Determinants of trends in loneliness among Dutch older people over the period 2005–2010. J Aging Health, *26*(3), 422–440

Hooghe, M., & Stolle, D. (Eds.). (2003). *Generating social capital: Civil society and institutions in comparative perspective.* Palgrave Macmillan.

Hunsaker, A., & Hargittai, E. (2018). A review of Internet use among older adults. *New Media & Society, 20*(10), 3937–3954.

Islam, M. K., Merlo, J., Kawachi, I., Lindström, M., & Gerdtham, U. G. (2006). Social capital and health: Does egalitarianism matter? A literature review. *International Journal for Equity in Health, 5*(1), 3.

Kääriäinen, J., & Lehtonen, H. (2006). The variety of social capital in welfare state regimes–a comparative study of 21 countries. *European Societies, 8*(1), 27–57.

Kawachi, I., Subramanian, S. V., & Kim, D. (Eds.). (2008). *Social capital and health.* Springer.

Knack, S., & Keefer, P. (1997). Does social capital have an economic payoff? A cross-country investigation. *The Quarterly Journal of Economics, 112*(4), 1251–1288.

Kuisma, M., & Nygård, M. (2015). The European Union and the Nordic models of welfares—path dependency or policy harmonisation? In Grøn, C. H., Nedergaard, P., & Wivel, A. (Eds.), *The Nordic countries and the European Union. Still the other European community?* (pp. 158–172). Routledge.

Kuitto, K. (2016). From social security to social investment? Compensating and social investment welfare policies in a life-course perspective. *Journal of European Social Policy, 26*(5), 442–459.

Kumlin, S., & Rothstein, B. (2005). Making and breaking social capital: The impact of welfare-state institutions. *Comparative Political Studies, 38*(4), 339–365.

Kumlin, S., Stadelmann-Steffen, I., & Haugsgjerd, A. (2018). Trust and the Welfare State. In E. M. Uslaner (Ed.), *The Oxford handbook of social and political trust* (pp. 385–408). Oxford University Press.

Litwin, H., & Shiovitz-Ezra, S. (2011). Social network type and subjective well-being in a national sample of older Americans. *The Gerontologist, 51*(3), 379–388.

Lykes, V. A., & Kemmelmeier, M. (2014). What predicts loneliness? Cultural difference between individualistic and collectivistic societies in Europe. *Journal of Cross-Cultural Psychology, 45*(3), 468–490.

Morel, N., Palier, B., & Palme, J. (2012). Beyond the welfare state as we knew it? In N. Morel, B. Palier, & J. Palme (Eds.), *Towards a social investment welfare state?* (pp. 1–32). Policy Press.

Muckenhuber, J., Stronegger, W. J., & Freidl, W. (2013). Social capital affects the health of older people more strongly than that of younger people. *Ageing & Society, 33*(5), 853–870.

Neira, I., Vázquez, E., & Portela, M. (2009). An empirical analysis of social capital and economic growth in Europe (1980–2000). *Social Indicators Research, 92*(1), 111–129.

Nygård, M., Kuisma, M., Krüger, N., & Campbell-Barr, V. (2015). Investing in our future? The influence of social investment ideas on family policy discourses in Finland, Germany and the UK. In U. Korkut, K. Mahendran, & G. Bucken-Knapp (Eds.), *Discursive governance in politics, policy, and the public sphere* (pp. 31–46). Palgrave Macmillan.

Nyqvist, F., Cattan, M., Conradsson, M., Näsman, M., & Gustafsson, Y. (2017). Prevalence of loneliness over ten years among the oldest old. *Scandinavian Journal of Public Health, 45*(4), 411–418.

Nyqvist, F., Victor, C. R., Forsman, A. K., & Cattan, M. (2016). The association between social capital and loneliness in different age groups: A population-based study in Western Finland. *BMC Public Health, 16*(1), 542.

Ólafsson, S., Daly, M., Kangas, O., & Palme, J. (Eds.). (2019). *Welfare and the great recession: A comparative study.* Oxford University Press.

Paxton, P. (1999). Is social capital declining in the United States? A multiple indicator assessment. *American Journal of Sociology, 105*(1), 88–127.

Pinquart, M., & Sorensen, S. (2001). Influences on loneliness in older adults: A meta-analysis. *Basic and Applied Social Psychology, 23*(4), 245–266.

Putnam, R. D. (1993). *Making democracy work: Civic traditions in modern Italy*. Princeton University Press.

Putnam, R. D. (2000). *Bowling alone*. Free Press.

Reeskens, T., & van Oorschot, W. (2014). European feelings of deprivation amidst the financial crisis: Effects of welfare state effort and informal social relations. *Acta Sociologica, 57*(3), 191–206.

Rothstein, B., & Stolle, D. (2008). The state and social capital: An institutional theory of generalized trust. *Comparative Politics, 40*(4), 441–459.

Sarracino, F., & Mikucka, M. (2017). Social capital in Europe from 1990 to 2012: Trends and convergence. *Social Indicators Research, 131*(1), 407–432.

Saxonberg, S., & Szelewa, D. (2007). The continuing legacy of the communist legacy? The development of family policies in Poland and the Czech Republic. *Social Politics, 14*(3), 351–379.

Scheepers, P., Grotenhuis, M. T., & Gelissen, J. (2002). Welfare states and dimensions of social capital: Cross-national comparisons of social contacts in European countries. *European Societies, 4*(2), 185–207.

Schuldi, M. (2005). *The reform of Bismarckian Pension Systems: A comparison of pension politics in Austria, France, Germany, Italy and Sweden*. Amsterdam University Press.

Siegert, D. (2009). Why no 'Dilemma of Simultaneousness'? The 'Great Transformation' in Eastern Central Europe considered from the point of view of post-socialist research. In R. Frank & S. Burghart (Eds.), *Driving forces of socialist transformation* (pp. 89–112). Praesens.

Sundström, G., Fransson, E., Malmberg, B., & Davey, A. (2009). Loneliness among older Europeans. *European Journal of Ageing, 6*(4), 267.

Taylor-Gooby, P., Leruth, B., & Chung, H. (2017). Where next for the UK welfare state? In Taylor-Gooby, P., Leruth, B., & Chung, L. (Eds.), *After Austerity. Welfare State transformation in Europe after the great recession* (pp. 48–66). Oxford University Press.

Vanderleyden, L., & Heylen, L. (2007). Ouderen, hun sociale contacten en de beleving ervan: continuïteit of verandering? [Elderly people, their social contacts and experiences: Stable or changing?] *Tijdschrift voor Sociologie, 28*(1), 52–78.

Victor, C. R., Scambler, S. J., Shah, S., Cook, D. G., Harris, T., Rink, E., & De Wilde, S. (2002). Has loneliness amongst older people increased? An investigation into variations between cohorts. *Ageing & Society, 22*(5), 585–597.

Yang, K., & Victor, C. (2011). Age and loneliness in 25 European nations. *Ageing & Society, 31*(8), 1368–1388.

Fredrica Nyqvist is a Senior lecturer in Social Policy at Åbo Akademi University, Finland. She is also an Associate professor/docent of Social Policy at University of Helsinki. She gained her Ph.D. in Social Policy from Åbo Akademi University in 2009 focusing then on social capital and health differences amongst Swedish and Finnish speakers in Finland. After her Ph.D. she worked as a Senior researcher at National Institute of Health and Welfare (THL) and accomplished a three year post-doctoral Fellowship within the FLARE (Future Leaders of Ageing Research) programme supported by members of the European Research Area in Ageing (ERA-AGE) and was financed by the Academy of Finland. Her current research is on active ageing, loneliness and on issues related to well-being of linguistic minorities.

Mikael Nygård is Professor of Social Policy at the Åbo Akademi University, Finland, with previous tenures as Academy lecturer of Social Policy at the same university, and Senior lecturer of Social Sciences at the Swedish Polytechnic, Finland. He is a board member of the Finnish Social Policy Association and a member of the editorial committee of Janus, the Finnish Journal of Social Policy and Social Work. He has held a position of Visiting Fellow at the Oxford Brooks University, UK, in 2013. His research interest ranges from research on societal participation of various groups, such as older adults, youth and people with disabilities, to health-related research and welfare state analysis.

Thomas Scharf is Professor of Social Gerontology in the Population Health Sciences Institute at Newcastle University, having previously been Director of the Irish Centre for Social Gerontology, NUI Galway, Ireland (2010–2015) and Director of the Centre for Social Gerontology, Keele University (2006–2010). He is a Fellow of the Academy of Social Sciences, has held visiting professorships at the universities of Manchester, Keele, Vienna and Galway, and is currently President of the British Society of Gerontology (2019–2022). His research focuses on topics broadly relating to social inclusion and exclusion in later life and to socio-spatial features of ageing.

Conclusion. What Comparative Studies Reveal About Social Capital and Well-Being?

Anna Almakaeva, Alejandro Moreno, and Rima Wilkes

The aim of this book was to help understand the nature of social capital and subjective well-being and to consider their interrelations in several world regions—Europe, including former USSR countries, Latin America and Asia. Although these two topics have received much attention in recent decades, the role of social, economic, and institutional context remains under investigated. The contributors analyze the impact of context using time and spatial perspectives. They examine similarity of social capital and well-being trends in different geographical locations and test stability of associations between social capital, well-being and their determinants across time-points, countries and regions. Cross-cultural survey data in combination with quantitative data analysis implemented as the main analytical tool in all chapters of the volume provide clear evidence that country setting indeed matters.

Overall, the book further contributes in the field in several directions. First, it allows to trace the impact of communist legacy on social capital in the long run. Second, it discovers the role of exogenous shocks and turbulent times on erosion and reviving of social capital and well-being. Third, it reveals how country conditions change the roots of social capital and shape relations between social capital and well-being.

A. Almakaeva (✉)
HSE University, Moscow, Russia
e-mail: aalmakaeva@hse.ru

A. Moreno
Instituto Tecnológico Autónomo de México (ITAM), Mexico City, Mexico
e-mail: amoreno@itam.mx

R. Wilkes
University of British Columbia, Vancouver, Canada
e-mail: wilkesr@mail.ubc.ca

A. Almakaeva et al. (eds.), *Social Capital and Subjective Well-Being*, Societies and Political Orders in Transition,
https://doi.org/10.1007/978-3-030-75813-4_13

1 Communist Legacy, Crisis and Transition

In this volume we follow a broad definition of social capital and interpret it as social ties, trust and pro-civic orientations which are efficient for reinforcing cooperation. Previous studies detected a detrimental effect of Communist past on generalized trust. In the opening chapter Mai Beilmann, Laur Lilleoja and Anu Realo investigate three former USSR countries—Estonia, Latvia, and Lithuania—and show that this effect is not universal. First, these countries were already diverse before the collapse of the Soviet Union. According to the second wave of the WVS only 19% of Latvian respondents answered that “most people can be trusted”. Estonia and Lithuania slightly outperformed Latvia as 28% and 31% of participants selected the same option. The gap between Estonia, Lithuania and the most trustful countries of the second wave (1989–1993)—Norway and Sweden—were rather huge and reached more than 30 percent points.

Second, after the dissolution of the Soviet Union Estonia and Lithuania demonstrated a small drop to 22%, but not Latvia where trust, on the contrary, increased to 25%. In the recent 7th wave of the WVS collected in 2017–2018 Estonia and Lithuania had trust levels only slightly higher than during Communist period (33% and 34% respectively). Unfortunately, Latvia missed the 6th and 7th waves of the WVS, but ESS data demonstrate that in 2018 it was still worse than its neighbors (see Fig. 3 in the Chapter “Learning to Trust: Trends in Generalized Social Trust in the Three Baltic Countries from 1990 to 2018”).

Third, the growth of trust in Norway over 30 years (between the 2nd to 7th waves of the WVS) was moderate. In the 7th wave trust reached only 73% compared to 61% in the 2nd wave. In Sweden the shift was even less—5 percent points. Figure 4 in the Chapter “Learning to Trust: Trends in Generalized Social Trust in the Three Baltic Countries from 1990 to 2018” shows that changes in trust between 1996 and 2018 hardly exceed 20 percent points. Therefore, generalized trust looks like a rather stable trait, especially in high trusting societies, but it is still subject for some fluctuations after traumatic periods of transition.

Tim Reeskens and Leen Vandecasteele in Chapter “The Impact of Economic Insecurity on Social Capital and Well-Being: An Analysis across Different Cohorts in Europe” as well as Fredrica Nyqvist, Mikael Nygård and Thomas Scharf in Chapter “Social Capital and Loneliness in Welfare State Regimes Before and After the Global Financial Crisis: Results Based on the European Social Survey” examine the impact of the world financial crisis of 2008. Their findings further confirm low elasticity of generalized trust since its shifts in Europe before and after crisis were significant only in some countries and these changes were rather small.

Fourth, institutional trust as indicator of linking social capital is a much more flexible phenomenon but not a linear function of exogenous shocks. Reeskens and Vandecasteele detected a negative effect of the 2008 economic crisis on the overall index of political trust but we observe mixed trends for three Baltic countries. A clear drop of political trust after the USSR disruption occurred only in Lithuania (see Chapter “Learning to Trust: Trends in Generalized Social Trust in the Three

Baltic Countries from 1990 to 2018"). It seems that the shape and velocity of changes depend on specific institutions under evaluation and do not necessarily go hand in hand with generalized trust.

Pro-civic orientations cover human values and tolerance. Analogously to institutional trust, tolerance is also quite volatile characteristic. David Sulmont and Kiara Castaman (Chapter "Rainbows in Latin America: Public Opinion and Societal Attitudes Towards Homosexuality"), Sotheeswari Somasundram, Muzafar Shah Habibullah, Murali Sambasivan and Ratneswary Rasiah (Chapter "Antecedents of Religious Tolerance in Southeast Asia Sotheeswari") show tangible dynamic of LBGT and religious tolerance in Latin America and Southeast Asia. In Europe the Great Recession followed after 2008 produced a detrimental effect on tolerance towards homosexuals. This effect was even more pronounced for younger Europeans (see Chapter "The Impact of Economic Insecurity on Social Capital and Well-Being: An Analysis across Different Cohorts in Europe ").

Value changes and value trends have been thoroughly investigated by the proponents of modernization theory of Inglehart and Welzel (Inglehart, 2018; Inglehart & Welzel, 2005; Welzel, 2013). They show that modern societies have been gradually evolving in the direction self-expression values. This trend is mostly produced by the generational shift as younger cohorts who take existential security for granted exhibit a significantly higher levels of postmaterialism. At the same time, little is known whether values can change over an individual's life span. Existing evidence on individual value trajectories is mixed. In the recent review Bardi and Goodwin (2011) note that published surveys simultaneously support plasticity and stability hypotheses. Two chapters in the book address the same issue.

Tim Reeskens and Leen Vandecasteele use a pseudo-panel design with matched socio-demographic groups of European citizens. They found very small and inconsistent effects of economic crisis on the four Schwartz value dimensions between 2008 and 2016. On the contrary, Silko Pfeil, Rico Bornschein, Eric Holdack (Chapter "Cultural Transition of Human Values—A Longitudinal Study on East-West Migration in Germany") demonstrate that values do adjust to the social context. Based on the SOEP panel data their study reveals the non-linear growth of postmaterialism among migrants from Eastern Germany after their relocation to the Western part. Pfeil, Bornschein, and Holdack also confirm the negative and persistent impact of Soviet legacy. Postmaterialist orientations in Eastern Germany grew comparatively slowly between 1996 and 2016 and its public remains less inclined towards those values than the West German public.

While Chapter "Cultural Transition of Human Values – A Longitudinal Study on East-West Migration in Germany" demonstrate plasticity of values we do not see the impact of financial crisis of 2008 on values of Europeans. Probably, the influence of crisis depends on the level of deprivation and its duration which vary across European countries. Pooled sample which Reeskens and Vandecasteele use for their analysis disguise these inter-country differences. In addition, the pseudo-panel design traces value shifts of socio-demographic groups. To uncover the impact of 2008 financial crisis on personal values scholars need classical panel data.

In sum, generalized trust and values seem to be more stable, while institutional trust and tolerance show a more fluctuating nature. In a similar vein, subjective well-being may shrink rapidly when exposed to negative traumatic events. Moreover, the levels of its disruption and recovery depend on the age cohort. For instance, in Russia, the collapse of the Soviet Union affected all groups, but the oldest cohort exhibited the most negative trend (Foa et al., 2018). Chapter "The Impact of Economic Insecurity on Social Capital and Well-Being: An Analysis across Different Cohorts in Europe" shows the same detrimental effect but, on the contrary, it was more salient among young Europeans. These findings go in line with Chapter "Social Capital and Loneliness in Welfare State Regimes Before and After the Global Financial Crisis: Results Based on the European Social Survey". Fredrica Nyqvist, Mikael Nygård and Thomas Scharf did not detect a sizeable rise of loneliness among older people.

2 Roots of Social Capital

Previous studies demonstrate that economic and social development, equality and lower levels of corruption amplify "good" social capital in a society (Rothstein & Uslaner, 2005; Uslaner, 2013; Whiteley, 2000; Zak & Knack, 2001). However, the greater part of evidence came from cross-sectional (cross-country) samples collected at one time-point and, therefore, is not free from spurious correlations. The study by Beilmann, Lilleoja and Realo covers longitudinal trends and partly overcomes this limitation. Beilmann, Lilleoja and Realo concentrate on Estonia, Latvia, and Lithuania and use data from 1991 to 2018. Contrary to expectations, these authors failed to find mutually correlating time trends between generalized trust, corruption and inequality. These results are similar to Fairbrother and Martin's study (2013) who found cross-sectional correlation between inequality and trust in the United States, but it disappeared in the longitudinal association. The promoting effect of human development was only detected in Estonia but not in Lithuania and Latvia. Most likely, relations between social capital, corruption, inequality and human development are rather complex and indirect. There are some studies which go in line with this hypothesis as they also reveal non-linear cross-sectional patterns between trust and development (Almakaeva et al., 2017; Peiró-Palomino & Tortosa-Ausina, 2013).

Chapter "Emigration and Trust: Evidence from Eastern Europe and Central Asia", written by Dragos Radu, Ekaterina Skoglund and Soomin Ma, continues investigation of macro conditions and focus on the role of emigration. Although there are dozens of papers on migration, little is known about changes of trust in sending societies. Radu, Skoglund and Ma propose two direct mechanisms of how migration affects trust: (1) self-selection and (2) network ties of migrants. The first mechanism implies that individuals with high trust and low risk aversion are more prone to emigrate. Therefore, their outflows should result in the "trust drain" in the country of origin. In contrast, the second mechanism should lead to the opposite outcome as it sees migrants as the least trusting group. Strong ingroup ties which are necessary for successful relocation work as bonding social capital and separate emigrants from outgroups in the country of destination and in the country of origin. In addition, emigrants are usually less satisfied with institutions in the sending society and have low institutional confidence. Low institutional confidence, in turn, reinforces the erosion of generalized social trust. The outflow of distrusting individuals lifts the levels of trust in the sending society.

The evidence, presented in the second chapter, confirms that migration do affect trust in sending countries. However, country-level correlations between generalized trust and overall migration rates demonstrate a u-shape pattern. Emigration of highly-educated citizens has a more clearly negative relationship with generalized social trust, but not in a linear way.

Individual data obtained from six post-Soviet countries show that this effect is hardly produced by self-selection. People with migration experience or migration plans have lower levels of generalized trust and lower levels of institutional trust. However, for institutional trust this pattern is not so pronounced. It is likely, that the second mechanism works better in the case of migrants but, at the same time, it does not increase the levels of trust in a society. These results are mostly descriptive but they certainly deserve more detailed investigation in future studies.

The last two chapters of the volume's first part are devoted to another dimension of social capital-tolerance. David Sulmont and Kiara Castaman (Chapter "Rainbows in Latin America: Public Opinion and Societal Attitudes Towards Homosexuality") deal with tolerance towards LGBT in Latin America (LA). Their chapter shows that although this region still has high levels of prejudice, it has changed significantly over the last 20 years. In line with the theory of intergenerational value change (Inglehart & Welzel, 2005), changes are associated with economic development and democratization. Progressive legislation introduced in some LA countries has enhanced acceptance of LGBT Community, although in some cases greater levels of acceptance have preceded more liberal legislation.

At the individual level, all elements of social capital are found to be closely connected with each other. Generalized trust, posmaterialism and tolerance have robust positive relations between them. Nonetheless, these results again demonstrate a mismatch with long-term time trends. While tolerance towards LGBT among LA countries has increased between 1994 and 2014, generalized trust and postmaterialism have either degraded or remained unchanged. It seems that Latin American societies have grown more tolerant towards gays despite the fact that they have not moved significantly towards self-expression values.

As noted in the previous studies, religiosity is one of the main antagonists of "open-minded" attitudes. In general, this holds true for LA societies but this effect varies depending on denomination. Catholics are more tolerant than other religious groups. Perhaps the Latin American branch of Catholicism identified as the Theology of Liberation, which was influential in the 1960s and 1970s, may have had something to do with this "openness", but that is just our speculation, as the surveys employed do not provide any way to check.

Sotheeswari Somasundram, Muzafar Shah Habibullah, Murali Sambasivan and Ratneswary Rasiah (Chapter "Antecedents of Religious Tolerance in Southeast Asia Sotheeswari") continue investigation of tolerance. They focus on religious tolerance in the four countries of Southeast Asia (Malaysia, Philippines, Thailand and Singapore) and draw a line between individual and social religiosity. They reveal a very robust impact of individual religiosity in all four countries but it is not universal. In Philippines, Thailand and Singapore individual religiosity promote tolerance, in Malaysia it works in the opposite direction. Social religiosity has a similar negative effect in Malaysia, but has nothing to do with tolerance in Philippines and Thailand. In Singapore its impact is positive but not robust. These authors assume that the eroding influence of religiosity in Malaysia may be rooted in its colonial heritage which produced settlement and occupation segregation between three largest ethnic and religious groups—Malay, Chinese and Indian. This legacy in combination with politicization of these intergroup differences have produced strong bonding social capital.

3 Social Capital as a Trigger of Subjective Well-Being

The second part of the volume examines the impact of social capital on subjective well-being at the micro and macro levels (see Fig. 1). Figure 1 shows that country or regional social capital functions as common property and informal institute which creates a specific normative environment in a community. Individual social capital encompasses social ties, trust and pro-civic orientations. It constitutes a personal resource which people utilize to achieve a better life and higher levels of well-being.

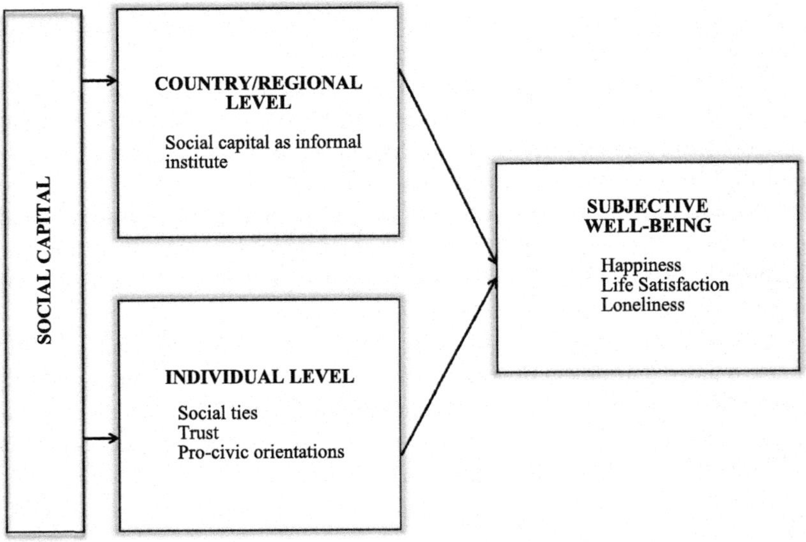

Fig. 1 Impact of social capital on subjective well-being

Some studies already have detected a positive association between social capital and well-being at the macro-level (Bjornskov, 2003; Elgar et al., 2011). Nevertheless, this approach has been criticized since it treats countries as units of analysis and ignores within-country diversity. Jesus Peiró-Palomino and Emili Tortosa-Ausina (Chapter "Formal and Informal Institutions as Drivers of Life Satisfaction in European Regions") handle this problem by using a sample of 166 European sub-regions. They show that both generalized trust and network support do amplify the level of life satisfaction in a sub-region. Yet, this effect is not universal. Positive influence of trust demonstrates linear dependence and becomes larger in the areas with low life satisfaction. The influence of social networks follows a u-shape pattern. It has the weakest positive impact in the regions with middle life satisfaction and totally vanishes in the areas with the highest well-being.

Chapter "The Effects of Democracy and Trust on Subjective Well-being: A Multi-level Study of Latin American Countries" written by Isabel Neira, Marta Portela and Maricruz Lacalle-Calderon confirms a relative role of social capital in the promoting of well-being. Neira, Portela and Lacalle-Calderon incorporate multi-level regression modeling and data from the Latin Barometer collected in 2016 in 18 Latin American countries. They reveal that neither individual no country's generalized trust result in a higher sense of well-being. Trust in government plays a more important role in promoting happiness and life satisfaction in Latin America.

Janine Jongbloed and Ashley Pullman investigate interrelations between subjective well-being, social and human capital in the Chapter "Degree of Benefit? The Interconnection Among Social Capital, Well-Being and Education". According to their analysis the amount of people with tertiary education in a country does not lift well-being of European citizens. Individual social and human capital are found to be significant triggers of personal happiness. Social and human capitals act in cooperation and compensate for the lack of each other. Therefore, generalized trust and social relatedness have stronger positive effect on well-being of less educated individuals. This effect is even more pronounced in the case of social relatedness which Jongbloed and Pullman use as a measure of network support.

Irina Vartanova and Vladimir Gritskov (Chapter "Occupation and Subjective Well-Being: A Knowledge Economy Perspective") continue this line of research and focus on the influence of knowledge work and other job characteristics. Vartanova and Gritskov assume that knowledge workers should exhibit higher levels of subjective well-being since they have more job autonomy, higher income and less exposed to the work-life conflict. They reveal that knowledge workers indeed outperform manual and service workers but these discrepancies exist only in the countries with less developed knowledge economy. Income, indeed, partly moderates this link, but a clear impact of job autonomy and work-life conflict was not detected. Explaining the absence of differences between service, manual and knowledge workers in the prosperous countries, Vartanova and Gritskov propose that advanced social policy and strong employment protection mitigate the negative effect of low-skilled job on well-being.

The study of Fredrica Nyqvist, Mikael Nygård, Thomas Scharf (Chapter "Social Capital and Loneliness in Welfare State Regimes Before and After the Global Financial Crisis: Results Based on the European Social Survey") show similar results. Nyqvist, Nygård and Scharf are interested in the consequences of financial crisis of 2008 for elderly Europeans and use the feeling of loneliness as the main indicator of subjective well-being. They demonstrate that Nordic, Anglo-Saxon and Continental welfare regimes produce less loneliness among older adults compared to Eastern and Southern regimes. Contrary to expectations, crisis of 2008 did not result in the decline in well-being and in 2014 most countries performed better than in 2006. Correlations between generalized trust, social contacts and well-being were positive but the impact of social capital became less salient after crisis of 2008. Overall, in 2014 in four out of five welfare models either generalized trust or social contacts promoted well-being among older adults. The only regime which totally absorbed the influence of social capital on well-being was Nordic welfare regime. These findings confirm that effective social policy reduce the importance of personal resources in obtaining higher levels of subjective well-being.

Acknowledgements The work of Anna Almakaeva on this chapter and the whole volume was supported by the HSE University Basic Research Program and the Russian Academic Excellence Project '5–100'. The editors thank Francesco Sarracino for his valuable comments and suggestions.

References

Almakaeva, A., Welzel, C., & Ponarin, E. (2017). Human empowerment and trust in strangers: The multilevel evidence. *Social Indicators Research*, 1–40. https://doi.org/10.1007/s11205-017-1724-z

Bardi, A., & Goodwin, R. (2011). The dual route to value change: Individual processes and cultural moderators. *Journal of Cross-Cultural Psychology, 42*(2), 271–287. https://doi.org/10.1177/0022022110396916

Bjornskov, C. (2003). The happy few: Cross-country evidence on social capital and life satisfaction. *Kyklos, 56*(1), 3–16. https://doi.org/10.1111/1467-6435.00207

Elgar, F. J., Davis, C. G., Wohl, M. J., Trites, S. J., Zelenski, J. M., & Martin, M. S. (2011). Social capital, health and life satisfaction in 50 countries. *Health & Place, 17*(5), 1044–1053. https://doi.org/10.1016/j.healthplace.2011.06.010

Fairbrother, M., & Martin, I. W. (2013). Does inequality erode social trust? Results from multilevel models of US states and counties. *Social Science Research, 42*(2), 347–360. https://doi.org/10.1016/j.ssresearch.2012.09.008

Foa, R. S., Inglehart, R., Ponarin, E., & Karabchuk, T. (2018). Set-point theory and societal collapse: The case of Russia. *Journal of Happiness Studies, 19*(6), 1639–1656. https://doi.org/10.1007/s10902-017-9888-4

Inglehart, R. F. (2018, March). Cultural evolution: People's motivations are changing, and reshaping the world. https://doi.org/10.1017/9781108613880

Inglehart, R., & Welzel, C. (2005). *Modernization, cultural change, and democracy: The human development sequence*. Cambridge University Press.

Peiró-Palomino, J., & Tortosa-Ausina, E. (2013). Can trust effects on development be generalized? A response by quantile. *European Journal of Political Economy, 32*, 377–390. https://doi.org/10.1016/j.ejpoleco.2013.09.008

Rothstein, B., & Uslaner, E. M. (2005). All for all: Equality, corruption, and social trust. *World Politics, 58*(01), 41–72. https://doi.org/10.1353/wp.2006.0022
Uslaner, E. M. (2013). Trust and corruption revisited: How and why trust and corruption shape each other. *Quality & Quantity, 47*(6), 3603–3608. https://doi.org/10.1007/s11135-012-9742-z
Welzel, C. (2013). *Freedom rising: Human empowerment and the contemporary quest for emancipation.* Cambridge University Press.
Whiteley, P. F. (2000). Economic growth and social capital. *Political Studies, 48*(3), 443–466. https://doi.org/10.1111/1467-9248.00269
Zak, P. J., & Knack, S. (2001). Trust and growth. *The Economic Journal, 111*(470), 295–321.

Anna Almakaeva (Ph.D. in Sociology) is a deputy head of the Ronald F. Inglehart Laboratory for Comparative Social Research at the Higher School of Economics (Russia). Her research interests include social capital, values, subjective well-being and comparative studies. She is a member of the World Value Survey Russian team and the European Values Study Russian team.

Alejandro Moreno got Ph.D. from the University of Michigan in 1997. He is a professor of political science at ITAM (Instituto Tecnológico Autónomo de México) since 1996. He has served as President of the World Association for Public Opinion Research, WAPOR (2013–2014), as Vice-president for the World Values Survey Association (since 2013), and as Managing Director of the Latinobarometro surveys (2010–2017). He has also been the Director of Public Opinion Polling for newspaper Reforma (1999–2015) and currently for newspaper El Financiero (since 2016). His main research and academic interests focus on public opinion elections and voting behavior, political culture and social values, comparative politics, and survey research methodologies.

Rima Wilkes (Ph.D.) is a professor at the department of Sociology at the University of British Columbia (Canada). In 2017–2018 she was president of the Canadian Sociological Association. Her research interests include political sociology, race and ethnicity, trust, immigration and social movements.

The manufacturer's authorised representative in the EU is Springer Nature Customer Service Centre GmbH, Europaplatz 3, 69115 Heidelberg, Germany. If you have any concerns regarding our products, please contact ProductSafety@springernature.com

Printed and bound by CPI Group (UK) Ltd, Croydon, CR0 4YY
30/09/2026
02225593-0004